AF426020

A Handbook of
NOBEL LAUREATES
IN MEDICINE

An Inspirational Journey in the Annals of medical science

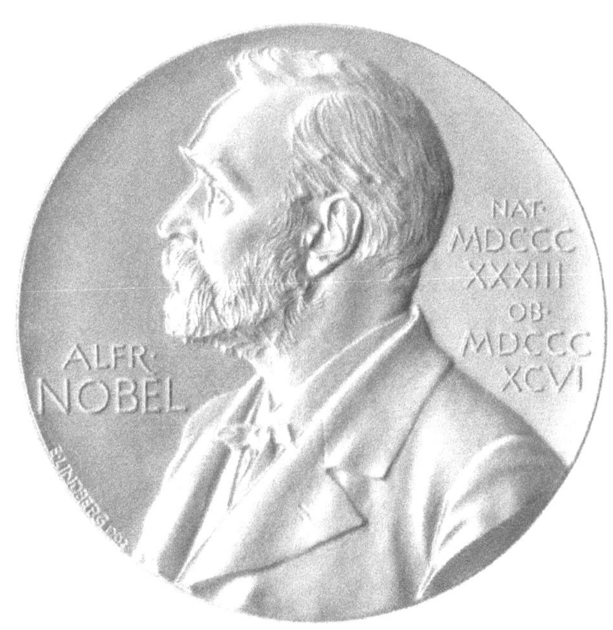

DR VENKATESAN SANGAREDDI MD
DR LATHA VENKATESAN MD

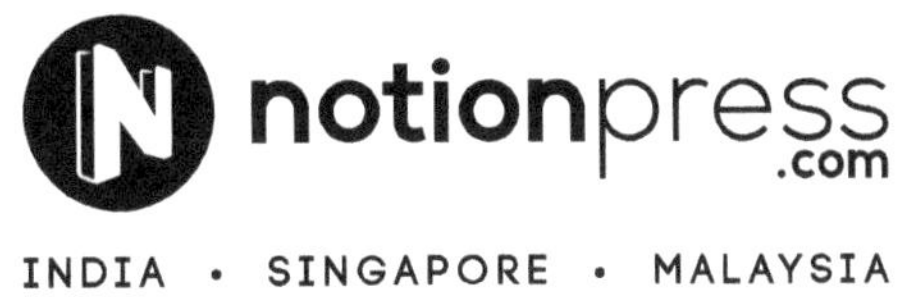

INDIA · SINGAPORE · MALAYSIA

ISBN 979-8-89544-552-5

CONTENTS

The Nobel Legacy

ABOUT THE AUTHOR

Dr. Venkatesan Sangareddi is a distinguished alumnus of Coimbatore Medical College, where he completed his graduation in 1987. With a career spanning nearly three decades as a Professor of Cardiology at Madras Medical College, Chennai, one of Asia's oldest and most esteemed medical institutions in India. He has made significant contributions to the field of cardiology. His commitment to education is evident in his role as a mentor to over 200 cardiologists who now have a global presence.

His academic contributions extend to his website, "Expressions in Cardiology," which has been a valuable resource for the medical community for over 15 years, attracting more than six million visits. This book aims to serve as a comprehensive guide to Nobel Prize winners in Medicine, offering insights into the history and struggles of the men and women who have pushed the boundaries of medical science. Through this work he encourages readers to appreciate the dedication and commitment of these scientists, and to recognize the hard-earned successes that the medical profession enjoys today.

Living in an era marked by rapid scientific advancement, Dr. Venkatesan is passionate about bridging the gap between laboratory research and clinical practice, especially in cardiology. He is keen to explore contemporary issues such as outcome analysis, cost-effectiveness, and ethical challenges in medicine, with the hope of finding innovative solutions.

His personal life is closely intertwined with the medical field, as evidenced by his spouse, Dr. Latha Venkatesan, a senior consultant obstetrician with over 25 years of experience at Sundaram Medical Foundation, Chennai. She has played a crucial role in gathering important illustrations for this book. The author also extends his gratitude to his daughter, Shreenila Venkatesan, a psychologist, for her invaluable support and input in the book's design.

Through his book, he not only aims to educate and inspire the next generation of medical professionals but also to pay tribute to the pioneers whose efforts have shaped the landscape of modern medicine.

PROLOGUE

Humans inhabited our planet for over 300,000 years. They are just one among the living organism amidst a millions of lives in a world of infinite biomass. But, humans became supreme over all other beings with their unique and continuously growing intellect. With only about 5,000 years of recorded history, we can only imagine how they dealt with tough environments and sickness. Whether it is right or wrong, feasible or not, humans are trying to take absolute control over their life.

How the mankind tackled disease over the years, form an impressive history. Since Hippocrates from Kos islands, Greece, challenged the idea that diseases come from evil spirits, modern science began. He believed each disease has a scientific reason, making him known as the father of modern medicine. It took over 2000 years to follow his ideas. In the last two centuries, incredible medical discoveries were made, like understanding genes and cells. We now have specific treatments for thousands of disease and go deep in to an organ, and repair the defect or even replace it. These stunning discoveries, along with improved living conditions has doubled the life expectancy from around 40 to 70 in the last two centuries. This has a direct coincidence with the thumping medical discoveries that happened in the same time span.

The book aims to record all the winners of the Nobel Prize in medicine, a special award created by the inventor of dynamite Alfred Nobel in the year 1901. It's interesting that, this man though, not belonging to medical profession, had a great foresight and initiated this prestigious prize thorough his will. The book would serve as a guide for understanding 120 years of scientific advancements and the progress of medical science as seen by the Nobel committee. The author hopes that this book would inspire the next generation, and help them pursue science for the good of humanity in a righteous manner.

ALFRED NOBEL AND THE CREATION OF THE NOBEL PRIZE

The beginning

Alfred Nobel's life is a tale that reads almost like fiction. Born in the mid-19th century in Stockholm, he was the kind of guy who was always thinking, always creating. He had a knack for invention and a mind for business. His most famous invention, dynamite, was a game-changer. It revolutionized industries like construction and mining, making hard jobs easier and opening up possibilities that were unthinkable before.

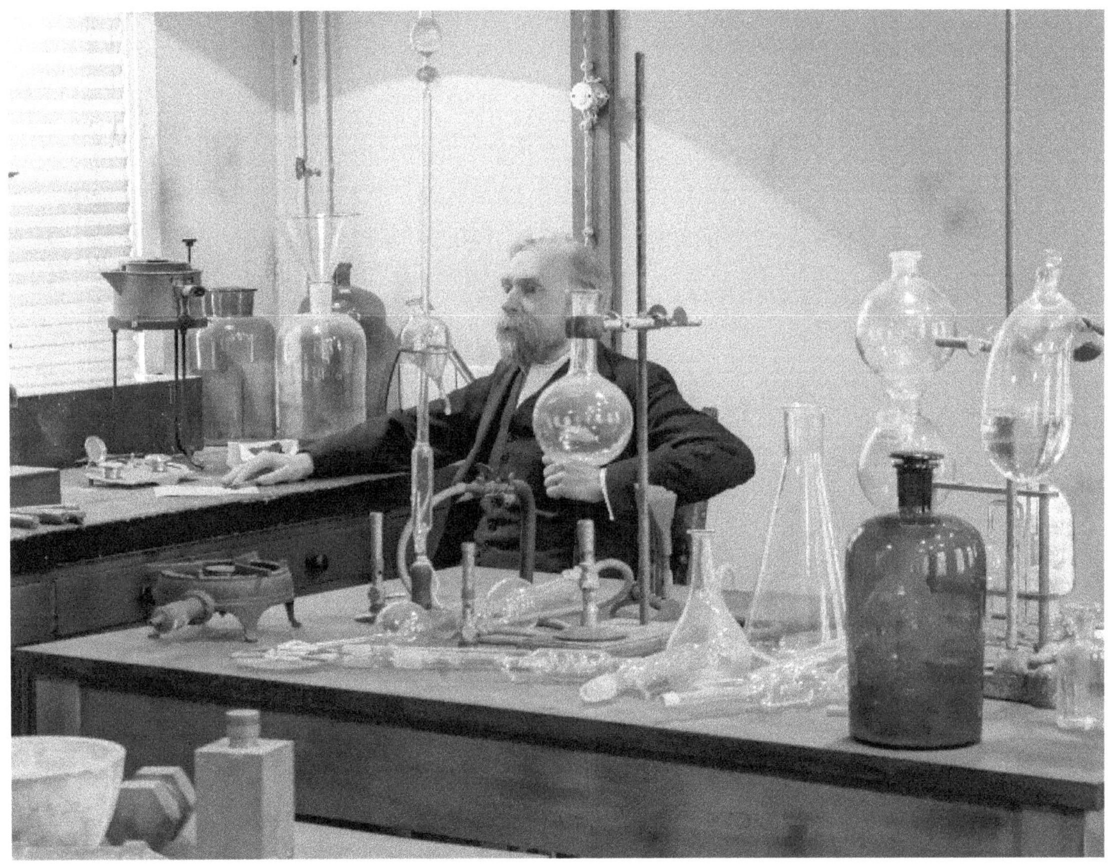

Alfred Nobel in his laboratory

However, there was a twist to the story. Nobel's remarkable invention, dynamite, served not only constructive purposes but also found its application in warfare, causing destruction. This unintended consequence was something Nobel had not anticipated. Reflect for a moment on the challenge of creating something with the intention of doing good, only to witness its misuse and the harm it brings. Undoubtedly, this would have posed a significant struggle for Nobel.

One fateful day, Nobel, who was very much alive, was taken aback when he caught sight of his own obituary in a newspaper. It was a mistake, but what it said really got to him. It called him the "merchant of death" because of his role in creating dynamite. Just picture that – being labeled like that when you're still around to read it. Nobel was deeply shaken. He began to think hard about what his life and work meant, and what he'd be leaving behind.

This moment of shock and reflection led Nobel to make a big decision. He didn't want to be remembered as the guy who made dynamite and nothing else. He wanted to leave a legacy that would be positive, that would help people. So, he came up with the idea of the Nobel Prizes. He saw these prizes as his chance to flip the script on his legacy. Instead of being remembered for dynamite and destruction, he wanted to be associated with celebrating great achievements that helped humanity. It was his way of saying, "Hey, I believe in the power of human creativity and goodness."

And so, the Nobel Prizes were born out of this mix of regret, reflection, and a desire to make things right. Nobel wanted these awards to shine a light on people who were making real, positive changes in the world. It was his way of encouraging and honoring those who were using their talents to benefit others. This was especially true for the Nobel Prize in Medicine or Physiology, which was all about recognizing the folks who were pushing boundaries to improve health and save lives.

In this story of Nobel, we find a reminder that our actions and creations can have impacts we never imagined. And sometimes, it takes a jolt to make us see the bigger picture and push us to leave a mark that's truly beneficial for the world.

— The Genesis of the Nobel Prize in Medicine

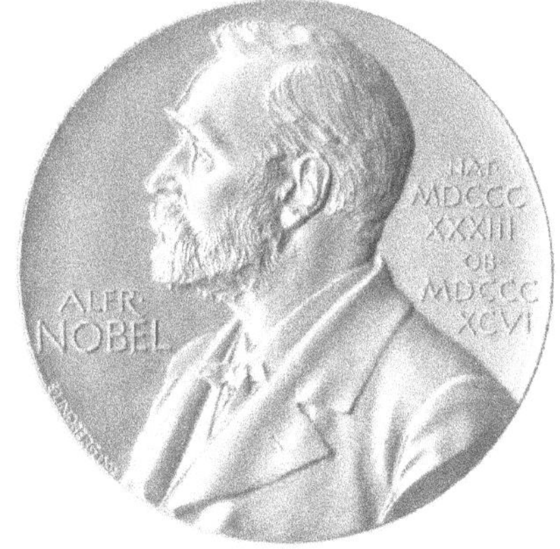
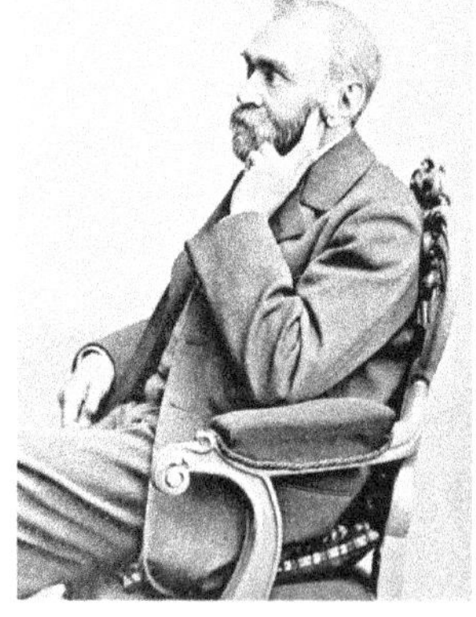
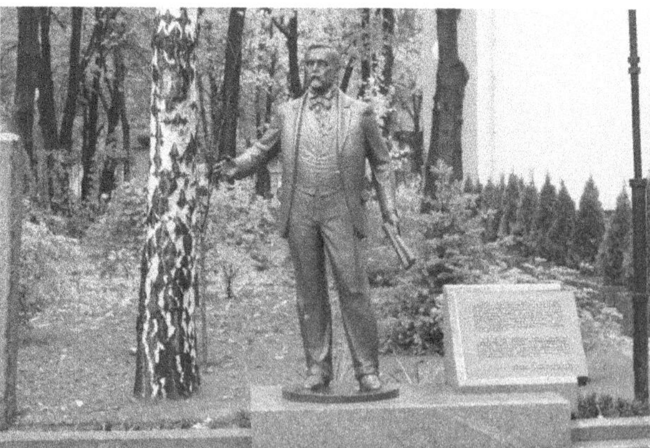

The glittering medal and his monument at St. Petersburg, Russia

When Alfred Nobel was mulling over the idea of the Nobel Prizes, he had a clear vision for the category of Medicine. He wasn't just thinking about rewarding smart people for their brainy achievements. Nobel was after something more. He wanted this prize to spotlight discoveries that would genuinely make life better, especially in the fields of medicine and health. You see, Nobel was really interested in science that touched lives, that made a difference in the everyday health and well-being of people.

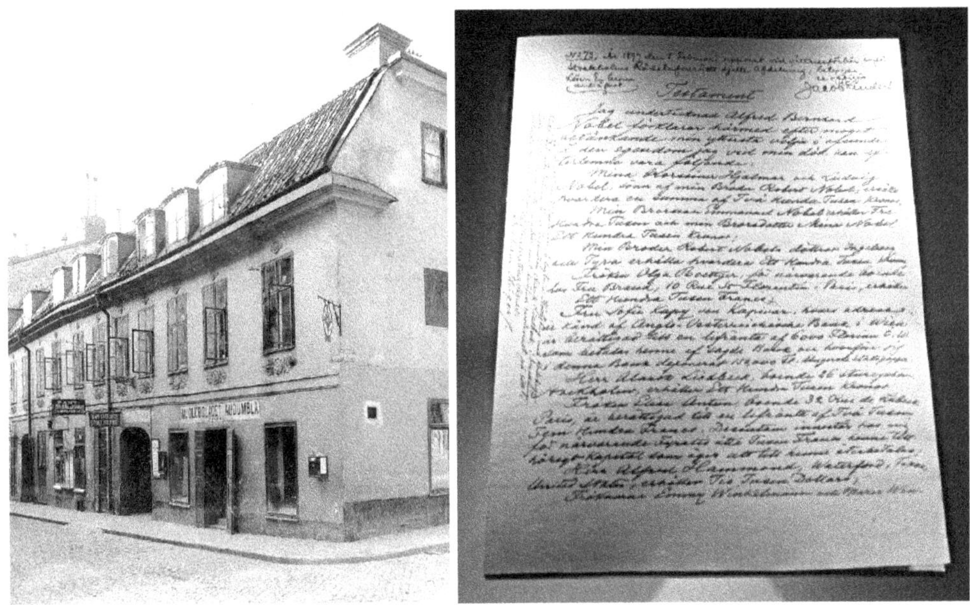

The house where Nobel lived and his famous statement of will

Why physiology is so closely associated with medicine is a question of both history and science. This association is not accidental; it reflects a deep and practical connection. Physiology, the study of how the body functions in its normal state, is fundamental in identifying and understanding diseases, or pathologies. This concept has guided medical breakthroughs in the past and remains a key element in contemporary medical research.

It's important to highlight, particularly for young people aspiring to careers in medicine, the enduring significance of physiology. From the beginning of medical education to the highest levels of research, an understanding of physiology is crucial. Knowing how the human body normally works is the first step in identifying and treating what goes wrong. This has been a core principle since the early days of the Nobel Prize in Medicine or Physiology, and it continues to be just as important in the ever-advancing field of medicine.

Think about it – in Nobel's time, the world of medicine was on the brink of some pretty exciting stuff. There were diseases that baffled doctors, conditions with no cures, and a whole lot of mystery about how the human body worked. Nobel saw an opportunity here. By creating a prize for Medicine or Physiology, he wanted to light a fire under the smartest minds of the world. He was challenging them to dig deeper, explore further, and come up with discoveries that could change the course of health and medicine.

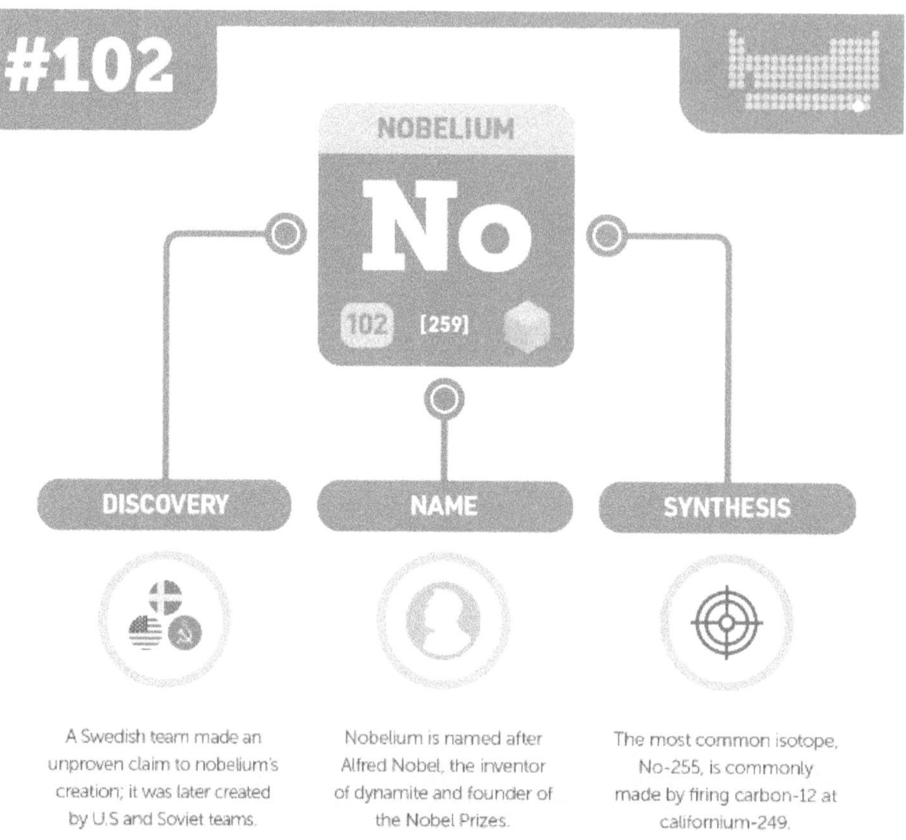

A metal was as named in the periodic table after his name

The first Nobel Prize in Medicine, awarded in 1901, is a perfect example of Nobel's dream turning into reality. The award went to Emil Adolf von Behring, a name you might not hear often, but one that left a significant mark. Von Behring was honored for his work on serum therapy, particularly for its use against diphtheria, which was a major killer of children at the time. Imagine being a parent in those days, living in fear of a disease that could take your child from you. Then comes along a person like von Behring with his life-saving therapy. That's the kind of impact Nobel was aiming for.

The reaction to this first award was a mix of excitement and awe within the scientific community and beyond. It wasn't just about the prize money; it was the honor and recognition. Scientists and doctors around the world saw the Nobel Prize as a new pinnacle of achievement. It was a game-changer. Suddenly, there was this prestigious international award acknowledging the hard work and genius of those striving to unravel the mysteries of medicine and the human body.

This inaugural prize set the tone for the future. It sent a message that the Nobel Prize in Medicine was serious business – a recognition of work that not only showcased scientific excellence but also brought tangible benefits to mankind. In a way, it helped shape the direction of medical research, steering it towards endeavors with real-world impact. The Nobel Prize wasn't just a pat on the back; it was a call to action for the world's brightest minds to apply their brilliance to solve the most pressing health challenges of humanity.

Impact of the World Wars

The two World Wars didn't just shape world history; they also left a profound mark on medical research and the Nobel Prizes. War, as grim as it is, has often been a catalyst for medical innovation. It's a time when the urgency of saving lives becomes more pressing than ever. During both World Wars, we saw an intense focus on developing medical solutions that directly adressed the injuries, diseases, and health conditions prevalent in war-torn environments.

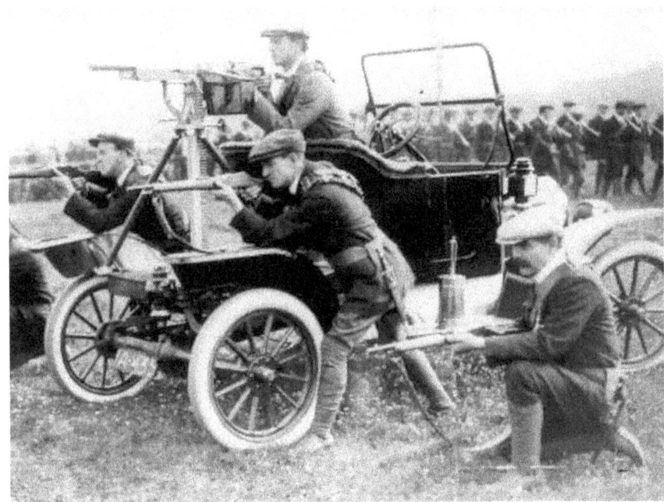
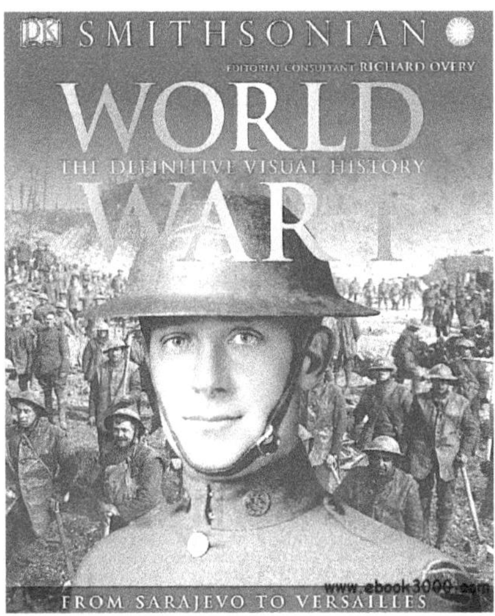

Several Nobel laureates during these times were recognized for work that either responded to or was heavily influenced by the needs of wartime. For instance, the discovery of penicillin by Alexander Fleming, Ernst Boris Chain, and Howard Florey, which earned them the Nobel Prize in 1945, revolutionized the treatment of infections, especially crucial during the war years. Their work is a classic example of how a dire situation can push scientific inquiry towards breakthroughs that continue to save millions of lives.

Post-war periods were marked by significant leaps in medical science. The devastation and the collective experience of the wars led to increased investment and interest in medical research. There was a greater push towards understanding diseases, leading to groundbreaking discoveries in various fields of medicine and physiology. The Nobel Prizes during these times reflected this surge in scientific innovation, honoring advances that might not have been achieved with such urgency if not for the demanding circumstances of war.

Evolution of the Prize Over Time

Over the years, the Nobel Prize in Medicine has evolved, both in its criteria and its scope. Initially, the focus was more on discoveries that had immediate practical applications in medicine. However, as our understanding of health and disease has grown, so has the scope of the Prize. It began encompassing a broader range of fields within medicine and physiology. This expansion reflects the evolving landscape of medical science, where new fields of study have emerged and gained prominence.

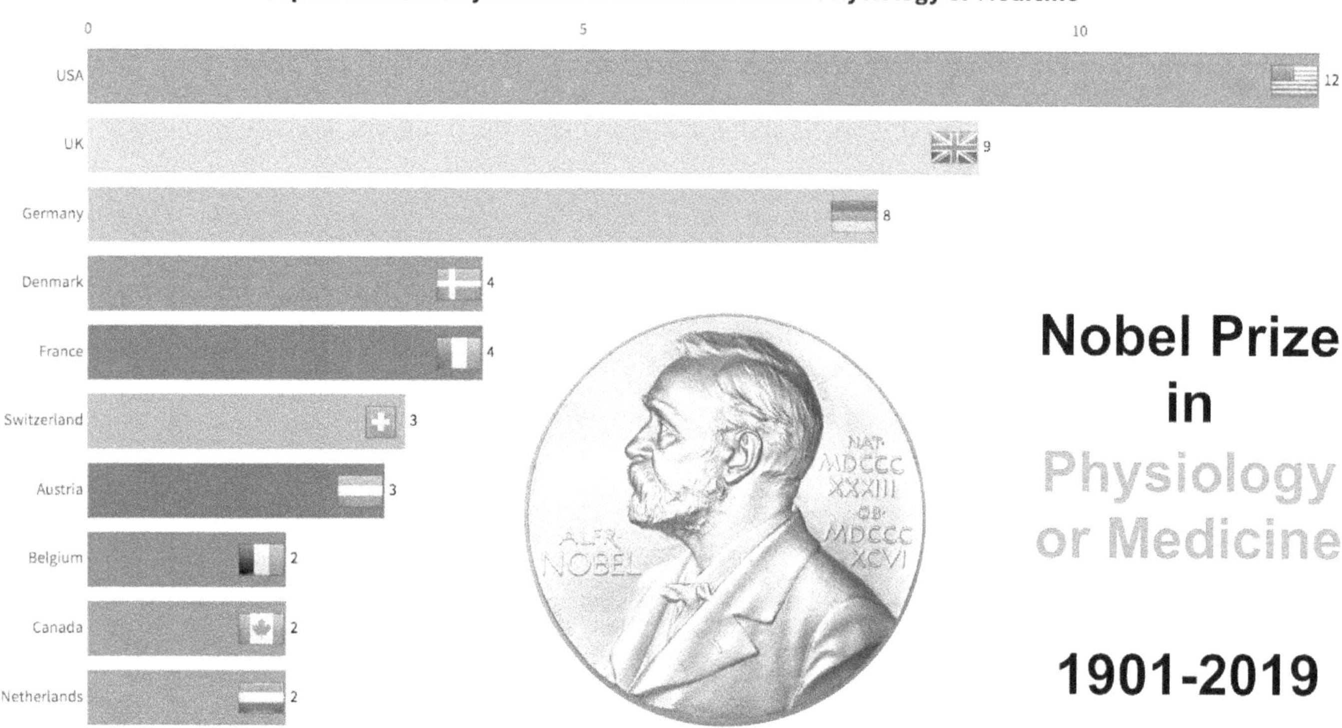

The selection process, too, has seen changes. In the early days, the Nobel Committee heavily relied on nominations from a select group of university professors and previous laureates. Over time, this process has become more inclusive and diverse. Now, a wider range of experts from around the world are invited to nominate, allowing the Committee to consider a broader spectrum of potential laureates. This change is crucial because it ensures that the Prize remains relevant and continues to recognize the most groundbreaking work in the field of medicine and physiology.

As we set off on this incredible journey, we're just scratching the surface. Get ready to meet the brilliant minds who were honored with the Nobel Prize in Medicine or Physiology. These amazing individuals revolutionized our understanding of the human body and health. Their stories are filled with dedication, groundbreaking discoveries, and pivotal moments that made a real impact. First up, let's dive into the life of Emil Adolf von Behring, a true Pioneer, whose groundbreaking work saved countless lives. Join us as we embark on an extraordinary exploration of medical breakthroughs!

EMIL VON BEHRING (1901)

The genesis of vaccine science

Behring's profound impact on medical science was internationally recognized when he was awarded the first Nobel Prize in Medicine in 1901 for his development of serum therapies against diphtheria.

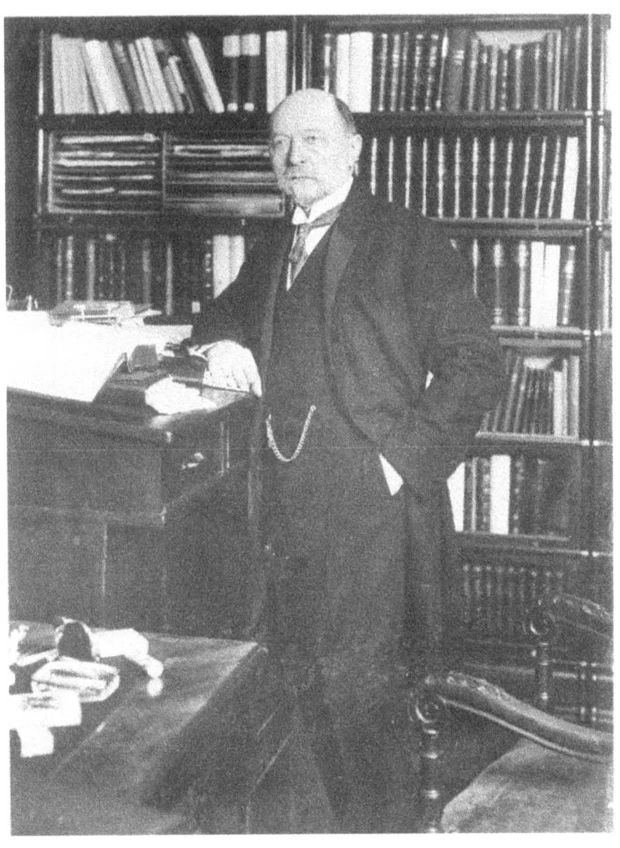

History

Emil von Behring, born on March 15, 1854, in Hansdorf, Prussia (now Ławice, Poland), embarked on his educational journey despite financial constraints. He joined the Army Medical College in Berlin in 1874, a move that enabled him to pursue his studies affordably while committing to military service. Behring earned his medical degree in 1878 and completed his State Examination in 1880.

During his military service in Poland, Behring began his foundational research into septic diseases. His work on the action of iodoform, published in 1882, hinted at its antitoxic properties without directly killing microbes. This research marked the start of his contributions to immunology and serum therapy.

Behring's potential led to further training in experimental methods with pharmacologist C. Binz in Bonn. In 1888, he was appointed as an assistant at the Institute of Hygiene in Berlin under the guidance of Robert Koch, a pivotal moment that aligned him with leading scientists like Paul Ehrlich. Behring became a Professor of Hygiene at Halle in 1894 and moved to Marburg in 1895 to hold a similar position.

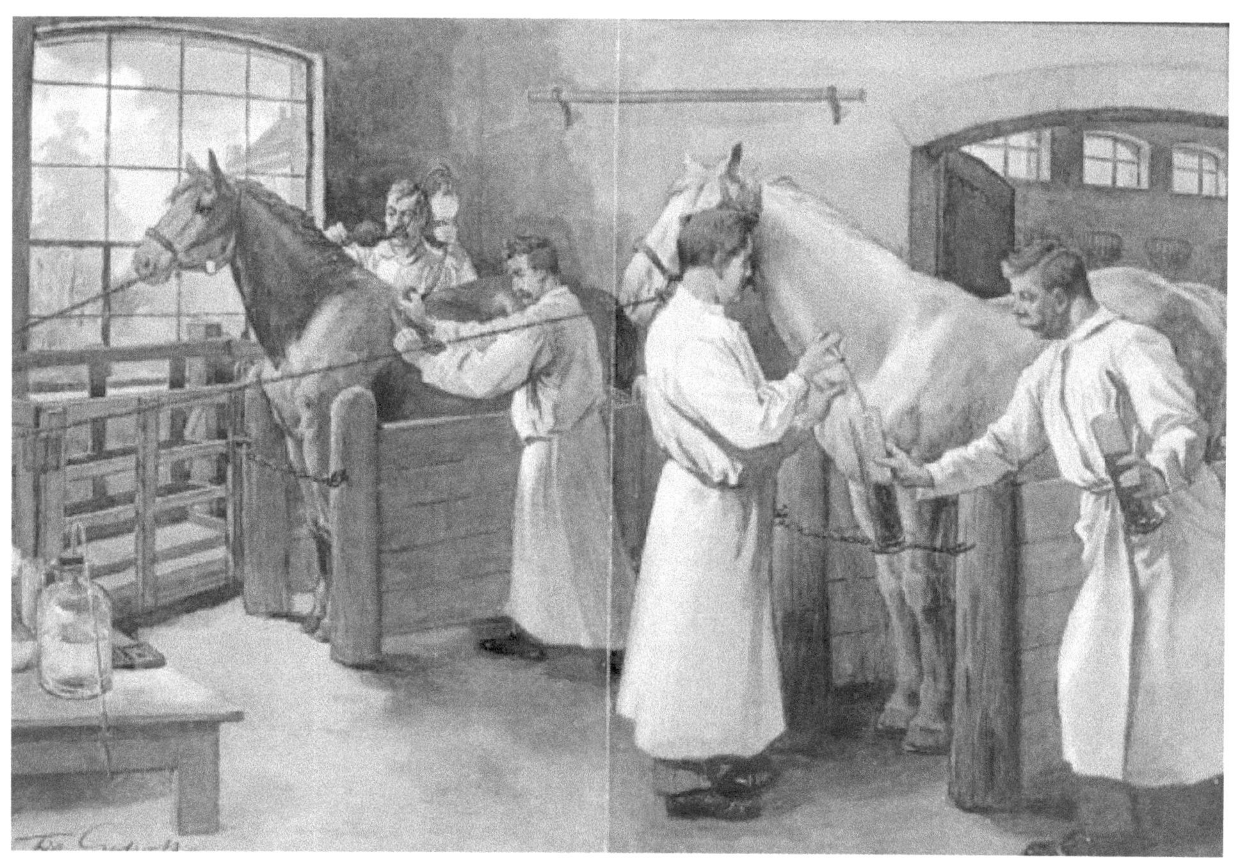

Behring's live animal lab where serum from Horses were prepared

Behring's research and academic career were significantly influenced by contemporaries such as Pasteur, Koch, Ehrlich, Löffler, Roux, and Yersin, positioning him at the forefront of scientific and medical advancement. In his personal life, he married Else Spinola in 1896 and had six sons. Behring passed away in Marburg on March 31, 1917. His legacy in immunology and therapeutic medicine remains a cornerstone of modern medical science.

Snippets

Diphtheria Antitoxin Development (Early 1890s)

In the early 1890s, Emil von Behring, working at the Institute for Infectious Diseases under Robert Koch, made a groundbreaking contribution to medical science by developing the first effective therapeutic serum against diphtheria, a major health menace of the era. His initial work on iodoform's antitoxic effects laid the groundwork for this discovery, significantly reducing the mortality rate of diphtheria.

Collaboration with Shibasaburo Kitasato (1890)

A crucial advancement in immunology came in 1890 when Behring teamed up with Shibasaburo Kitasato. Kitasato, a distinguished Japanese bacteriologist, brought valuable expertise and insights to their joint research. Their work together led to the discovery that injecting animals with sterilized cultures of diphtheria or tetanus could induce the production of antitoxins in the blood. This groundbreaking research not only introduced the concept of passive immunity but also set a landmark in combating infectious diseases.

Serum Therapy Introduction (1891 and Beyond)

In 1891, Behring successfully treated a child suffering from diphtheria with the therapeutic serum, marking the beginning of a new era in managing infectious diseases. Overcoming initial challenges in the concentration and standardization of antitoxins, with the help of bacteriologist Paul Ehrlich, Behring's serum therapy gained traction and became a critical remedy for diphtheria.

Tuberculosis Research

Behring also explored tuberculosis, seeking an effective therapeutic agent. Although his attempts in finding a healing serum for tuberculosis were not as successful, he made significant contributions to preventive vaccination and the broader field of infectious disease research.

Influence

Emil von Behring's development of serum therapy was greatly influenced by collaborations with key figures and groups. He worked with Erich Wernicke, a medical researcher, developing the first effective therapeutic serum against diphtheria. Another significant collaboration was with Shibasaburo Kitasato, leading to the creation of a serum for tetanus, instrumental in the development of passive immunization.

Paul Ehrlich, a colleague at Robert Koch's institute, played a crucial role in enhancing the diphtheria antitoxin by developing enrichment techniques and standardizing the antitoxins. This collaboration facilitated the establishment of a laboratory in Berlin for mass production of serum, primarily using horses.

Behring's career also benefited from the support of influential individuals like Friedrich Althoff from the Prussian Ministry of Education and Cultural Affairs, who aided in advancing Behring's academic career and his appointment at Philipps Marburg University.

Additionally, Behring was part of "The Marburg Circle," a group of eminent scientists, including Eugen Korschelt, Paul Friedrich, Arthur Meyer, Friedrich Schenk, Carl August Beneke, and August

Gürber. The collective discussions and collaborations within this group significantly contributed to the scientific environment that fostered Behring's groundbreaking research.

Current Implications

Pioneering Serum Therapy: Foundations of Passive Immunotherapy

The groundbreaking work of Emil von Behring in serum therapy has had a monumental impact on modern medicine. His innovations in the late 19th and early 20th centuries established the basic principles of passive immunotherapy, which continues to shape medical practices and research today.

Breakthroughs in Antitoxins: Treating Diphtheria and Tetanus

Behring's key contributions to the treatment of diphtheria and tetanus with antitoxins marked the first practical use of immune sera for infectious diseases. Originating from the transfer of sera between immunized and infected animals, this concept has greatly evolved and enhanced the field of immunology.

Monoclonal Antibody Therapy: A Modern Medical Foundation

Currently, passive immunity principles are integral in treating various non-communicable diseases like cancer, autoimmune disorders, and cardiovascular diseases through monoclonal antibody therapy. This technique offers precise, targeted treatments, a concept that was unimaginable during Behring's era.

Addressing Contemporary Viral Infections

The idea of transferring antibodies from one individual to another is being researched as a potential solution for modern viral infections, such as ebola virus and SARS-CoV-2. This method mirrors Behring's initial experiments and underscores the enduring importance of his contributions.

Enhancing Understanding of Humoral Immunity and Vaccination

Behring's discoveries laid the groundwork for a deeper comprehension of humoral immunity and the advancement of active vaccinations against infectious diseases. His exploration of the therapeutic potential of antibodies paved the way for contemporary advanced antibody-based immunotherapies.

Impact and Products

Diphtheria Serum Breakthrough

In the early 1890s, Emil von Behring, with Erich Wernicke, developed the first effective serum for diphtheria. This serum, utilizing antibodies from immunized animals, neutralized the diphtheria toxin and marked a significant advance in treating this deadly disease.

Tetanus Serum Development

Behring's work extended to tetanus, where in collaboration with Shibasaburo Kitasato, he created a serum that similarly countered the tetanus toxin. This innovation was vital in understanding and managing another life-threatening infectious disease.

Serum Therapy Advancement and Industrial Production

The first application of Behring's diphtheria serum in 1891 set a new precedent in medical treatment. Paul Ehrlich later enhanced the serum's efficacy through concentration and standardization techniques. Partnering with Hoechst, Behring facilitated the serum's mass production, significantly reducing diphtheria mortality and establishing serum therapy as a key medical treatment.

Role During World War I

Behring's tetanus serum was crucial during World War I, saving soldiers' lives by preventing and treating tetanus infections. Its initial cautious reception gave way to widespread adoption in military medicine.

Foundation for Modern Immunotherapy

Emil von Behring's research in serum therapy was a major stepping stone for today's vaccines and immune treatments. By demonstrating serum therapy's therapeutic potential, he inspired further research into immune system manipulation, significantly impacting the course of immunological research and treatment.

"Emil von Behring's development of a vaccine against diphtheria stands as a landmark achievement in medicine. Often referred to as a life-saving breakthrough, his discovery significantly changed the course of healthcare and is credited with saving millions of children's lives."

RONALD ROSS (1902)

The man with a mission

In 1902, Ronald Ross achieved a milestone in medical history by receiving the Nobel Prize in Medicine for his groundbreaking work on malaria. Ross's discovery that the Anopheles mosquito transmitted the malarial parasite laid the foundation for modern methods of combating the disease, a contribution that has had enduring implications in the field of medicine.

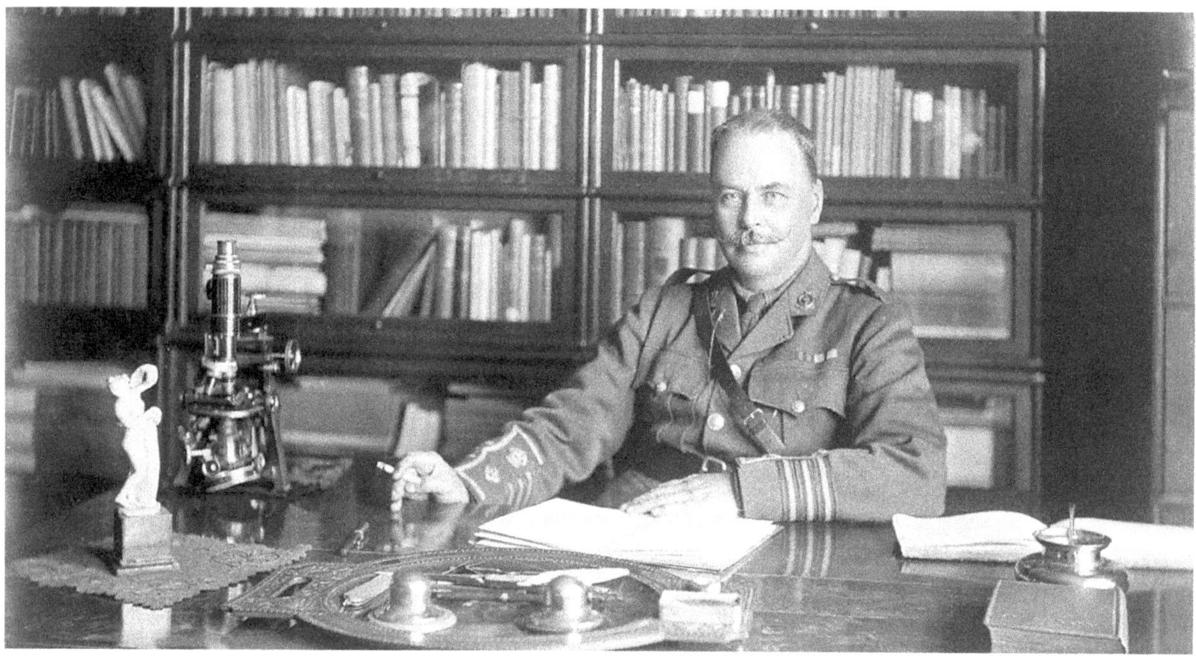

History

Ronald Ross, born on May 13, 1857, in Almora, India, was the eldest child of Sir Campbell Claye Grant Ross, a general in the British Indian Army, and Matilda Charlotte Elderton. At the age of eight, he was sent to England to live with his aunt and uncle on the Isle of Wight. Ross attended primary schools at Ryde and later, a boarding school in Springhill near Southampton. His early education was marked by an inclination towards literature, music, and mathematics.

Despite Ross's aspiration to become a writer, his father influenced his decision to enroll at St Bartholomew's Hospital Medical College in London in 1874. Though he was not fully committed to medicine initially and spent much of his time composing music and writing poems and plays, he passed the examinations for the Royal College of Surgeons of England in 1879. He further qualified from the Society of Apothecaries in 1881, after a four-month training at the Army Medical School.

Ross's career in the Indian Medical Service began in 1881, leading him to various postings across India. His time in Bangalore was particularly significant, where he first observed the potential of controlling mosquitoes to combat malaria. His return to India in 1895, after studying bacteriology in London, marked the beginning of his focused research on malaria, prompted by his interactions with Sir Patrick Manson, who believed India was the ideal place for such studies.

Ross's discovery of the malarial parasite in the gastrointestinal tract of the Anopheles mosquito in 1897 in Secunderabad was a pivotal moment in his career. This discovery proved the hypothesis of Laveran and Manson and established the method for combating malaria. Ross's subsequent work in India and later in West Africa at the Liverpool School of Tropical Medicine expanded upon these findings, significantly contributing to the field of tropical medicine and the global fight against malaria.

Snippets:

The Indian connection

Ronald Ross's journey into malaria research began in earnest in 1895 in India. His initial observation of the early stages of the malaria parasite inside a mosquito's stomach set the stage for his future discoveries. Despite facing challenges, including a transfer to a malaria-free region, Ross remained focused on his research goals.

Breakthrough in Secunderabad

Ross's persistence paid off in July 1897 in Secunderabad. After culturing 20 adult "brown" mosquitoes from larvae, he successfully infected these mosquitoes with the blood of a malaria patient.

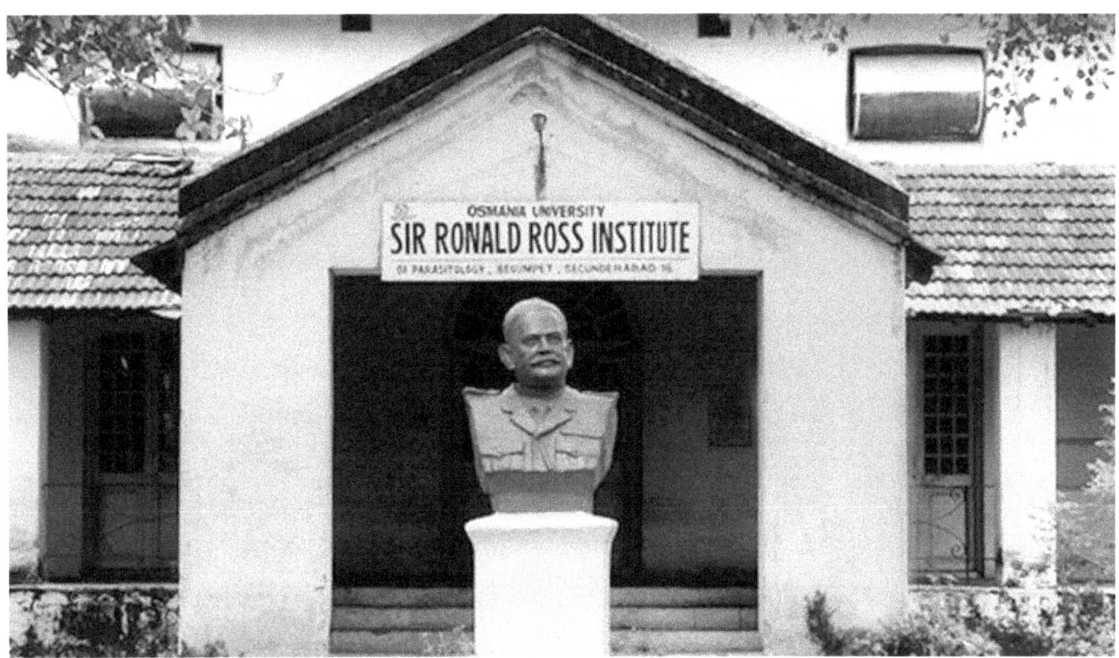

The Ronald Ross Institute at Secunderabad India

This critical experiment led to his historic discovery when, upon dissecting the mosquitoes, he found the malarial parasite. This finding conclusively demonstrated that mosquitoes transmitted malaria, a breakthrough that reshaped the scientific approach to combating the disease.

Global Research and Impact

After resigning from the Indian Medical Service in 1899, Ross joined the Liverpool School of Tropical Medicine. His role here was not just academic; he actively devised anti-malaria schemes in West Africa, marking one of many expeditions to develop malaria control measures. His research extended to places like Egypt, Panama, Greece, and Mauritius, reflecting the global significance of his work.

Predecessors

Before Ronald Ross's discovery, several scientists made significant strides in understanding malaria, laying the groundwork for Ross's eventual breakthrough.

Vassily Danilewsky's Early Observations

Vassily Danilewsky, a Russian physiologist, was a crucial figure in early malaria research. In the 1880s, he studied blood parasites in birds and reptiles and discovered several parasites, including trypanosomes and what he identified as 'pseudovacoules.' His description of these 'pseudovacules' aligns with what we now recognize as unstained malaria parasites. Danilewsky's work, much of which was initially published in Russian, only became widely known after the French publication of his book "La Parasitologie Comparée du Sang" in 1889.

The Role of William MacCallum

In North America, medical student William MacCallum and his colleague Eugene Opie, while examining birds infected with Haemoproteus columbae, a relative of malaria parasites, observed flagellated structures and proposed a process of sexual reproduction in these parasites. MacCallum's insight was critical in understanding the malaria life cycle, though its full significance was initially overlooked by Ross.

Current Implications

Ronald Ross's discovery that mosquitoes transmit malaria parasites has had a profound and lasting impact on the fight against malaria. His work not only provided crucial insights into the disease's transmission but also laid the groundwork for the development of effective control strategies.

Global Health Strategies

Since Ross's discovery, there has been a significant global effort to control and eradicate malaria. Strategies include mosquito control measures, such as the use of insecticide-treated nets and indoor residual spraying, and the development of antimalarial drugs. These methods have collectively contributed to a substantial decrease in malaria cases and deaths worldwide.

Modern Research and Challenges

Ross's work continues to inspire current research on malaria. Scientists have made advances in understanding the complex life cycle of malaria parasites and are working on developing effective vaccines. However, challenges such as drug resistance and the adaptability of the Anopheles mosquito remain.

Education and Awareness

Ross's contributions have also emphasized the importance of public health education and awareness in combating malaria. Efforts to educate communities in malaria-endemic areas about prevention and treatment have been crucial in reducing the disease's impact.

Continuing the Fight Against Malaria

The ongoing battle against malaria is a testament to the significance of Ross's work. While great strides have been made, continued research, innovation, and global cooperation are essential to ultimately eradicate this disease.

Impact and Products

Advances in Malaria Prevention

Ross's work led to a better understanding of the malaria life cycle, guiding public health efforts to target the mosquito vector. This has resulted in effective mosquito control measures, such as the use of insecticide-treated bed nets and indoor residual spraying, which have played a crucial role in reducing malaria transmission.

Development of Antimalarial Drugs

Ross's research paved the way for the development of antimalarial drugs, further enhancing the ability to treat and prevent malaria infections. These drugs have been vital in reducing the disease's impact, especially in endemic regions.

Global Health Initiatives

Ross's discoveries have been integral to shaping global health policies and initiatives aimed at eradicating malaria. His work underpins the efforts of organizations like the World Health Organization in their ongoing battle against this disease.

Educational and Awareness Programs

Ross's legacy also extends to educational and awareness programs that focus on malaria prevention and control, emphasizing the importance of community participation in combating the disease. Ronald Ross's contributions to malaria research have not only advanced scientific understanding but have also saved countless lives, making him an enduring figure in the archives of medical history.

NIELS RYBERG FINSEN (1903)

The enlightened man and his phototherapy for skin infections

In 1903, Niels Ryberg Finsen, a Danish physician, was awarded the Nobel Prize in Medicine for his significant contributions to medical science through the development of phototherapy.

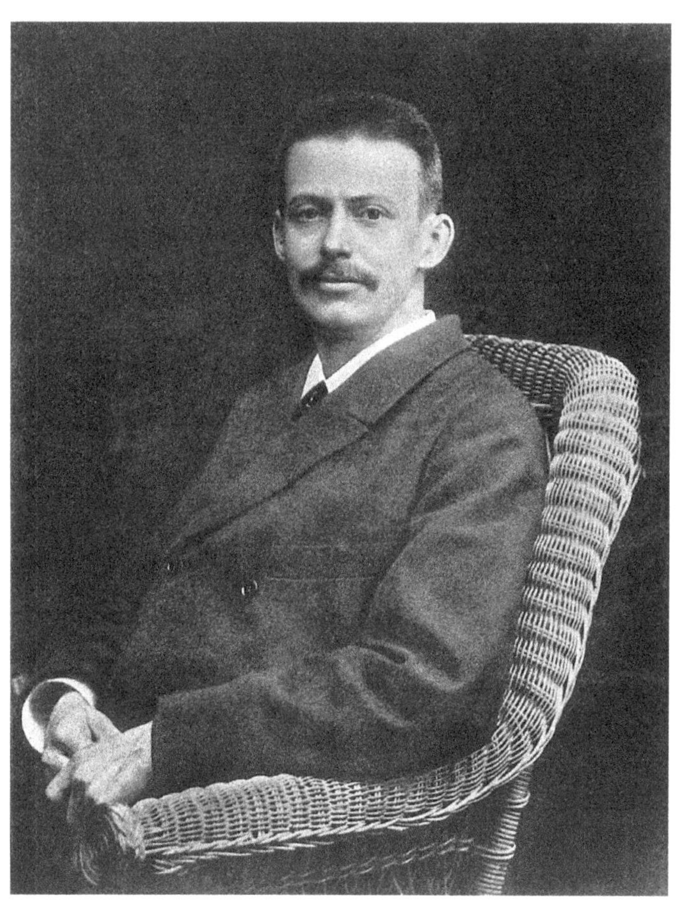

History

Niels Ryberg Finsen, born on December 15, 1860, in the Faroe Islands, was a pioneer in the field of phototherapy. Despite challenges in his early education, including a transfer to Iceland due to difficulties with the Danish language, Finsen overcame these obstacles and excelled in his studies. In 1882, he moved to Copenhagen to study medicine, graduating in 1890. He then became a prosecutor of anatomy at the University of Copenhagen. Finsen's personal battle with Niemann–Pick disease, a condition that affects the organs, was a key factor that led him to investigate the therapeutic effects of light.

Snippets

Finsen's significant contributions began with his study of the effects of light on living organisms. In 1893, he made a crucial discovery that exposure to certain wavelengths of light prevented the pustules in smallpox from becoming infected, reducing scarring. Building on this, he developed an ultraviolet light treatment for lupus vulgaris, a form of skin tuberculosis, which achieved remarkable success.

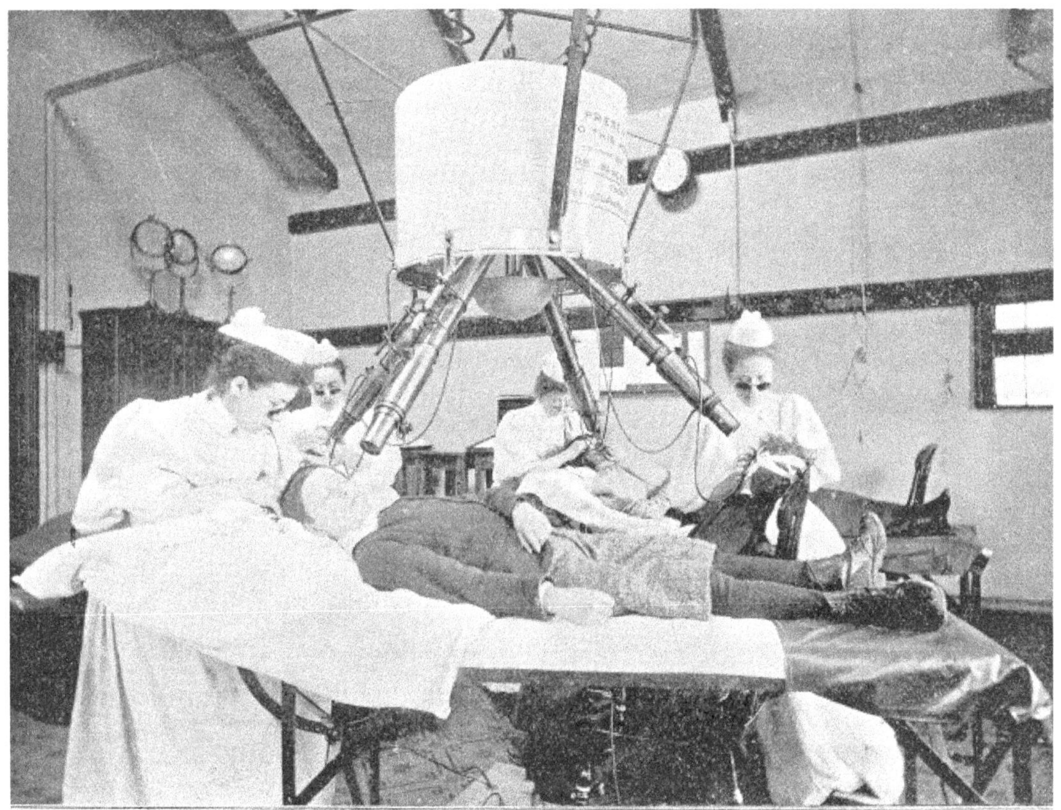

Fig. 4.—The Treatment by the Electric Light.

Current Implications

Today, Finsen's legacy in phototherapy continues to influence modern medicine. His research opened avenues for the development of various light-based treatments, including the use of ultraviolet light for skin conditions and other medical applications.

Impact and Products

Finsen's work led to the establishment of the Finsen Institute in 1896, which specialized in light therapy for skin diseases. This institute set a precedent for similar centers globally, significantly advancing the field of dermatological treatment. Finsen's methods and findings have greatly influenced the development and application of light therapy in modern medicine.

IVAN PAVLOV (1904)

A pioneer who stunned the scientific world with his simple dog experiments

Ivan Pavlov's journey from a prospective theological student to a Nobel laureate in medicine highlights his remarkable transformation and contributions to the field of physiological research.

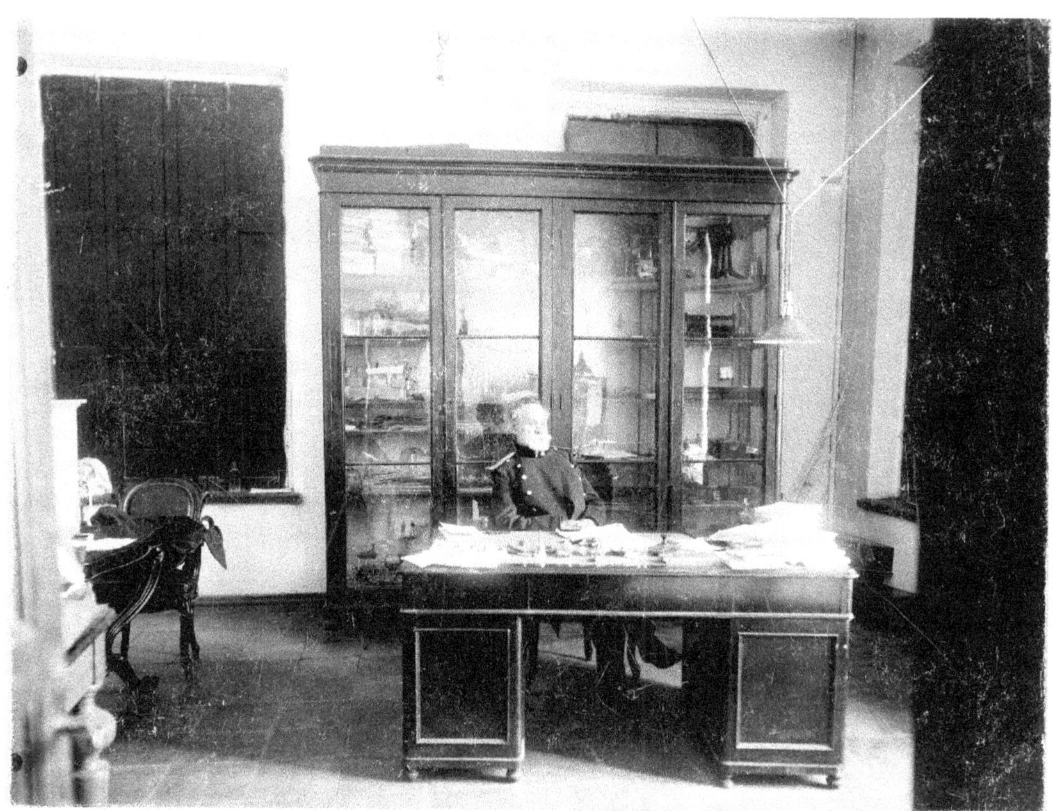

History

Ivan Petrovich Pavlov, a Russian and Soviet experimental neurologist and physiologist, was born on September 26, 1849, in Ryazan, Russia. Initially setting out to study theology, Pavlov was inspired by the scientific ideas of Dmitry Pisarev and Ivan Sechenov, leading him to pursue natural sciences at the University of St. Petersburg. He received his M.D. from the Imperial Medical Academy in St. Petersburg and further honed his skills in Germany under cardiovascular physiologist Carl Ludwig and gastrointestinal physiologist Rudolf Heidenhain.

Pavlov's early research focused on the physiology of the circulatory system. From 1888 to 1890, he investigated cardiac physiology and blood pressure regulation, developing expertise in surgical techniques. His transition to the study of the physiology of digestion marked the beginning of his most famous work. Pavlov's innovative approach and techniques in his digestive research laid the groundwork for his discovery of the conditioned reflex.

Pavlov's academic career was marked by tenacity and excellence. After returning to Russia in 1886, his initial applications for academic positions faced setbacks. However, in 1890, he was appointed professor of Pharmacology at the Military Medical Academy, and in 1891, he organized and directed the Department of Physiology at the Institute of Experimental Medicine in St. Petersburg. Under his leadership, the institute became a significant center of physiological research.

Snippets

The Birth of Classical Conditioning

Pavlov's most influential work emerged from his experiments with dogs in the 1890s. He observed that dogs salivated not only when they tasted food but also when they heard the footsteps of the lab assistant who fed them. This observation led to his famous experiment with the bell and the food, where he trained dogs to associate the sound of a bell with food, causing them to salivate at the sound alone. This phenomenon, termed 'classical conditioning,' became a foundational concept in behavioral psychology.

The Pavlovian Dog Experiments

In his well-known experiment, Pavlov paired the presentation of food with the sound of a metronome. After repeated pairings, the dogs started to salivate in response to the metronome alone, even when no food was presented. This experiment demonstrated the principle of associative learning and showed how a neutral stimulus, when associated with a significant one, could elicit a conditioned response.

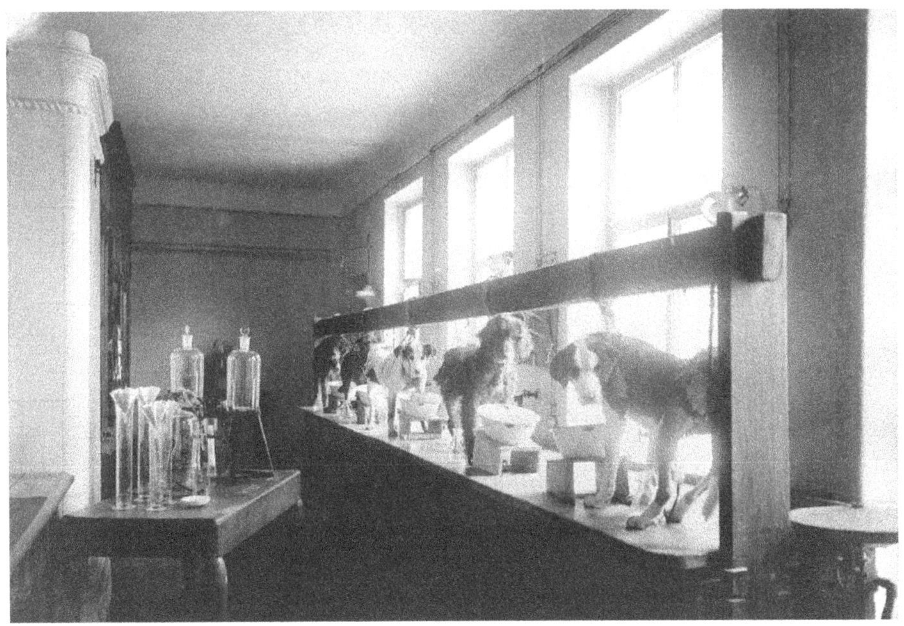

The humble research associates of Pavlov in his lab

Broadening the Scope of Conditioning

Pavlov's experiments went beyond just the salivary response. He explored various conditioning types, including temporal conditioning (where time intervals play a role) and differential conditioning (differentiating between similar stimuli). These studies expanded the understanding of learning and reflexes, demonstrating that behavior could be significantly influenced by the environment.

Innovations in Research Methods

Pavlov's experimental approach was meticulous and innovative. He developed surgical techniques to measure salivary responses accurately and used rigorous scientific methods, setting high standards for experimental psychology and physiology research.

From Physiology to Psychology

While Pavlov started his experiments focusing on digestion physiology, his findings had a profound impact on psychology, particularly in understanding how organisms learn and adapt to their environment. His work bridged the gap between physiological processes and psychological phenomena.

Predecessors in the Study of Reflexes and Digestion

Before Ivan Pavlov's landmark work on classical conditioning, several other scientists and thinkers had delved into the exploration of reflexes and the digestive process, setting the stage for Pavlov's discoveries.

One notable figure in the field of reflexology was Ivan Mikhaylovich Sechenov, a prominent Russian physiologist, who significantly influenced the field. Sechenov is often recognized as the father of Russian physiology, whose materialistic views on reflexes greatly influenced Pavlov. Sechenov's work transformed the understanding of conditional reflexes and the functioning of the brain, laying a theoretical foundation that Pavlov built upon.

Current Implications

The Impact on Psychology and Neuroscience

Ivan Pavlov's research, especially his classical conditioning experiments, has significantly impacted modern psychology and neuroscience. His concept of conditioned reflexes has provided a fundamental understanding of learning processes and behavior.

Advancements in Behavioral Studies

Pavlov's work has led to advancements in behavioral psychology, enhancing the understanding of how environmental factors can shape behaviors. His conditioning experiments serve as a model for studying associative learning not just in animals, but also in humans.

Applications in Therapy and Education

Pavlov's principles have been applied in various therapeutic approaches and educational settings. Techniques derived from his theories are used in behavior modification, cognitive-behavioral therapy, and in developing teaching methods.

Neuroscientific Explorations

In neuroscience, Pavlov's work has prompted further exploration into the neural mechanisms underlying learning and memory. This has contributed to a more comprehensive understanding of the brain's function and plasticity.

Impact and Products

Advances in Behavioral Neuroscience and Psychology

Ivan Pavlov's studies on classical conditioning have had a lasting impact on both neuroscience and psychology. His experiments, originally aimed at understanding digestion, inadvertently uncovered fundamental principles of learning and behavior. The concept of classical conditioning, demonstrated through his bell and food experiment with dogs, became a cornerstone in behavioral science. It underpins various psychological theories, especially behaviorism, and has significantly contributed to the understanding of how associative learning shapes behavior.

Influence Beyond Psychology

Pavlov's principles are integral to modern therapeutic techniques. For instance, exposure therapy, a common treatment for phobias and anxiety disorders, is based on the principles of conditioning. By gradually exposing individuals to their fears in a controlled environment, this therapy aims to desensitize and condition new, non-fearful responses.

Pavlov's Legacy in Neuroscience

Pavlov's work also contributed significantly to neuroscience, particularly in understanding the link between the nervous system and behavior. His research provided insights into how the brain processes and responds to environmental stimuli.

Cultural Impact

Pavlov's work has also permeated popular culture, with the term "Pavlovian" often used to describe instinctive or conditioned responses to stimuli. His research has enhanced the public's understanding of how environment and conditioning can influence behavior, an insight that continues to resonate in various social and cultural contexts. Pavlov's pioneering work not only advanced the field of behavioral science but also provided a framework for understanding and addressing human and animal behavior in a multitude of contexts.

ROBERT KOCH (1905)

The relentless warrior, who tamed the invincible tuberculous bacilli

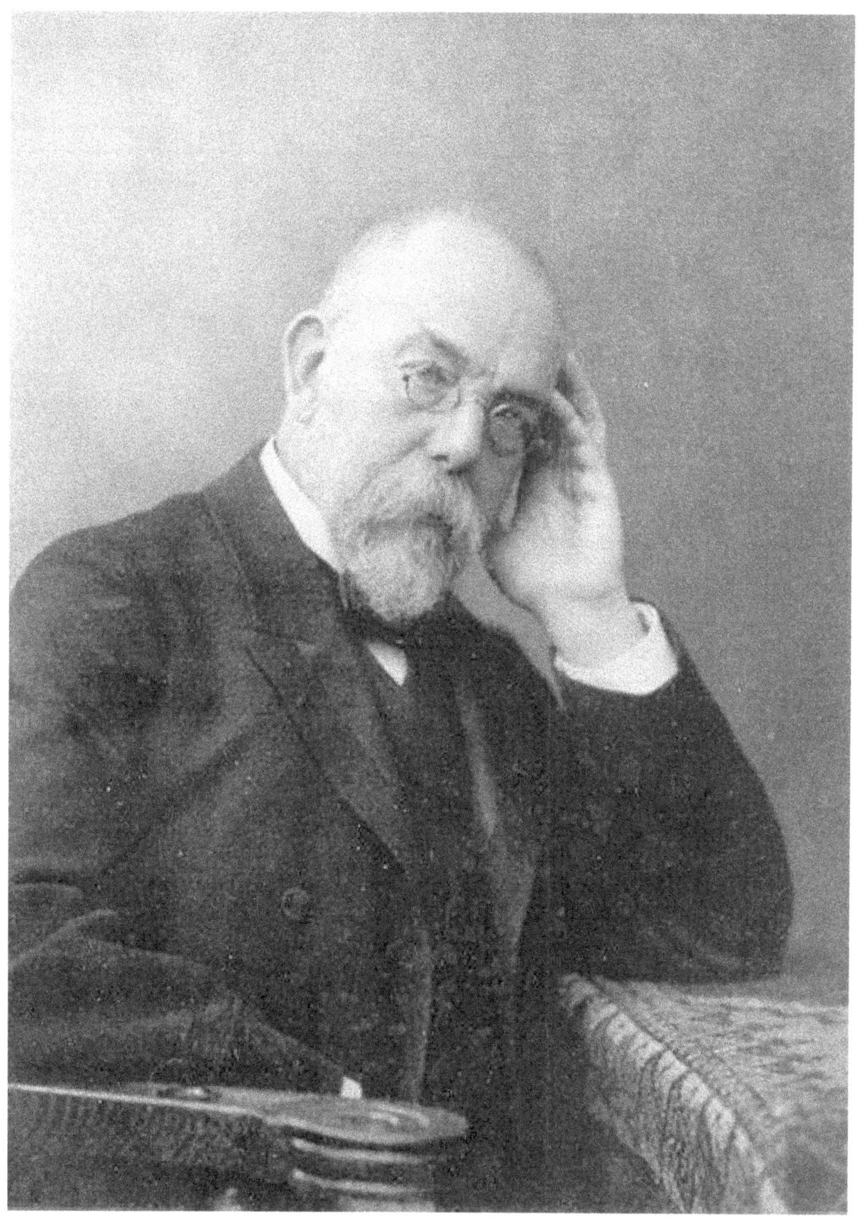

History

Robert Koch, born on December 11, 1843, in Clausthal, Germany, began his journey in medicine at the University of Göttingen in 1862. Influenced by the Professor of Anatomy, Jacob Henle, and later by Rudolf Virchow, Koch was deeply engaged in the study of infectious diseases. After obtaining his M.D. degree in 1866, Koch served in various medical roles, including as a district medical officer in Wollstein, where he conducted his groundbreaking research on anthrax. His early work in bacteriology, conducted in a humble home laboratory with basic equipment, set the stage for his later monumental achievements.

During his time in Wollstein, Koch focused on anthrax, a prevalent disease among farm animals in the region. His innovative research methods led to the discovery of the anthrax bacillus and the development of a new bacteriological technique, laying the foundation for modern microbiology. Koch's work on anthrax, as well as his discoveries of the bacteria responsible for tuberculosis in 1882 and cholera in 1883, solidified his reputation as one of the founding fathers of bacteriology.

In recognition of his contributions, Koch was appointed to various prestigious positions, including as a member of the Imperial Health Bureau in Berlin, Professor of Hygiene at the University of Berlin, and Director of the newly established Institute of Hygiene. His later career saw him conducting research on other infectious diseases, including malaria and rinderpest in Africa and India.

Koch's legacy extends beyond his scientific discoveries. He formulated Koch's postulates, criteria used to establish the causative relationship between a microorganism and a disease. His work not only brought about new scientific understanding but also significantly impacted public health, shaping the approach to controlling and preventing infectious diseases.

Snippets

Groundbreaking Work on Anthrax

Robert Koch's earliest significant contribution to bacteriology was his research on anthrax. In 1876, he isolated and identified Bacillus anthracis, the bacterium responsible for the disease. His work not only demonstrated the presence of this bacterium in the blood and tissues of infected animals but also established a causal relationship between the microorganism and the disease. Koch's findings on anthrax transmission, particularly regarding spore formation and contamination of soil, were crucial in developing preventive measures, including vaccination programs.

Tuberculosis and Cholera Discoveries

Koch's research on tuberculosis led to the identification and isolation of Mycobacterium tuberculosis in 1882. His innovative laboratory techniques, including acid-fast staining, were pivotal in visualizing and identifying this bacterium. Koch's studies extended to understanding the mechanisms of transmission, significantly influencing public health measures like sanatoriums and vaccination programs.

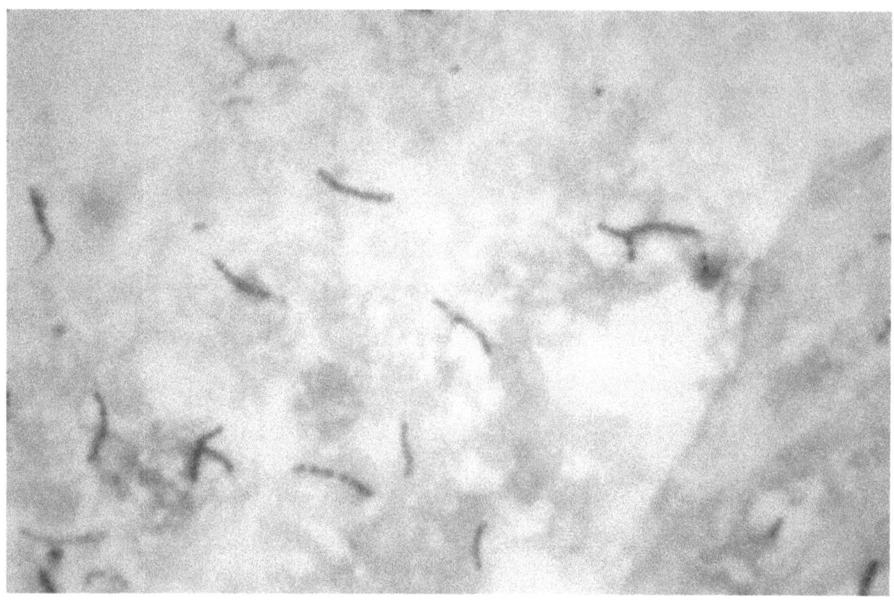

These Innocent looking Tuberculous bacilli, still able to wage a war with humanity

In addition to tuberculosis, Koch's work on cholera was noteworthy. He identified Vibrio cholerae as the causative agent of the disease, which revolutionized the understanding and approach to managing cholera outbreaks. His methodologies in studying cholera set new standards in microbiological research.

Development of Koch's Postulates

One of Koch's most enduring contributions is the formulation of Koch's postulates. These criteria became the gold standard for establishing a causal relationship between a specific microorganism and a disease. His postulates are fundamental to the field of bacteriology and infectious disease research.

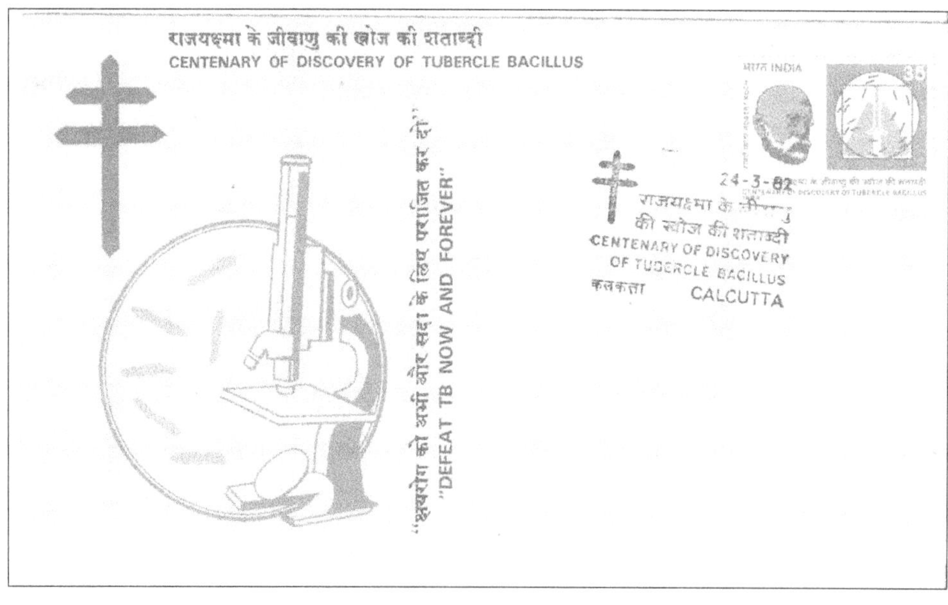

Advances in Laboratory Techniques

Koch's development of innovative laboratory techniques, such as agar plate cultures and the use of solid media, greatly enhanced the study of microorganisms. These techniques allowed for the accurate isolation, cultivation, and identification of bacteria, setting new standards for scientific investigation in bacteriology.

Koch's research and discoveries transformed the understanding of infectious diseases and laid the foundation for the field of medical bacteriology. His meticulous approach to research and emphasis on laboratory techniques set a new precedent for scientific investigation.

Influence in Microbiology and Bacteriology

Before Robert Koch's significant contributions to microbiology and bacteriology, several key figures laid important groundwork in these fields.

Antonie van Leeuwenhoek (1670s)

Dutch scientist Antonie van Leeuwenhoek is often celebrated as the father of microbiology. He was the first to observe microorganisms, which he called "animalcules," using microscopes that he designed himself. His meticulous observations and descriptions in the late 17th century provided the first glimpses into the microbial world.

Ignaz Semmelweis (1840s)

Ignaz Semmelweis, a Hungarian physician, made groundbreaking discoveries in the 1840s regarding the prevention of puerperal fever in maternity wards. He introduced handwashing practices in clinics, significantly reducing mortality rates. His work predated the germ theory of disease and emphasized the importance of cleanliness in medical settings.

John Snow (1850s)

An English physician, John Snow, is known as one of the founders of modern epidemiology. In the 1850s, he mapped cholera outbreaks in London and identified contaminated water as a transmission method for the disease. This work was instrumental in establishing the relationship between pathogens and disease.

Louis Pasteur (1860s)

French chemist and microbiologist Louis Pasteur made critical contributions to the development of germ theory. His work in the 1860s on fermentation and putrefaction led to the understanding that microorganisms are responsible for these processes, which was a key step in developing the germ theory.

These early contributors to germ theory and bacteriology created a foundation upon which scientists like Robert Koch could build. Their collective efforts were crucial in shaping our understanding of infectious diseases and the role of microorganisms.

Current Implications

Enduring Influence of Koch's Postulates

The most significant and lasting impact of Robert Koch's work in modern microbiology is the formulation of Koch's Postulates. These criteria, established for linking specific microbes to specific diseases, revolutionized the scientific method in infectious disease research. They provided a systematic way to establish causation, moving beyond mere association and elevating scientific rigor in the field. Koch's Postulates continue to be the gold standard in microbiology, shaping diagnostic methods and informing disease prevention and treatment strategies.

Tuberculosis and Public Health Advances

Koch's discovery of Mycobacterium tuberculosis, the bacterium responsible for tuberculosis, in 1882 was a monumental achievement. It marked the first time a specific microorganism was definitively linked to an infectious disease. This breakthrough had far-reaching implications for public health, leading to more precise diagnostic tools and interventions. It also significantly contributed to immunology, informing the development of vaccines and therapeutic strategies.

Global Impact in Cholera Research

Koch's work extended beyond tuberculosis to other diseases, including cholera. His research expeditions in regions affected by cholera, such as Egypt and India, were crucial in identifying Vibrio cholerae as the causative agent. This finding was pivotal for developing accurate detection and diagnostic methods and implementing effective preventive measures. His commitment to global health challenges underlined his vision of applying scientific advancements universally for humanity's benefit.

Anthrax Research and Immunization

Koch's identification of Bacillus anthracis as the cause of anthrax laid the groundwork for vaccine development against this disease. His ability to translate scientific findings into practical applications showcased his commitment to advancing public health through preventive measures.

Ethical Reflections

While Koch's scientific contributions are significant, it's important to reflect on the ethical complexities of his involvement in eugenics. This aspect of his legacy invites a nuanced examination of the relationship between scientific achievements and ethical responsibility, emphasizing the importance of critically assessing historical figures and learning from the past to shape a more responsible scientific future.

Impact and Products

Tuberculosis and Mycobacterium tuberculosis Discovery (1882)

Koch's identification of Mycobacterium tuberculosis as the causative agent of tuberculosis was a pivotal moment in medical history. This discovery laid the groundwork for developing targeted diagnostic tools and interventions, crucial for controlling and preventing tuberculosis.

Development of Koch's Postulates

Koch established a systematic framework for linking specific microbes to diseases. These postulates became foundational in microbiology, guiding the identification of pathogens and influencing public health policies and diagnostic strategies.

Global Impact on Cholera Research

Koch's research on cholera, particularly his identification of Vibrio cholerae, had a significant global impact. His work informed public health strategies and led to the development of effective prevention and control measures against cholera.

Influence on Immunology and Public Health

Beyond identifying pathogens, Koch contributed to immunology, notably through his work on anthrax and the development of vaccines. His methodological rigor in research set a standard in medical microbiology, shaping contemporary approaches to infectious diseases.

SANTIAGO RAMÓN Y CAJAL AND CAMILLO GOLGI (1906)

Laid the foundations of neuroscience by his magical neuronal vison

Santiago Ramón y Cajal and Camillo Golgi, two giants in the field of neuroscience, were jointly awarded the Nobel Prize in Medicine. This accolade was a testament to their groundbreaking work in unraveling the complexities of the nervous system.

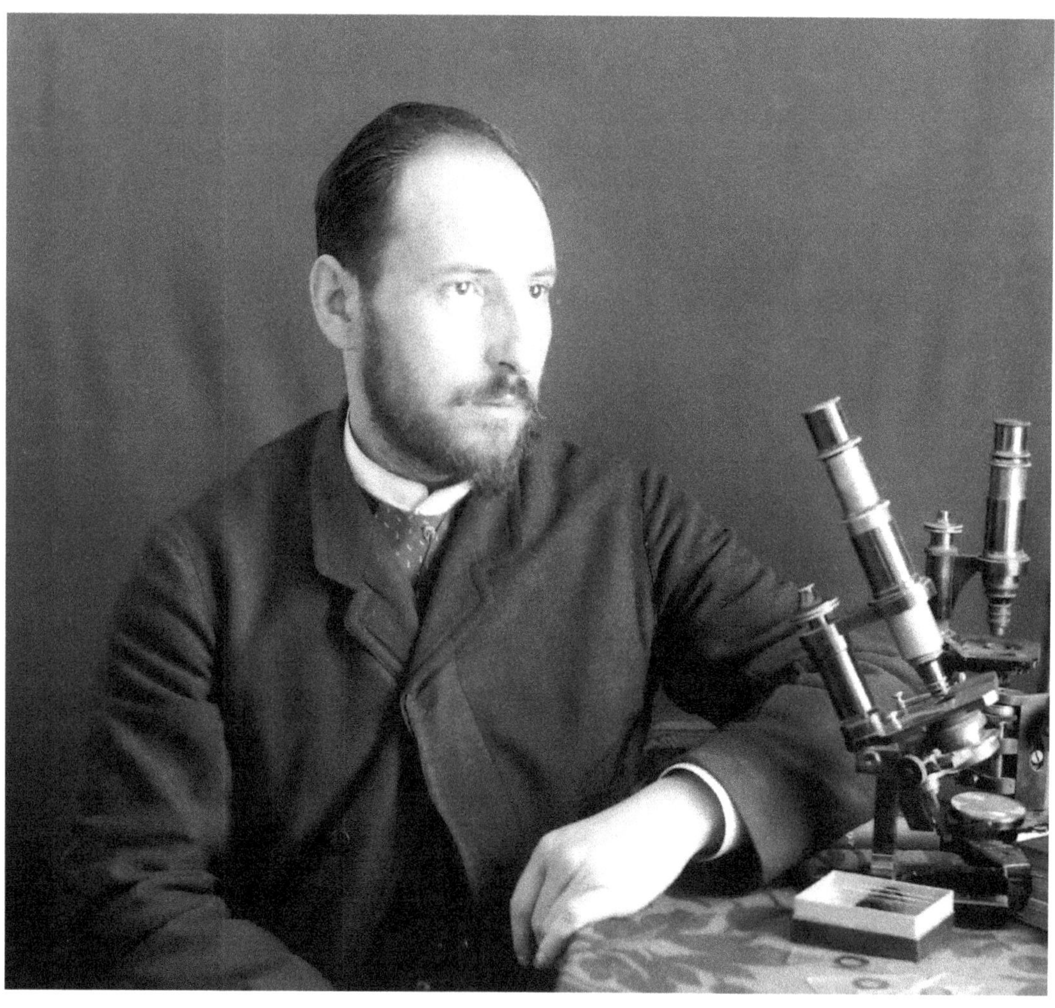

History

Santiago Ramón y Cajal's journey into the world of science was as unique as his discoveries. Born on May 1, 1852, in Petilla de Aragón, Spain, Cajal's initial interests were far from the scientific world. As a rebellious and artistic child, he was more inclined towards painting and gymnastics, showing little interest in conventional education. This rebellious streak even led to a mischievous incident at age eleven, where he was imprisoned for damaging a neighbor's gate with a homemade cannon. Despite these early inclinations, his father, a professor of applied anatomy, guided him towards the study of medicine, mainly under his direction at the University of Zaragoza.

Cajal's medical journey was marked by challenges and shifts. After obtaining his Licentiate in Medicine in 1873, he served as an army doctor, including a stint in Cuba where he contracted malaria and tuberculosis. His return to Spain marked the beginning of his serious engagement with the scientific world. He worked as an assistant in the School of Anatomy in Zaragoza, later becoming the Director of the Saragossa Museum. His academic career progressed with appointments in Valencia, Barcelona, and eventually Madrid, where he served as a professor of histology and pathological anatomy. Cajal's work in these roles was foundational, particularly his improvements to Golgi's silver nitrate stain, which revolutionized the study of neurons and the nervous system.

Camillo Golgi, born in July 1843 in Italy, contributed significantly to neuroscience with his unique staining technique that allowed for the visualization of intricate structures within the nervous system. Golgi's method, which involved using potassium dichromate and silver nitrate to stain neurons, was pivotal in enabling the detailed study of individual neurons within the dense network of the brain and spinal cord.

The contrasting backgrounds of Cajal and Golgi – one a rebellious artist turned scientist, the other a methodical and technical mind – converged in their shared pursuit of understanding the nervous system. Their discoveries and methods laid the groundwork for modern neuroscience, changing the way we understand the brain and its functions.

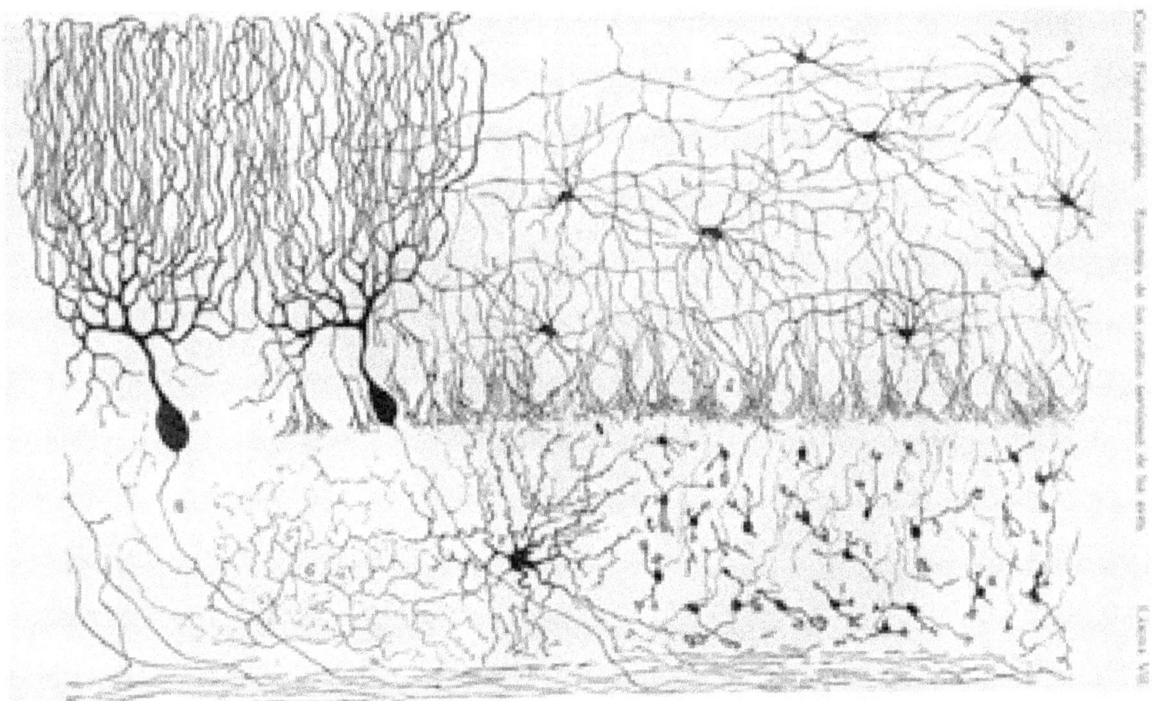

Cajal golgi neurone doctrine defined the function of nervous system

Snippets

Santiago Ramón y Cajal

Santiago Ramón y Cajal's scientific achievements are one of relentless curiosity and innovation. His journey began when he encountered Golgi's staining method, which he not only embraced but also refined. This technique was crucial for his studies, as it allowed him to observe neurons in unprecedented detail.

Cajal's work fundamentally changed the understanding of the nervous system. He passionately argued against the prevailing belief of a continuous neural network, proposing instead that the nervous system comprised billions of individual nerve cells. This groundbreaking concept, known as the "neuron doctrine," was a pivotal moment in neuroscience, establishing the neuron as the fundamental unit of the nervous system.

One of Cajal's most significant contributions was his detailed study of various parts of the brain and nervous system, including the retina, cerebellum, and spinal cord. His work in these areas, particularly his descriptions and illustrations, formed the basis of modern neuroanatomy. His seminal text, "Textura del Sistema Nervioso del Hombre y los Vertebrados," provided comprehensive insights into the structure of the nervous system and has been a cornerstone in the field for over a century.

Camillo Golgi

Camillo Golgi, an Italian scientist, was instrumental in the development of a staining technique using potassium dichromate and silver nitrate. This method, known as the Golgi stain, was revolutionary in its ability to reveal the intricate structures of the nervous system, previously a daunting task due to the density and complexity of neural networks.

Golgi himself, however, held a different view of the nervous system's organization, believing in the concept of a continuous neural network. This belief, contrary to Cajal's neuron doctrine, posited that the nervous system was made of interconnected networks. Despite this difference in views, Golgi's method was crucial in advancing the study of neuroanatomy and provided a foundation for Cajal's transformative discoveries.

Together, the contributions of Santiago Ramón y Cajal and Camillo Golgi represent a monumental advancement in the understanding of the nervous system.

Predecessors and Contemporaries in Neuroanatomy and Histology

Joseph von Gerlach: Gerlach's work, advocating a continuous neural network, influenced the scientific community before Cajal and Golgi's time. He was a proponent of the idea that the nervous system was made up of interconnected networks, a view later challenged by Cajal.

Rudolf Albert von Kölliker: A Swiss historian, Kölliker became a supporter of Cajal and the neuron doctrine after initially being influenced by Golgi's work. His change in stance was significant, as he was a well-respected authority in the field.

Wilhelm Waldeyer: He officially enunciated the neuron doctrine in 1891, a concept critical to modern neuroscience. Waldeyer played a key role in cementing the idea of the neuron as the basic structural and functional unit of the nervous system.

Aldo Perroncito: Working in Golgi's laboratory, Perroncito conducted studies on peripheral nerve regeneration that paralleled Cajal's work. However, his findings did not seem to influence Golgi's thinking on the Neuron Doctrine, highlighting the diversity of views even within the same research environment.

Current Implications

Neuron Doctrine Adoption: The neuron doctrine, championed by Cajal, which proposed that the nervous system is made of billions of separate nerve cells, has become the basic principle of the organization of the nervous system. This doctrine is a cornerstone of modern neuroscience, forming the basis for our understanding of how the brain and nervous system function.

Advancements in Histological Techniques: The staining techniques developed by Golgi and improved upon by Cajal significantly advanced the study of nervous tissue. Before these developments, the intricate details of nerve cells were virtually invisible to microscopes. Their methods allowed for a clearer visualization of neurons, paving the way for more detailed and accurate studies.

Influence on Subsequent Research: The work of Cajal and Golgi influenced a multitude of subsequent research in neuroscience. Their discoveries have been instrumental in the development of various theories and models concerning the brain and nervous system.

Educational and Research Value: Cajal's detailed descriptions and illustrations of the nervous system continue to be a valuable resource in neuroscience education and research. His drawings and observations have been reproduced in textbooks and remain relevant for understanding the structure and function of the nervous system.

Cell Theory Application to Neuroscience: The application of cell theory to the brain, an idea that became clear during their era, was a significant step forward. It helped in understanding that the brain, like other body tissues, is composed of individual cells, which was a paradigm shift in how we perceive and study the brain.

Impact and Products

Refinement of Staining Techniques: Cajal improved upon Golgi's original staining method, optimizing it for better visualization of nervous fibers. His modifications enabled clearer observations of nerve tissues in various organisms, including birds and mammalian embryos, which lacked myelin. This advancement was critical for understanding the detailed structure of nerve cells.

Contributions to Neuroanatomy: Cajal's comprehensive work, "Textura del Sistema Nervioso del Hombre y los Vertebrados," which was later translated and made available internationally, laid the foundation of modern neuroanatomy. It detailed the organization of nerve cells in the central and peripheral nervous system across various species.

Discovery of Neuronal Structures: Cajal's use of modified staining techniques led to several important discoveries, such as the identification of dendritic spines and the concept of axonal growth cones in developing neurons. These discoveries challenged the existing reticular theory and supported the neuron doctrine.

Influence on Current Neuroscience: Their work influenced current theories on brain function and learning, speculating on the relationship between intelligence and the efficiency of neural connections. This idea aligns with contemporary understanding in neuroscience.

Artistic Contributions: Both scientists were also skilled in drawing, a crucial skill in an era before cameras could be attached to microscopes. Their ability to accurately depict microscopic observations played a vital role in communicating their findings to the scientific community.

ALPHONSE LAVERAN (1907)

The extraordinary French, who first picked the protozoal pigments in RBC from Malaria patients

In 1907, Alphonse Laveran was awarded the Nobel Prize in Medicine for his discovery, which continues to be a cornerstone in the study and treatment of malaria and other protozoal diseases.

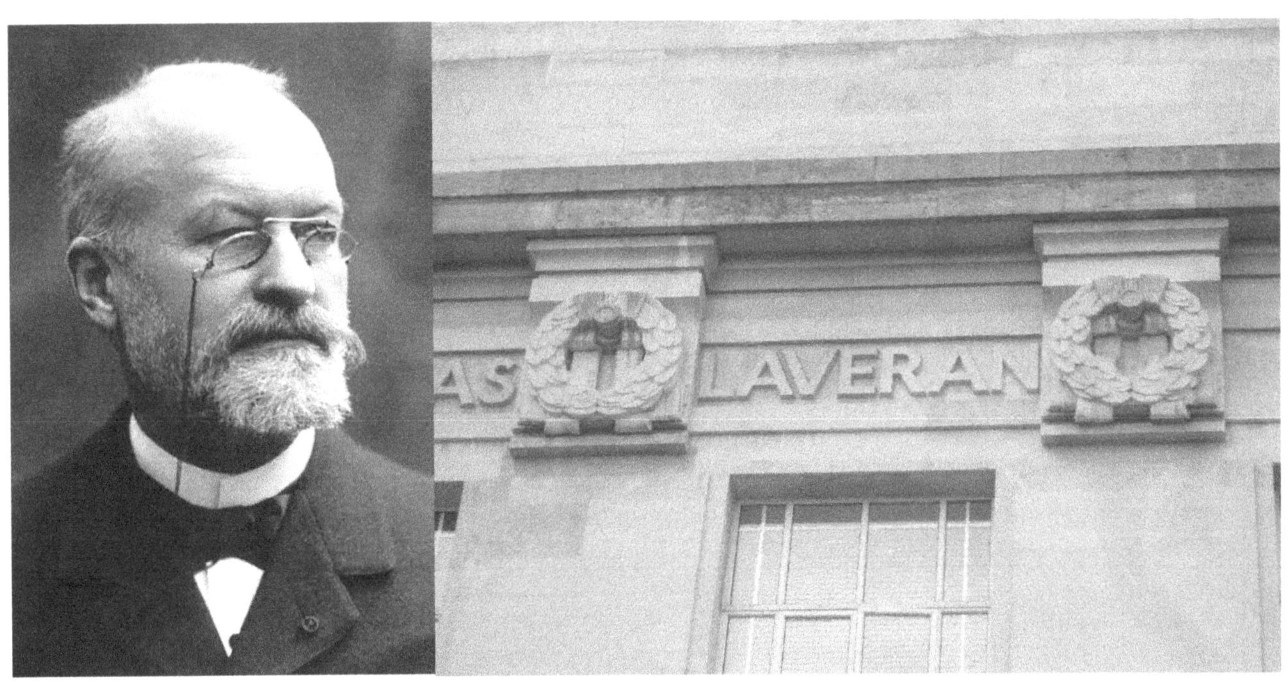

Laveran's name is etched in the walls of London school of tropical medicine

History

Alphonse Laveran, a French physician born in Paris in 1845, followed in his family's military medical footsteps. Educated at prestigious institutions like the Collège Sainte-Barbe and Lycée Louis-le-Grand, he chose a career in military medicine. During the Franco-Prussian War, he served as a Medical Assistant-Major. His key contributions to medicine began during his tenure in Algeria, where he was exposed to malaria's ravages in the military.

Snippets

Laveran's most groundbreaking discovery occurred in 1880 at a military hospital in Constantine, Algeria. Here, he identified pigmented cells in the blood of malaria patients, leading to his revolutionary finding: malaria is caused by protozoan parasites. This contradicted the common belief that malaria was caused by "bad air" or bacteria. His observations, meticulously noted in various forms and stages, unveiled the Plasmodium parasite as the true reason behind malaria.

Predecessors

Prior to Laveran, German physician Rudolf Virchow had observed the malarial pigment in 1849, providing early insights into blood infection related to malaria. However, Virchow misidentified the pigmented cells, mistaking them for endothelial cells and white blood cells. Laveran's insights corrected these earlier misconceptions, laying the foundation for modern understanding of malaria.

Current Implications

Laveran's discovery had profound implications for public health, particularly in tropical regions where malaria is endemic. His work paved the way for better understanding, treatment, and prevention strategies for malaria, a disease that continues to affect millions worldwide.

Impact and Products

Laveran's work led to significant developments in antiprotozoal drugs and strategies for disease control. His insights into protozoan-caused diseases expanded the field of tropical medicine and were instrumental in shaping modern strategies to combat diseases like malaria. The Société de Pathologie Exotique, founded using part of his Nobel Prize money, continues to contribute to tropical disease research.

In recognition of his contributions, Laveran was elected to the French Academy of Sciences in 1893 and was made Commander of the National Order of the Legion of Honour in 1912.

ILYA ILYICH MECHNIKOV AND PAUL EHRLICH (1908)

This Russian duo's dramatic discovery of human Immune system

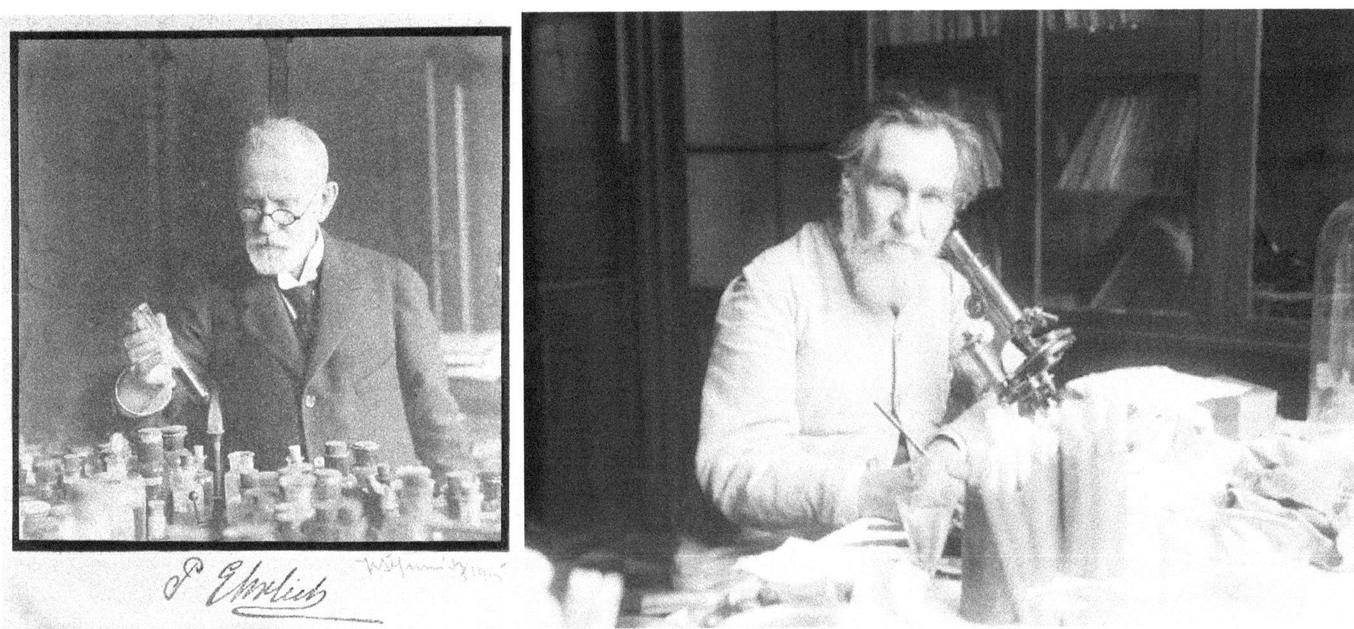

Ilya Ilyich Mechnikov and Paul Ehrlich were jointly awarded the Nobel Prize in 1908 for their pioneering work on immunity. Their research laid the foundation for the field of immunology, uncovering mechanisms of the immune system that protect against disease.

History

Ilya Mechnikov

Born on May 16, 1845, near Kharkov, in the Russian Empire, Mechnikov was the youngest of five children. His mother, of Jewish descent, played a significant role in his education, particularly in science. Mechnikov's passion for natural history was evident from a young age.

He entered the Kharkov Lycée, developing an interest in biology. Later, at the University of Kharkov, he completed a four-year degree in natural sciences in just two years. He then studied marine fauna in Heligoland and worked under Rudolf Leuckart at the University of Giessen, where he made his first scientific discovery related to intracellular digestion in flatworms.

Mechnikov's career was marked by challenges, including conflicts with colleagues and personal health issues. Despite these, he made significant contributions to immunology, notably his discovery of phagocytosis in 1882. His work at the Pasteur Institute in Paris, where he spent the latter part of his life, included treatises on senescence, disease, and death.

In his 1903 work, "The Nature of Man: Studies in Optimistic Philosophy," Mechnikov argued for the role of science in advancing civilization and improving human life.

Paul Ehrlich

Paul Ehrlich, born on March 14, 1854, in Strehlen, Prussia (now Strzelin, Poland), was a pioneering figure in the fields of hematology, immunology, and antimicrobial chemotherapy. His early exposure to the world of science was significantly influenced by his family. His mother's cousin, the pathologist Carl Weigert, introduced Ehrlich to the technique of staining cells with chemical dyes, which was crucial for viewing cells under a microscope. This experience during his medical studies at various universities including Breslau, Strasbourg, Freiburg, and Leipzig, sparked his lifelong fascination with cellular staining and its medical implications.

Ehrlich's major contributions were in understanding how antibodies neutralize toxins. He collaborated with Emil von Behring on treating diphtheria using blood serum containing antibodies. His theory that cells have receptors to bind harmful substances was a monumental contribution to immunology.

Snippets

Ilya Mechnikov's Phagocytosis Theory

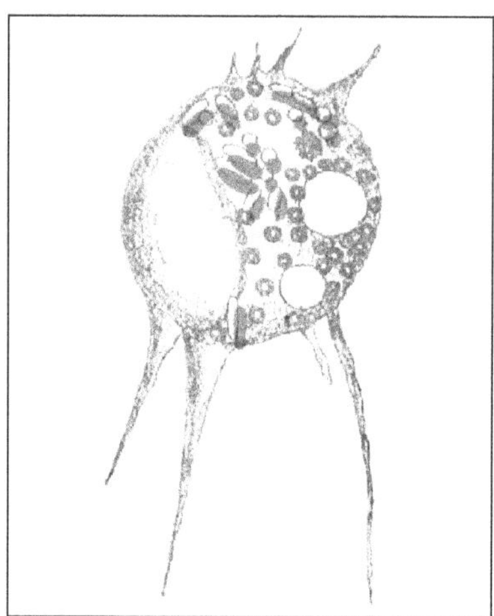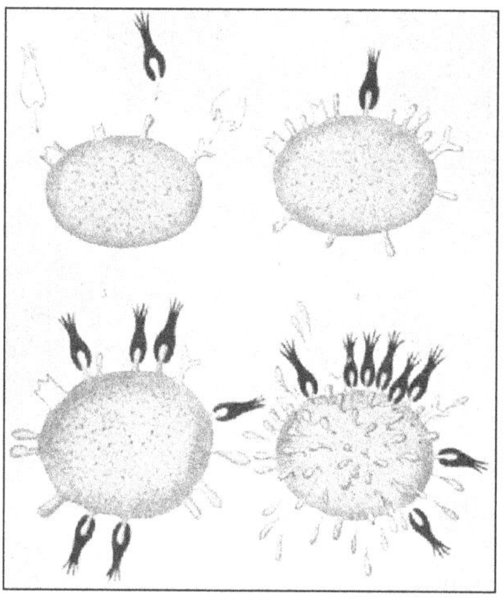

His cartoon of Neutrophils engulfing the Invading micro organisms

Discovery of Phagocytosis: Mechnikov discovered phagocytosis while studying starfish larvae in 1882. He observed that certain cells, which he later identified as macrophages and neutrophils, engulfed and destroyed invading pathogens.

Principle of Innate Immunity: This discovery laid the foundation for understanding the principle mechanism of innate immunity. Mechnikov's theory proposed that phagocytes play a crucial role in the body's defense against infection.

Extension to Organismal Harmony: Mechnikov's theory went beyond host defense, suggesting a broader role for phagocytosis in maintaining organismal harmony.

Paul Ehrlich's Side-Chain Theory

Antibodies and Receptors: Ehrlich's theory postulated that antibodies are produced by white blood cells and act as side chains (receptors) on the cell membrane.

Specificity and Binding: The theory emphasized the specificity of antibodies for interaction with particular antigens, occurring through precise binding via side chains.

Formation and Release of Antibodies: Ehrlich suggested that a cell under threat produces additional side chains to bind toxins. These extra side chains then break off to become antibodies, circulating through the body to target specific toxins or pathogens.

Magic Bullets: Ehrlich described these antibodies as "magic bullets" – agents that specifically target toxins or pathogens without harming the body.

Earlier Contributors

The early development of immunology was significantly shaped by several pioneering scientists whose work laid the foundations for our modern understanding of the immune system.

Louis Pasteur, renowned for his work on microorganisms, was a pivotal figure in early immunology. His research not only enhanced our understanding of infectious diseases but also provided insights into the immune response. Robert Koch's groundbreaking work, particularly on tuberculosis, contributed immensely to microbiology and immunology.

Jules Bordet's studies advanced our knowledge of the immune response, focusing on aspects like the complement system and the principles of humoral and cellular immunology. His work played a crucial role in shaping the field's future direction.

Emil Behring, alongside his work with Paul Ehrlich, made significant strides in serum therapies, particularly for diphtheria and tetanus. This work was instrumental in developing passive immunization techniques, which have had lasting impacts on medical science.

Current Implications:

The groundbreaking work of Ilya Mechnikov and Paul Ehrlich in the field of immunology has had a profound and lasting impact on modern medicine, particularly in the areas of immunology and vaccine development:

Phagocytosis and Cellular Immunity: Mechnikov's discovery of phagocytes and phagocytosis laid the groundwork for understanding the cellular mechanisms of the immune system. His concept of "self and not self" as the prerequisite for physiological inflammation and self-maintenance of the organism forms a critical component of modern immunology.

Antibody Standardization and Functions: Ehrlich developed methods for standardizing antibody activity in immune sera and described the neutralizing and complement-dependent effects of antibodies. His "side-chain" theory of antibody formation was pivotal in understanding how the immune system recognizes and neutralizes foreign substances.

Impact on Vaccine Development: Their discoveries have informed the development of vaccines, contributing to the understanding of how the immune system responds to pathogens and how this response can be harnessed to prevent diseases.

Foundations of Infection Biology: Mechnikov and Ehrlich were also the first to envision infection biology as the result of an interaction between host and pathogen, a concept that continues to guide contemporary research in immunology and microbiology.

Impact and Products

The principles set forth by Mechnikov and Ehrlich have played a crucial role in the evolution of vaccines. For instance, the concept of generating an immune response to a pathogen, a key aspect of vaccination, is deeply rooted in their theories. Over the years, various types of vaccines, such as live, non-live, and newer platforms like viral vectors and nucleic acid-based vaccines, have been developed.

This methodological advancement led to the creation of several key vaccines, including those for polio, measles, mumps, and rubella. The development of these vaccines was based on the understanding that specific immune responses, particularly antibodies, could protect against these diseases.

The legacy of Mechnikov and Ehrlich in immunology is not just confined to their time; it continues to shape and inspire current and future developments in vaccine and therapy creation, underscoring the transformative power of their scientific endeavors.

EMIL THEODOR KOCHER (1909)

This swaggy Swiss surgeon who conquered the world with unique thyroidectomy skills

Emil Theodor Kocher was awarded the Nobel Prize in Medicine in 1909, a testament to his monumental contributions to the medical field, particularly in surgery.

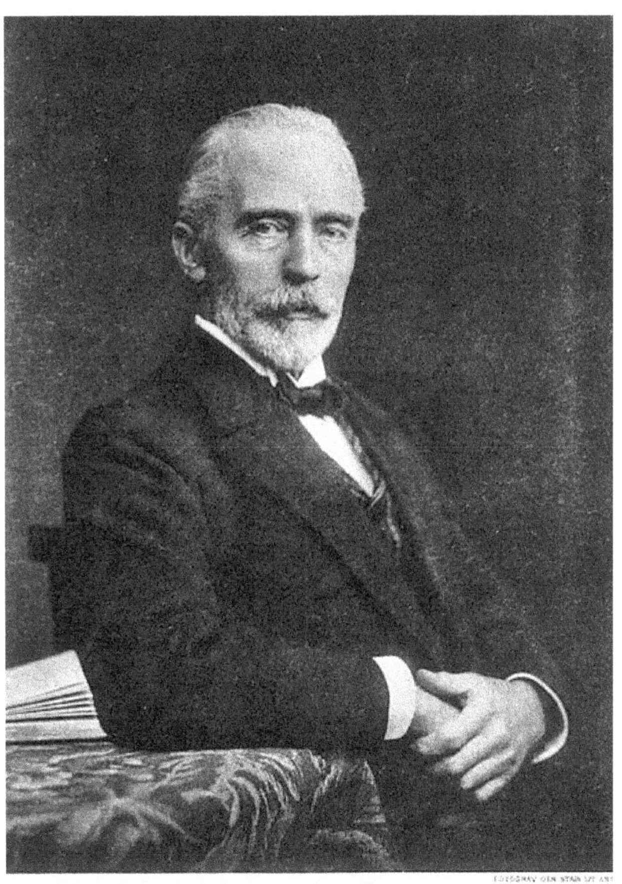

History

Emil Theodor Kocher, born on August 25, 1841, in Bern, Switzerland, was a revolutionary figure in surgery. After completing his medical studies at the University of Bern in 1865, Kocher expanded his knowledge across Europe, learning from leading figures in medicine. By 1872, he was appointed professor of surgery at the University of Bern, where he dedicated his career to surgical advancements, particularly in thyroidectomy.

Snippets

Kocher's most significant contribution to medicine was his work on thyroidectomy. He developed a safer technique for thyroid removal, significantly reducing the surgery's mortality rate. Moreover, Kocher was the first to describe the physiological effects of thyroidectomy, notably identifying the development of cretinism and hypothyroidism in patients from whom the thyroid had been completely removed. His observations led to the practice of leaving a part of the thyroid gland intact to prevent such complications.

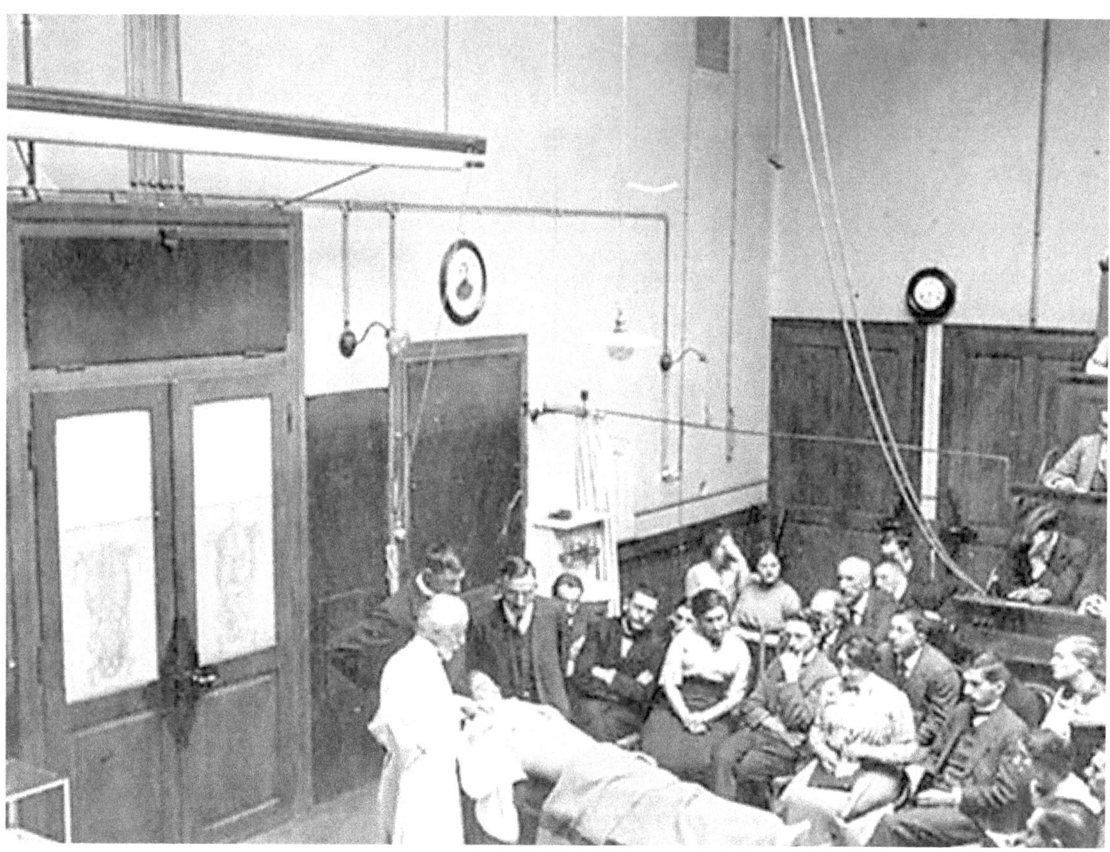

Kocher's teaching live classes from Theater

Earlier Contributors

Surgeons and scientists like Theodor Billroth and others made initial strides in understanding the thyroid gland and surgical infections, setting the stage for Kocher's breakthroughs. Their collaborative efforts and exchange of ideas were pivotal in advancing the field.

Current Implications

Kocher's work has left a lasting impact on modern surgical techniques and the field of endocrinology. His principles of asepsis and meticulous surgical methods are still in practice today, underscoring the importance of patient safety and precision in surgery. Furthermore, his research on the thyroid gland has influenced the current understanding and treatment of thyroid diseases.

Impact and Products

Kocher's advancements have led to significant progress in surgical techniques, anesthesia, and the management of thyroid diseases. The "Kocher incision" remains a standard approach for thyroid surgery, and his emphasis on preserving thyroid function has improved outcomes for patients undergoing thyroidectomy. His legacy is also evident in the continued innovation in surgical practices and endocrinology research.

"Seldom in the history of medicine has the recognition of the most effective cure followed as swiftly on the heels of the discovery of a disease as the establishment of the complete effectiveness of Iodothyrin and thyroidin followed the recognition of cachexia thyreopriva."

ALBRECHT KOSSEL (1910)

The great German who unlocked the secrets of nucleic acids

Albrecht Kossel was awarded the Nobel Prize in Medicine in 1910 for his contributions to our understanding of cell chemistry, particularly for his research on proteins and nucleic acids. His work laid foundational knowledge for the field of genetics.

History

Born in 1853 in Rostock, Germany, Kossel pursued medicine, driven by a keen interest in physiological chemistry. He studied under prominent scientists like Ernst Haeckel and Felix Hoppe-Seyler, which shaped his future research trajectory. Kossel's journey saw him holding positions at several German universities, where he dedicated his career to unraveling the complexities of cell chemistry.

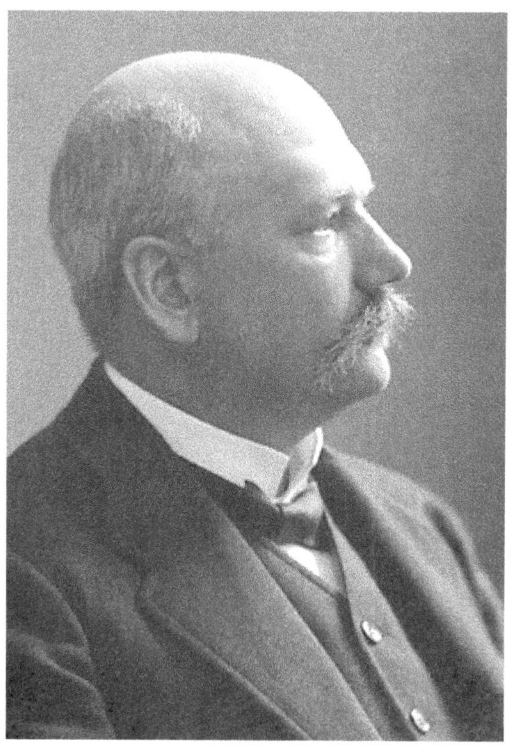

Kossel's studies under Felix Hoppe-Seyler at Strassburg were critical in shaping his future research directions. Hoppe-Seyler, head of the biochemistry department, was a pioneer in the field, and his focus on the chemical aspects of biology deeply influenced Kossel. After completing his education, which included a period at the University of Rostock where he passed his medical license exam in 1877, Kossel embarked on a career that would see him contributing foundational knowledge to biochemistry and genetics.

Kossel's dedication to his field was also evident in his editorial work for the Zeitschrift für Physiologische Chemie (Journal of Physiological Chemistry), a role he assumed following Hoppe-Seyler's death in 1895 and held until his own death in 1927. This position allowed him to influence the direction of research in physiological chemistry significantly.

Snippets

Discovery of Nucleic Acid Components

Kossel's groundbreaking work in biochemistry led to the isolation and characterization of the five nucleotide bases essential for life: adenine, cytosine, guanine, thymine, and uracil. These discoveries between 1885 and 1901 provided the chemical basis for understanding DNA and RNA's structure and function. Kossel's identification of these nucleobases laid the foundation for modern genetics, highlighting the molecular complexity of heredity and genetic information.

Protein Composition and Function

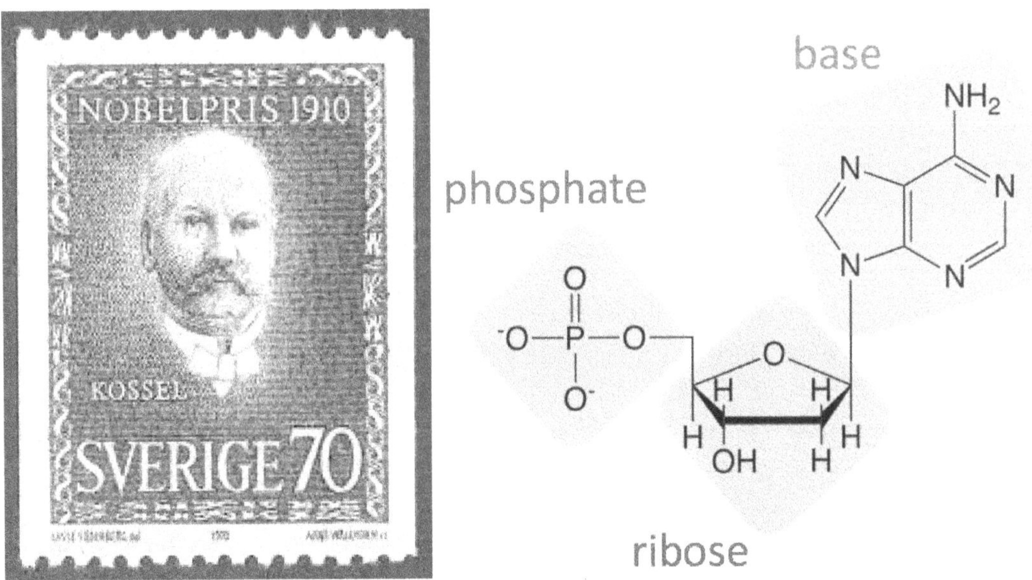

Kossel extended his research to proteins, uncovering their complex nature and vital roles within biological systems. He was particularly focused on the protein components of nucleins, demonstrating their composition of both a protein portion and a non-protein portion, which he identified as nucleic acid.

Impact on Molecular Biology

Kossel contributed to the foundational knowledge necessary for the development of molecular genetics, including the elucidation of the genetic code and the mechanisms of gene expression and regulation.

Early Researchers in Biochemistry and Molecular Biology

The narrative of early biochemistry and molecular biology is enriched by the contributions of several pioneering researchers, among whom Friedrich Miescher stands out for his foundational discovery of nucleic acids. In 1869, while working under Ernst Hoppe-Seyler at the University of Tübingen, Miescher isolated a substance from the nuclei of white blood cells found in pus, which he initially named "nuclein." This substance, later recognized as nucleic acid and eventually identified as deoxyribonucleic acid (DNA), marked a significant milestone in the understanding of the chemical basis of heredity.

Miescher's work did not stop at the discovery of nucleic acids. He also discovered protamine in salmon spermatozoa in 1874, an alkaline substance that interacts closely with nucleic acids and plays a role in the stabilization of insulin and as a reversal agent for heparin. This discovery further illustrates the complex interplay between proteins and nucleic acids in biological systems.

Current Implications

Foundation for Modern Genetics and Molecular Biology

Kossel's research on nucleic acids and proteins provided essential insights into the chemical basis of life. His identification of nucleotide bases laid the groundwork for understanding DNA and RNA's structure, crucial for the development of genetics and molecular biology.

Advancements in Genetic Engineering

The understanding of nucleic acids and proteins, stemming from Kossel's work, has significantly impacted genetic engineering. Techniques like CRISPR-Cas9 gene editing have become possible, allowing for precise modifications in the genetic makeup of organisms.

Contributions to Biotechnology and Medicine

Kossel's findings have paved the way for numerous applications in biotechnology and medicine, including the development of new drugs, therapies for genetic disorders, and the synthesis of artificial genes. His work has had a profound effect on medical research, diagnostics, and treatments.

Influence on Synthetic Biology

The elucidation of nucleic acid components and their functions has been instrumental in the emergence of synthetic biology, a field dedicated to redesigning organisms for useful purposes. Kossel's discoveries have enabled scientists to engineer biological systems for producing biofuels, pharmaceuticals, and other chemicals.

Impact on Understanding Human Genome

Kossel's research contributed to the foundational knowledge necessary for the Human Genome Project and other genomic studies. Understanding the structure and function of DNA has been critical in identifying genetic markers for diseases and understanding human evolution and diversity.

Impact and Products

Albrecht Kossel's work has had far-reaching implications in various fields, from genetic research to biotechnology, influencing both theoretical frameworks and practical applications.

Advances in DNA Research

Kossel's identification of the nucleotide bases—adenine, guanine, cytosine, thymine, and uracil—provided the chemical foundation necessary for the later discovery of the DNA double helix by Watson and Crick. This breakthrough has enabled a deeper understanding of genetic structures and mechanisms, facilitating advances in genetic testing, forensics, and our understanding of genetic diseases.

Genetic Engineering

The knowledge of nucleic acid components has been pivotal for the development of genetic engineering technologies. Techniques such as CRISPR-Cas9, which allows for precise editing of the DNA sequence in living organisms, owe their existence to the foundational work laid by Kossel and his contemporaries.

Biotechnology and Medicine

In biotechnology and medicine, Kossel's discoveries have led to the development of new therapeutic drugs and treatments. Understanding the molecular structure of DNA and proteins has been crucial in the field of pharmacogenomics, the study of how genes affect a person's response to drugs.

The impact of Kossel's work is evident in the Albrecht Kossel Institute for Neuroregeneration at the University of Rostock, named in his honor. It symbolizes his enduring influence on scientific research and his contributions to understanding the chemistry of life.

ALLVAR GULLSTRAND (1911)

The Swedish visionary's insight took us in a deep journey into human eyes

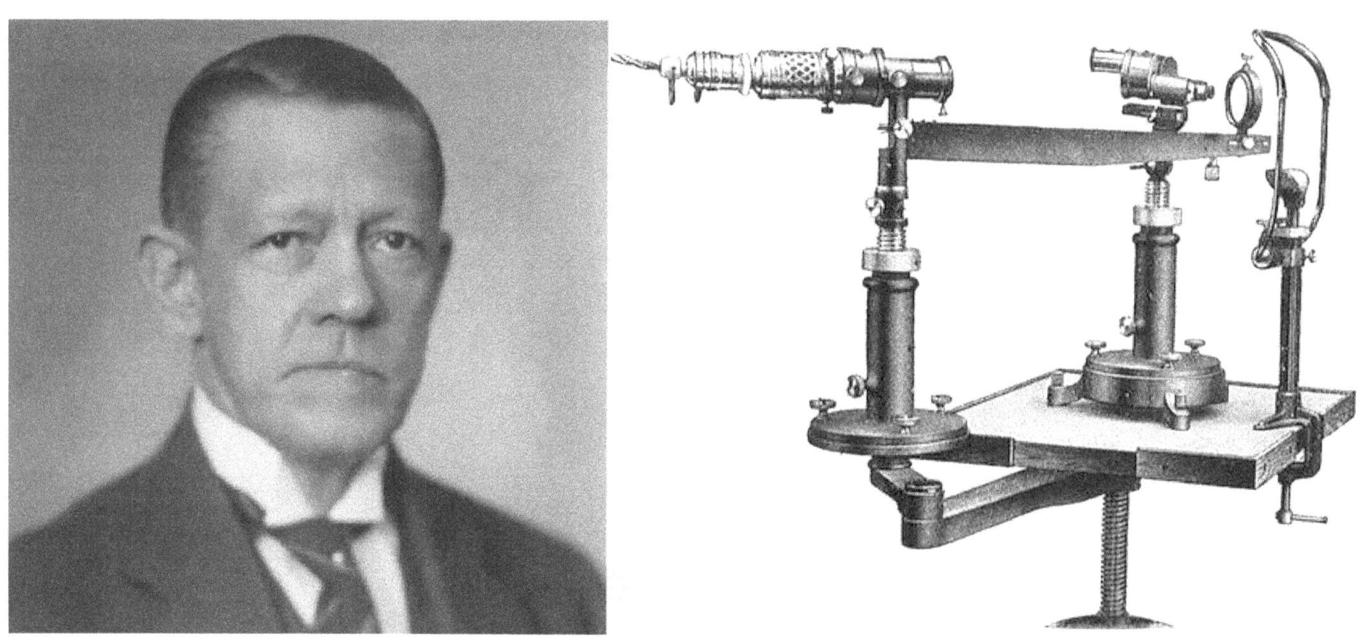

Allvar Gullstrand, the 1911 Nobel Prize laureate in Medicine, significantly advanced our understanding of the human eye's optics. His meticulous work, recognized for its contribution to ophthalmology, remains a cornerstone of optical and vision science.

History

Born in Landskrona, Sweden, in 1862, Gullstrand's path to becoming a pivotal figure in ophthalmology began with his education at Uppsala University. His academic and research pursuits there laid the groundwork for his future discoveries.

Snippets

Gullstrand's legacy is best remembered for his exploration of the eye as an optical system, presenting a mathematical model that describes how the eye focuses light to produce vision. This work has had a profound impact on the field, influencing both theoretical understanding and practical applications in eye care.

Current Implications

The principles uncovered by Gullstrand have directly informed the development of modern techniques in vision correction and eye surgery. His mathematical models are integral to the design of corrective lenses and the refinement of surgical methods that have improved the lives of millions.

Impact and Products

Developments in optical instruments and corrective lenses owe much to Gullstrand's pioneering research. The Gullstrand slit lamp remains a staple in ophthalmological diagnostics, and his work on improving corrective lenses has significantly advanced the field of vision correction. Today, Gullstrand's legacy is evident in the precision and care with which eye diseases are diagnosed and treated, affirming his lasting influence on the field of ophthalmology.

In conclusion, Gullstrand's contributions to medicine and physiology have had a lasting impact, paving the way for advancements in ophthalmology and optical science. His dedication to understanding the complexities of the eye has enhanced our ability to correct and improve vision, benefiting countless individuals around the world.

ALEXIS CARREL (1912)

The father of vascular surgery, who also sowed the seeds of organ transplantation

Alexis Carrel was awarded the Nobel Prize in Medicine in 1912 for his pioneering work in vascular suturing techniques. His innovative methods laid the groundwork for modern surgical practices, particularly in the fields of vascular surgery and organ transplantation.

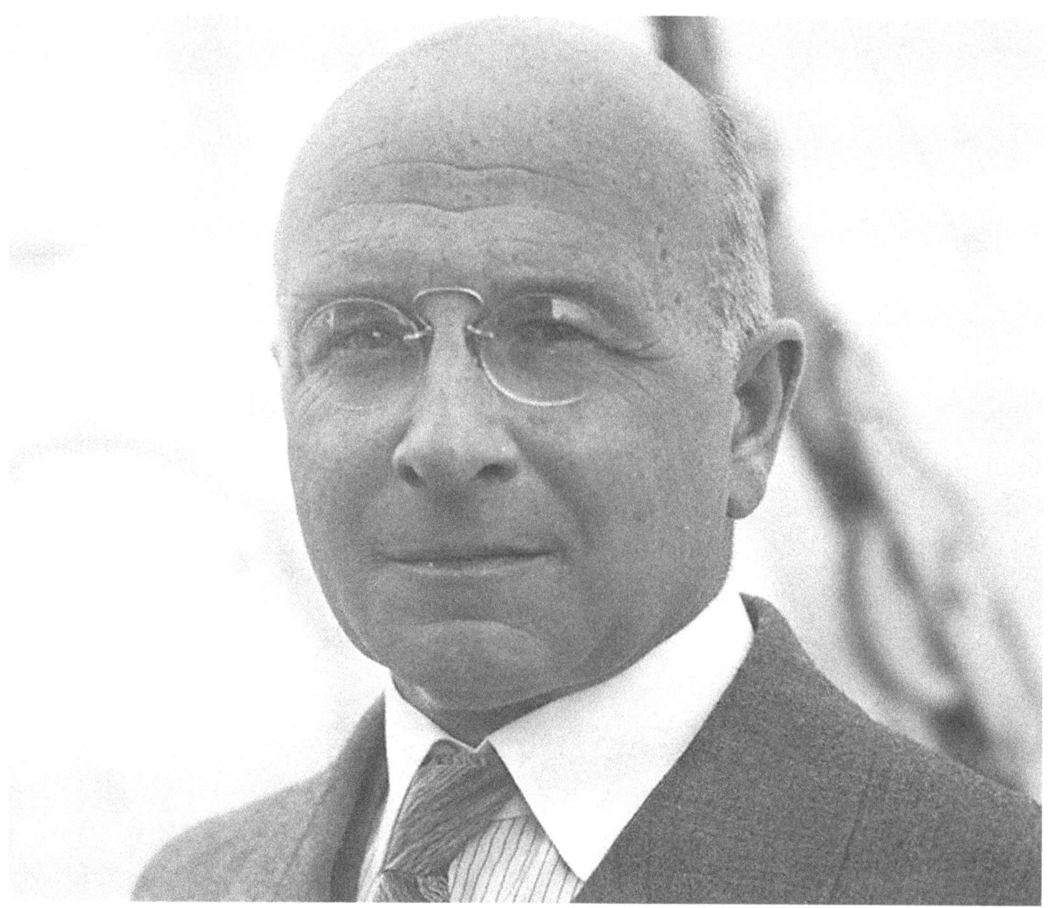

History

Alexis Carrel was born on June 28, 1873, in Sainte-Foy-lès-Lyon, Rhône, France. Raised in a devout Catholic family and educated by Jesuits, Carrel's early life in France set the stage for his future achievements. Despite facing challenges such as not being able to secure a hospital appointment in France due to pervasive anticlericalism, Carrel's determination led him to move to North America, where his career took a pivotal turn.

He was deeply affected by the assassination of French President Sadi Carnot, who died from a severed portal vein—a tragedy that inspired him to develop new techniques for suturing blood vessels. Carrel's "triangulation" technique, which minimized damage to the vascular wall during suturing, was revolutionary.

Snippets

Triangulation Technique for Suturing Blood Vessels

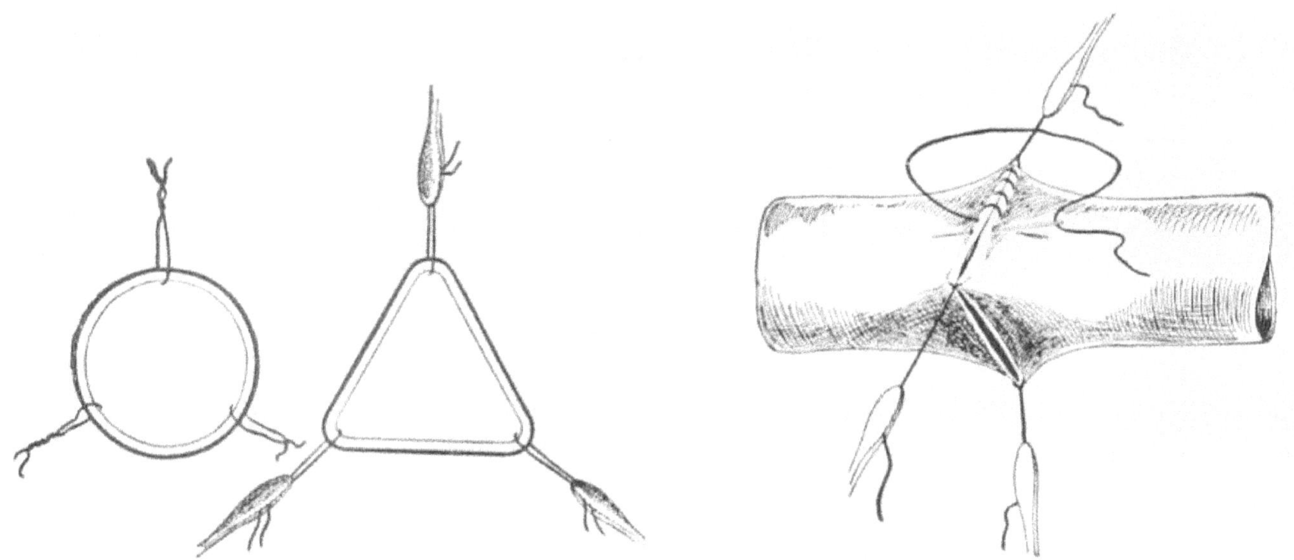

Carell's Method of Circular Arteriorrhaphy

Alexis Carrel's development of the triangulation technique revolutionized vascular surgery. By using three stay-sutures to minimize damage to the vascular wall during suturing, Carrel enabled more successful and precise connections of blood vessels.

Development of the Perfusion Pump

In collaboration with Charles Lindbergh, Carrel invented the first perfusion pump, marking a significant advancement in organ transplantation. This device allowed organs to remain viable outside the body for extended periods, facilitating complex surgeries including organ transplants and open-heart surgery.

Carrel-Dakin Method of Wound Irrigation

During World War I, Carrel, together with English chemist Henry Drysdale Dakin, developed the Carrel-Dakin method of treating wounds with an antiseptic solution. This method involved the mechanical irrigation of wounds with a high volume of antiseptic fluid, significantly improving wound care in the absence of antibiotics.

Influence on Organ Transplantation and Tissue Culture

Carrel's work extended beyond vascular surgery to include pivotal contributions to organ transplantation and tissue culture. His collaboration with Lindbergh on the Culture of Organs book and their development of the perfusion pump laid the groundwork for modern transplantation and surgical procedures.

Influence Vascular surgery and Organ transplantation.

Ancient accounts, dating as far back as 800 B.C., suggest that Indian doctors were among the first to practice skin grafting, utilizing skin from one part of the body to repair wounds and burns elsewhere. This early form of transplantation showcases the foundational understanding of bodily repair mechanisms that would evolve significantly over time.

The Renaissance period saw further advances with Italian surgeon Gasparo Tagliacozzi, often cited as the father of plastic surgery, who reconstructed noses and ears using patients' own skin, recognizing the issues with using skin from different donors due to immune response—a concept that would later become central to organ transplantation.

The early 20th century marked a pivotal era with surgeons like Eduard Zirm achieving the world's first successful corneal transplant in 1905, and Alexis Carrel, who was awarded the Nobel Prize in 1912 for developing techniques for connecting blood vessels, laying the groundwork for future organ transplants.

However, it wasn't until the mid-20th century that organ transplantation began to see more consistent success, with significant contributions from surgeons such as Joseph Murray and teams at Boston's Peter Bent Brigham Hospital. Their efforts in kidney transplantation, particularly between identical twins, demonstrated the importance of genetic compatibility in transplant success.

Current Implications

Advancements in Surgical Methods

Carrel's techniques for vascular anastomosis, where blood vessels are united end-to-end, remain integral to cardiovascular surgery today. These methods have been refined over the years but still echo the principles Carrel introduced in the early 20th century. The precision and effectiveness of these techniques have significantly reduced complications and improved outcomes in surgeries involving delicate vascular work.

Organ Preservation and Transplantation

The perfusion pump developed by Carrel and Lindbergh has evolved into sophisticated organ preservation systems that are critical for transplant surgery. Today's organ preservation technologies enable longer storage times and better condition of organs between donation and transplantation, directly contributing to the success rates of organ transplants.

Impact on Tissue Culture and Regenerative Medicine

Beyond his direct contributions to surgery, Carrel's early work in tissue culture has paved the way for advances in regenerative medicine. By demonstrating the potential for tissues to be cultured outside the body, Carrel contributed to the development of techniques that are now fundamental in tissue engineering and the cultivation of organs for transplantation.

Teaching and Training

Carrel's insistence on the importance of absolute asepsis and meticulous surgical technique has influenced the training of countless surgeons. The principles he championed are now fundamental components of surgical education, emphasizing the critical importance of technique and environment in successful surgical outcomes.

Impact and Products

Advancements in Surgical Methods

Carrel's introduction of the triangulation technique for suturing blood vessels significantly improved the success rates of vascular surgeries and was a key factor in making organ transplants possible. This technique minimized damage to the vascular wall during suturing, a practice that continues to influence modern surgical procedures.

Organ Preservation and Transplantation

The perfusion pump developed by Carrel and Lindbergh marked the beginning of organ preservation technology, allowing organs to remain viable outside of the body for longer periods. This invention paved the way for the development of the artificial heart and other critical advancements in organ transplantation.

Impact on Tissue Culture and Regenerative Medicine

Beyond his direct contributions to surgery, Carrel's work in tissue culture laid the groundwork for regenerative medicine, influencing current practices in tissue engineering and the cultivation of organs for transplantation.

CHARLES RICHET (1913)

A deserving Nobel for the discoverer of the dreaded acute Anaphylactic reaction

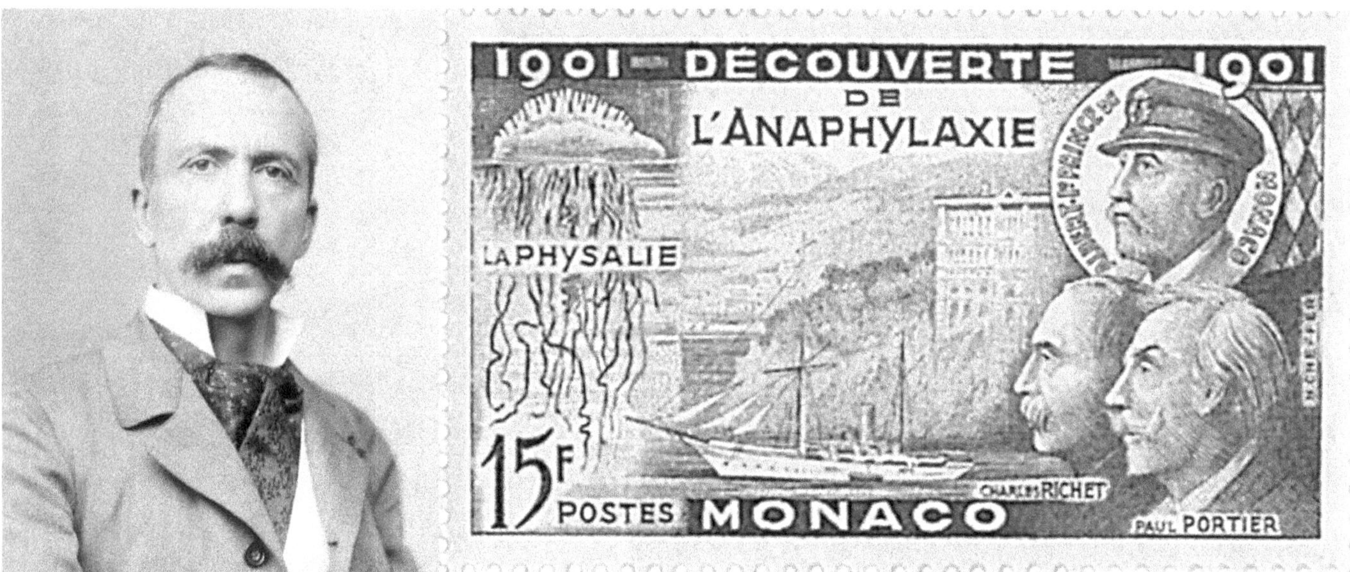

Charles Richet, a French physiologist, was awarded the Nobel Prize in Medicine in 1913 for his pioneering work on anaphylaxis, a term he coined to describe the severe allergic reactions that can occur when the immune system encounters a previously encountered antigen. This discovery was a monumental step forward in the field of immunology, highlighting the body's complex response to foreign substances.

History

Born in Paris in 1850, Richet's intellectual journey began with his medical degree, followed by a Doctorate in Sciences, eventually leading him to become a Professor of Physiology. His career was marked by extensive research across various fields of physiology, demonstrating his broad scientific interests and contributions to medical science.

Snippets

In 1902, alongside Paul Portier, Richet first observed anaphylaxis in dogs injected with jellyfish toxins, observing that a second dose of the toxin could provoke a severe reaction, even death. This observation was crucial for understanding the immune system's complexity and its sometimes counterintuitive reactions to foreign substances.

Current Implications

Today, Richet's discovery of anaphylaxis remains fundamental in allergy and immunology, informing how we treat and understand allergic reactions, from food allergies to drug sensitivities. His work has paved the way for lifesaving interventions and treatments in allergic reactions and anaphylactic shock.

Impact and Products

Richet's research has significantly influenced the development of treatments for allergic reactions, including the use of epinephrine for anaphylactic shock. Richet's work on anaphylaxis, his extensive contributions to physiology, and his interdisciplinary approach to science exemplify the profound impact one individual can have on advancing our understanding of human health and disease.

The man who solved the mysterious coil puzzle inside the mind boggling vestibular system

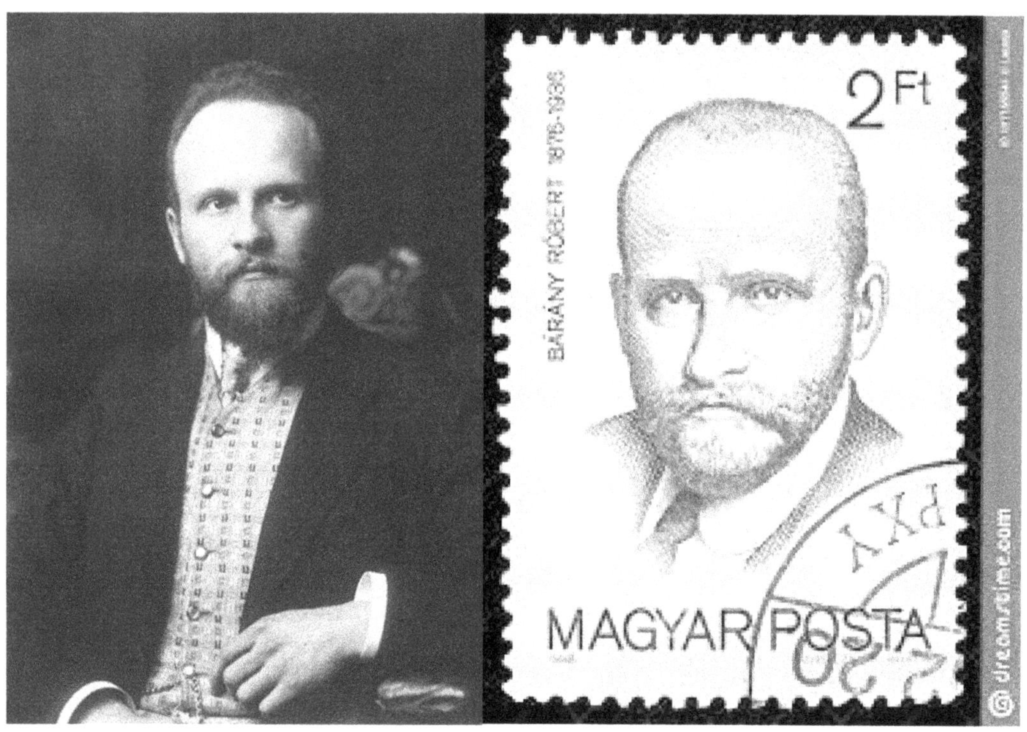

Robert Bárány, was awarded the Nobel Prize in Medicine in 1914 for his pioneering research on the physiology and pathology of the vestibular apparatus of the inner ear. His work significantly advanced the understanding of the mechanisms behind balance and orientation.

History

Robert Bárány, born on April 22, 1876, in Vienna, Austria-Hungary, emerged as a pivotal figure in the medical field due to his groundbreaking work on the vestibular apparatus of the inner ear, which plays a crucial role in balance and spatial orientation. Graduating with a medical degree from the University of Vienna in 1900, Bárány dedicated his early career to otology, the study of the ear and its diseases. His significant contributions in this field were recognized with the Nobel Prize in Medicine in 1914.

Bárány's path was marked by his innovative approach to understanding and diagnosing vestibular diseases. A serendipitous observation made while syringing a patient's ear with fluid led him to theorize about the endolymph's movement within the vestibular system, laying the groundwork for the caloric test, a method still used today to evaluate the vestibular system. This work not only advanced the diagnosis and treatment of vestibular disorders but also opened new avenues for surgical treatment of diseases affecting the vestibular organ.

Snippets

Understanding the Vestibular System

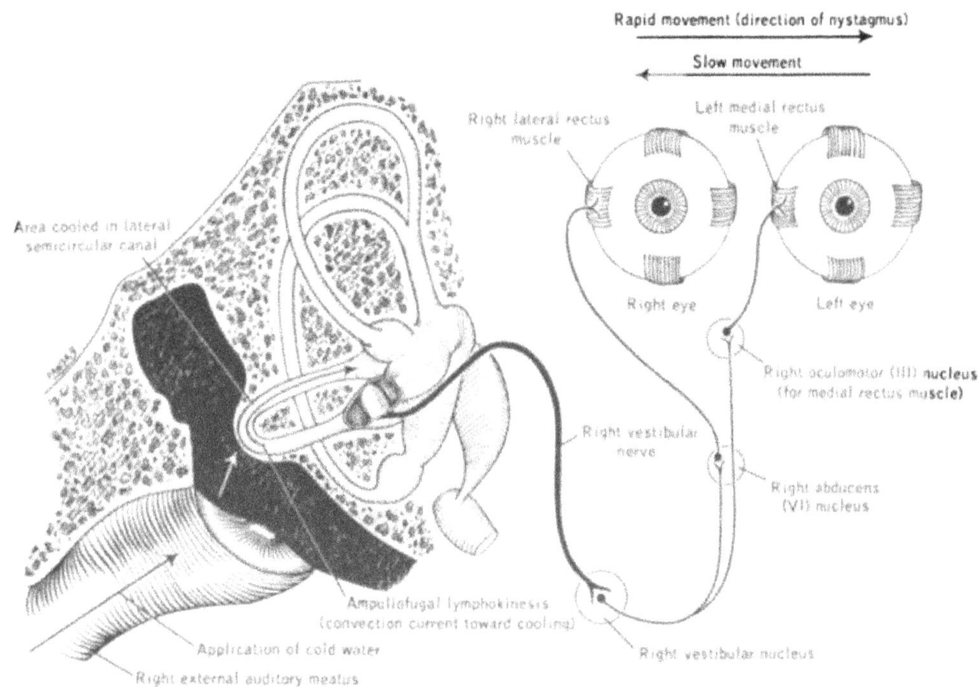

Robert Bárány's groundbreaking research focused on the vestibular system within the inner ear, crucial for maintaining balance and spatial orientation. He provided detailed insights into how this system helps organisms navigate their environment, emphasizing its role in equilibrium.

Diagnostic Tests for Vestibular Function

Bárány developed several diagnostic tests to assess vestibular function accurately. These tests were innovative at the time and have since become standard procedures in diagnosing balance disorders. Among these, the caloric test is notable for its effectiveness in inducing nystagmus and assessing the inner ear's response to temperature-induced fluid dynamics changes.

Impact on Otology and Neurology

The methodologies introduced by Bárány in studying the vestibular system have had a lasting impact on the fields of otology and neurology. His work laid the foundation for modern approaches to diagnosing and treating disorders related to balance and orientation, influencing clinical practices and patient care protocols.

Influence

The landscape of otology and neurology was shaped by visionaries long before modern achievements. In 1549, Jason Pratensis made early strides by discussing neurological diseases in his volume "De Cerebri Morbis," setting a precedent for the field. The monumental "Anatomy of the Brain" by Thomas Willis in 1664, alongside his introduction of the term "neurology," laid foundational knowledge of brain function and diseases like epilepsy and paralysis. The duo of Charles Bell and François Magendie in the 19th century differentiated motor and sensory pathways in the spinal cord, a breakthrough in understanding neural functions. Their work, along with pioneers like Luigi Galvani who demonstrated the electrical nature of nerve signals, and Santiago Ramón y Cajal's histological studies of neurons, were crucial in developing neurology as a scientific discipline.

Current Implications

Advancements in Diagnostic Techniques

Bárány's caloric vestibular stimulation method remains a cornerstone in diagnosing vestibular disorders. It has fostered experimental vestibular research crucial for understanding human locomotion and the vestibular influence on bodily perceptions, cognition, and emotions.

Integration with Modern Technology

In the last two decades, this method has been combined with brain imaging to precisely locate the human vestibular cortex, enhancing our understanding of vestibular system functioning.

Broadening Research Horizons

Bárány's tests are integral in neuroscience for exploring how vestibular signals impact bodily perceptions, cognition, and emotions, contributing significantly to multidisciplinary studies.

Impact and Products

Diagnostic Innovations

Bárány's research introduced precise diagnostic techniques for vestibular disorders, significantly improving the accuracy of diagnoses.

Therapeutic Advancements

His work led to the development of new treatments and rehabilitation exercises for patients suffering from vertigo and balance issues.

Educational Contributions

Bárány's findings have been crucial in educating healthcare professionals about the vestibular system's complexities, enhancing the overall approach to balance-related disorders.

Global Health Impact

His discoveries have informed public health strategies and clinical practices worldwide, contributing to the enhanced management of vestibular disorders.

JULES BORDET (1919)

The Belgian bacteriologist who spotted the curious complement system in Immunology

Jules Bordet, a Belgian physician, bacteriologist, and immunologist, was awarded the Nobel Prize in Medicine in 1919 for his seminal work on immunity, particularly his discovery of the components in blood serum that destroy bacteria.

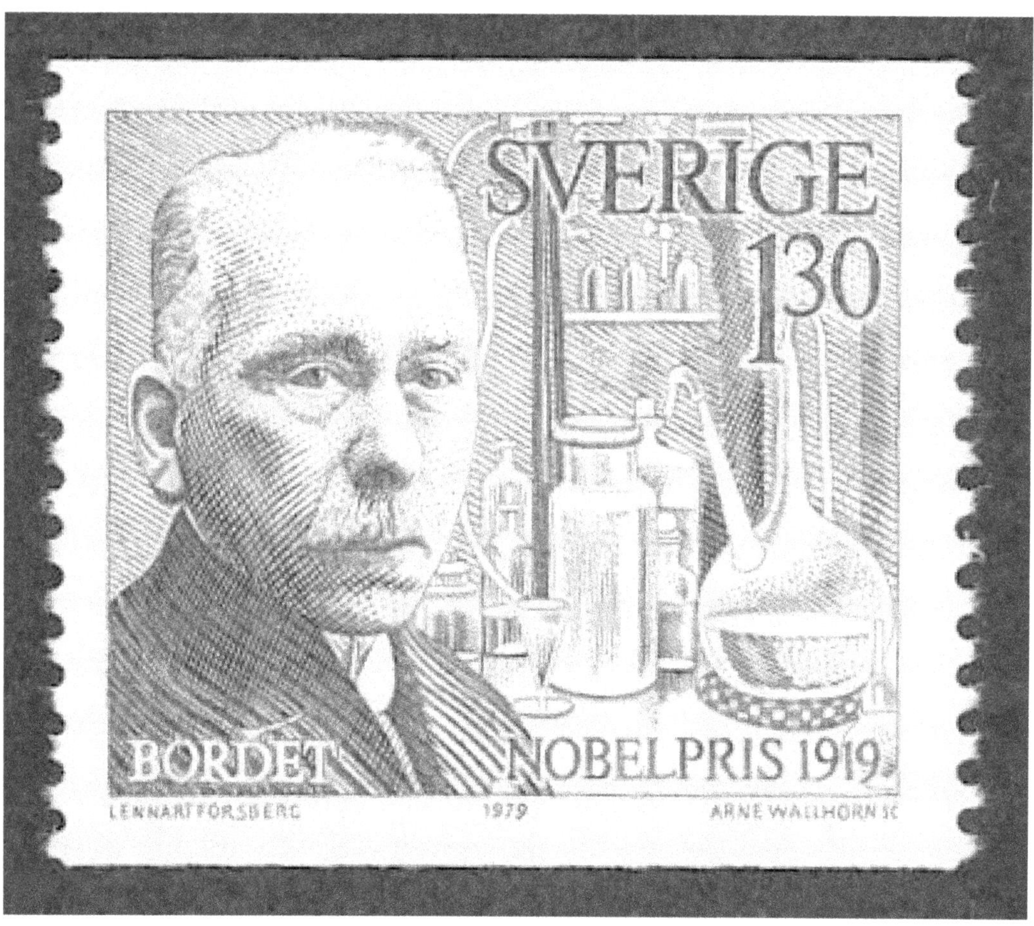

History

Born in Soignies, Belgium, in 1870, Bordet's early fascination with chemistry led him to a distinguished career in microbiology and immunology. After earning his M.D. from the Free University of Brussels, Bordet further honed his skills at the Pasteur Institute in Paris. He later returned to Brussels to head the newly formed Anti-Rabies and Bacteriological Institute, which he renamed the Pasteur Institute in honor of Louis Pasteur.

Snippets

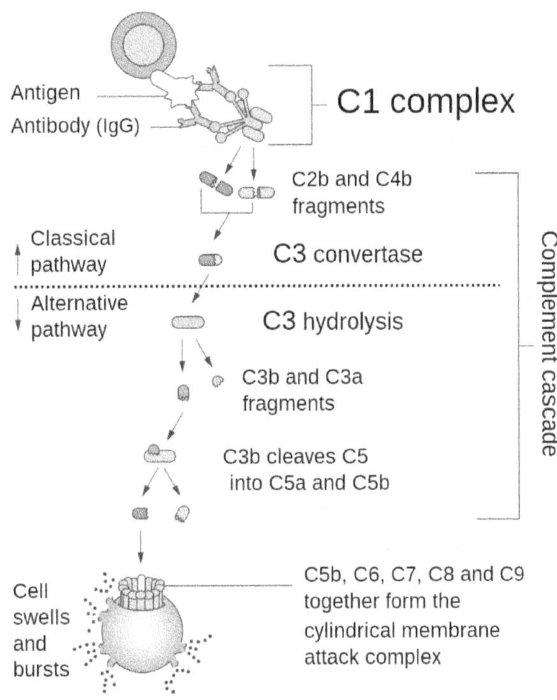

Our current understanding of complement system

Bordet's pioneering work included the discovery of the complement system, a key part of our immune defense that works alongside antibodies to destroy pathogens. He also developed complement fixation tests, which have become essential tools in diagnosing diseases. Additionally, Bordet identified the bacterium Bordetella pertussis, the causative agent of whooping cough, marking a significant milestone in medical microbiology.

Current Implications

Bordet's discoveries have had a profound impact on the development of vaccines, particularly for whooping cough, and the understanding of immune system reactions. His work on the complement system has also informed current research into immunological disorders, providing a basis for new therapeutic approaches.

Impact and Products

The identification of Bordetella pertussis was instrumental in the development of the whooping cough vaccine, significantly reducing the incidence of this potentially fatal disease. Bordet's work on complement and antibodies has furthered our understanding of the immune system's role in health and disease, influencing the development of various immunotherapies and vaccines.

Bordet's insights into the immune system's workings have paved the way for countless advances in medicine, making him a towering figure in the records of science.

AUGUST KROGH (1920)

Drew the first blue print of capillary circulation to reach the Nobel summit

August Krogh, a Danish physiologist, was awarded the Nobel Prize in Medicine in 1920 for his groundbreaking discovery of the capillary motor regulating mechanism

History

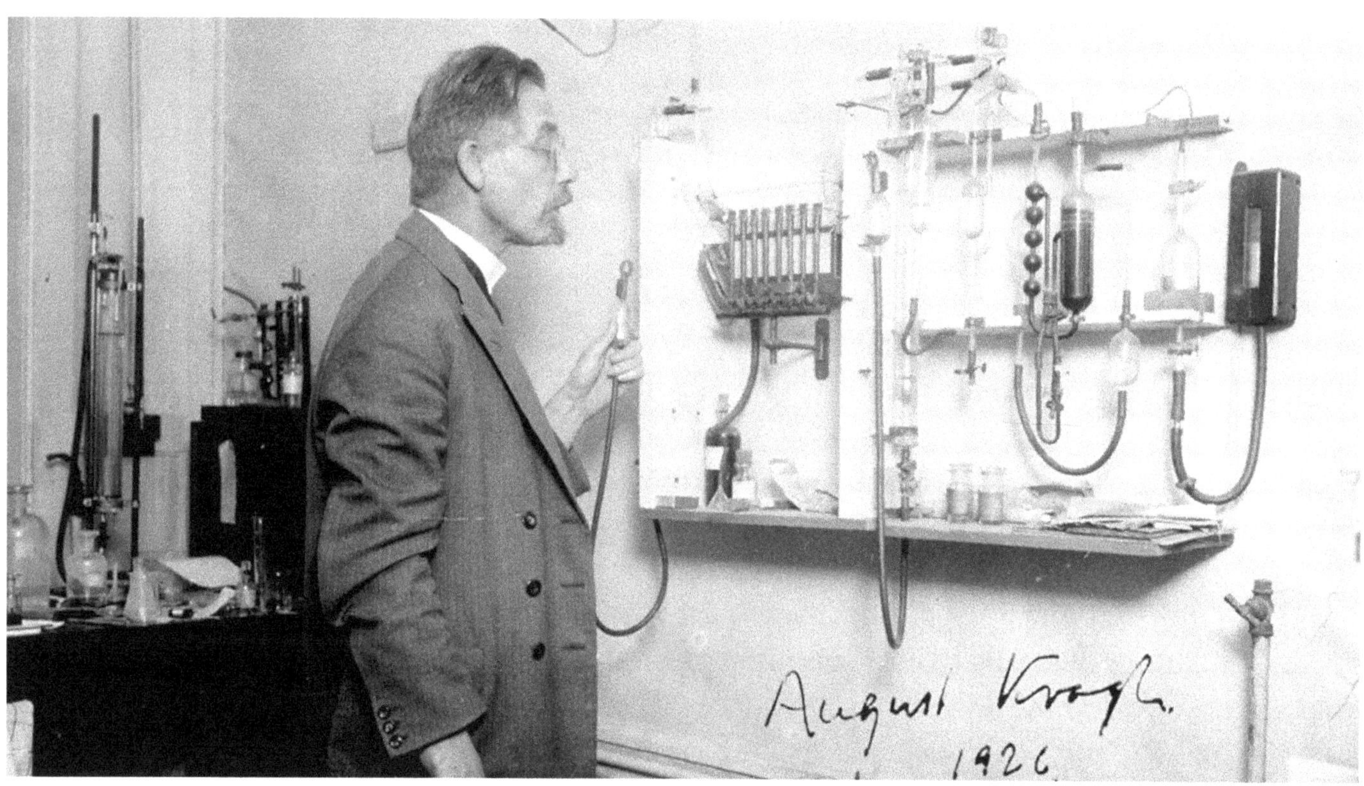

Born in Grenå, Denmark, Krogh's early interest in science led him to study medicine and zoology at the University of Copenhagen. His career was marked by a prolific partnership with his wife, Marie Krogh, also a scientist, with whom he conducted much of his notable research.

Snippets

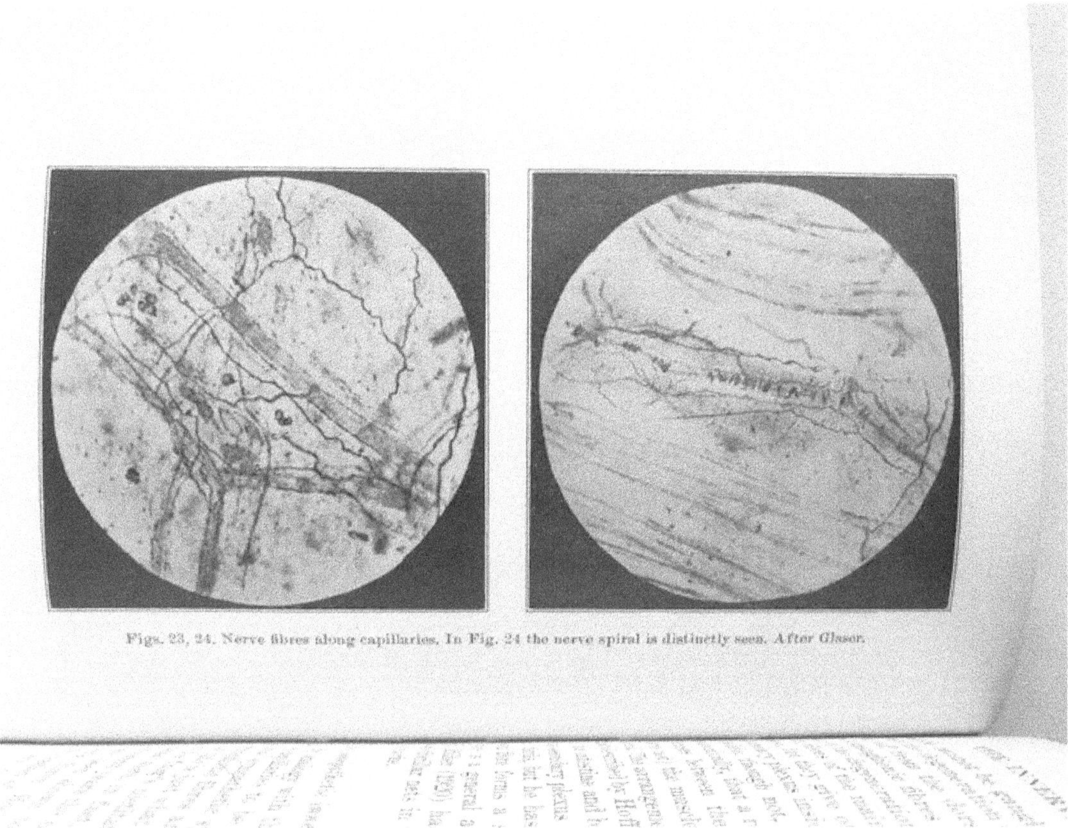

Krogh model : The interaction between nerve fibers and capillaries.

Krogh's work revolutionized our understanding of how blood oxygen levels are regulated and how the opening of capillaries is controlled to meet oxygen demand during muscle activity. His innovative methods for measuring blood gas levels laid the groundwork for modern respiratory physiology and exercise science.

Current Implications

Krogh's insights into capillary function and gas exchange have profound implications for medical and sports science, enhancing our understanding of respiratory disorders and informing training regimes for athletes to optimize performance and recovery.

Impact and Products

The principles discovered by Krogh have informed the development of therapeutic strategies for managing respiratory conditions and have supported advances in exercise physiology, benefiting countless individuals by improving health outcomes and athletic performance.

ARCHIBALD HILL AND OTTO MEYERHOF (1922)

This British-German duo's monumental concepts about metabolism of muscles is still live

In 1922, Archibald Hill and Otto Meyerhof were awarded the Nobel Prize in Medicine for their pioneering work on the metabolism of muscles. Their research laid the foundation for understanding how muscles convert energy, a topic that has profound implications for both medicine and biology.

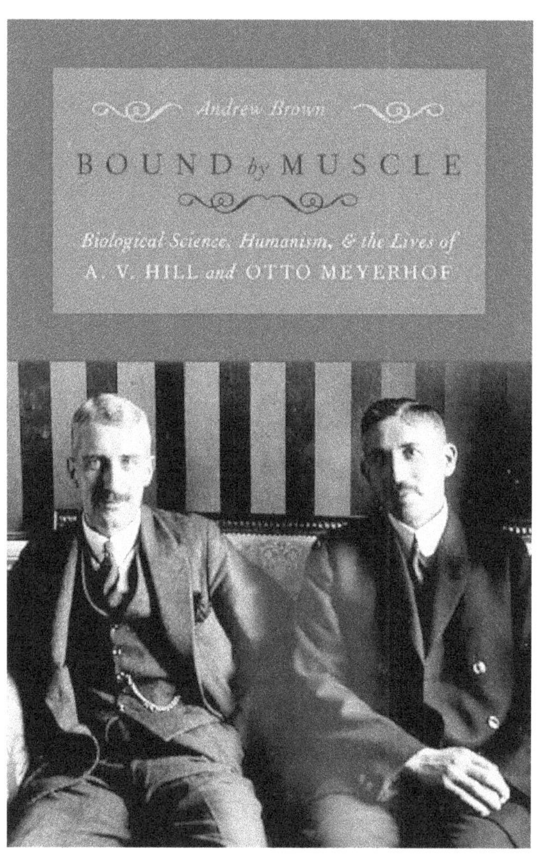

History

Archibald Vivian Hill was born in Bristol, England, on September 26, 1886. His educational journey took him from Blundell's School to Trinity College, Cambridge, where he initially studied mathematics. However, under the influence of Dr. Walter Morley Fletcher, Hill transitioned to physiology, marking the beginning of his illustrious career in this field. During World War I, Hill's skills were diverted to military efforts, where he innovated methods for anti-aircraft gunnery. Post-war, he returned to his physiological studies, collaborating closely with Otto Meyerhof, who was conducting parallel research in Germany.

Hill was not only a pioneering scientist but also a significant figure in the academic and public life, contributing to the defense scientific policy during World War II and serving in the British Parliament. Hill passed away on June 3, 1977, leaving behind a legacy celebrated for its profound impact on physiology and biophysics.

Otto Fritz Meyerhof was born on April 12, 1884, in Hannover, Germany, and later moved to Berlin with his family. His early interest in medicine led him to study at several prestigious universities, including Freiburg, Berlin, Strasbourg, and Heidelberg, where he graduated in 1909. Initially drawn to psychology and philosophy, Meyerhof's career took a decisive turn towards physiology under the influence of Otto Warburg, a prominent figure at Heidelberg.

The rise of the Nazi regime in Germany forced Meyerhof to emigrate, first to Paris in 1938 and then to the United States in 1940, amid the turmoil of World War II. In the U.S., he continued his research at the University of Pennsylvania, where he furthered the understanding of cellular metabolism until his death in 1951.

Early Influence

Early researchers in this field laid the foundational knowledge that enabled Hill and Meyerhof to make their groundbreaking discoveries. These pioneers in muscle research contributed significantly to our understanding of muscle function and biochemistry.

One of the earliest significant contributions came from the work on myosin, a key muscle protein. In 1864, Kühne extracted a viscous protein from muscle using concentrated salt solutions, which he named "myosin," considering it responsible for muscle's rigor state. This early work marked the beginning of a deeper understanding of muscle biochemistry.

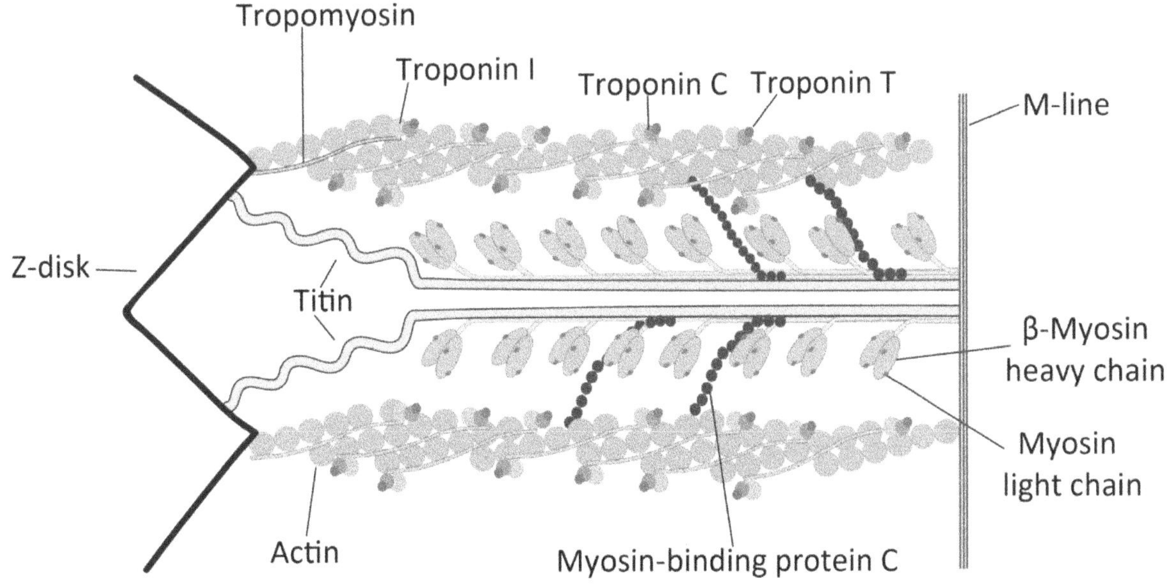

The myosin was first discovered by Meyerhof

The significance of ATP in muscle contraction was highlighted by Engelhardt and Lyubimova in 1939, who reported that myosin exhibited ATPase activity. This discovery was pivotal, aligning with Lohmann's suggestion in 1934 that ATP was likely the energy source for muscle contraction. Despite skepticism due to the prevailing belief that enzymes were small globular proteins, which myosin clearly was not, this finding underscored ATP's central role in muscle biochemistry.

Current Implications

Sports Medicine

Hill's concept of "oxygen debt" and the metabolic pathways illuminated by Meyerhof's research into glycolysis have been instrumental in developing training regimes and recovery strategies for athletes. Understanding how muscles produce and use energy during aerobic and anaerobic activities has allowed sports scientists and coaches to optimize performance and reduce the risk of injury. It has led to the development of targeted training programs that improve endurance, strength, and recovery times by scientifically managing the balance between exercise intensity and recovery. Techniques such as interval training, which alternates periods of intense exertion with periods of rest or low activity, directly derive from these principles.

Metabolic Diseases

The insights into the biochemical pathways of muscle metabolism have also had significant implications for understanding and treating metabolic diseases. The relationship between glycogen storage, lactic acid production, and oxygen consumption elucidated by Hill and Meyerhof's work is critical in conditions like diabetes, where glucose metabolism is impaired. Treatments that improve insulin sensitivity and promote efficient glucose usage in muscles can be traced back to an understanding of these fundamental metabolic processes. Furthermore, research into muscular dystrophies and other genetic conditions affecting muscle function continues to build on the foundational knowledge established by Hill and Meyerhof.

Impact and Products

In Metabolic Disorders:

Hill and Meyerhof's discoveries have led to significant insights into metabolic diseases, especially those related to muscle function and energy metabolism. By elucidating the roles of oxygen consumption and lactic acid metabolism in muscle, their research has informed strategies for managing conditions such as diabetes, where glucose metabolism is disrupted. Understanding these metabolic pathways is crucial for developing treatments that improve insulin sensitivity and promote efficient glucose usage in muscles, offering better management and potentially reducing the impact of such diseases.

In Athletic Training

The principles uncovered by Hill and Meyerhof have also been instrumental in the field of sports medicine, particularly in developing training programs that maximize athletic performance while minimizing the risk of injury. Their work on the production of heat in muscles, the oxygen debt concept, and the glycogen-lactic acid cycle has enabled a more scientific approach to training. This includes strategies for optimizing endurance, strength, and recovery through targeted exercise regimens that consider the aerobic and anaerobic metabolic capacities of athletes. Interval training, which leverages the body's aerobic and anaerobic systems, can be directly traced back to the metabolic principles they discovered.

Legacy and Continued Influence

Their research has continued to inspire scientists and clinicians to explore new treatments for metabolic disorders and to refine athletic training methods. The advancements in wearable technology that monitor physiological and metabolic parameters during exercise are a testament to the enduring impact of their discoveries.

FREDERICK BANTING AND JOHN MACLEOD (1923)

Insulin, one of the greatest Invention of 20th century with an inspiring script

In 1923, Frederick Banting and John Macleod were awarded the Nobel Prize in Medicine for their discovery of insulin. This groundbreaking work, conducted at the University of Toronto, Canada, revolutionized the treatment of diabetes, transforming it from a fatal disease to a manageable condition.

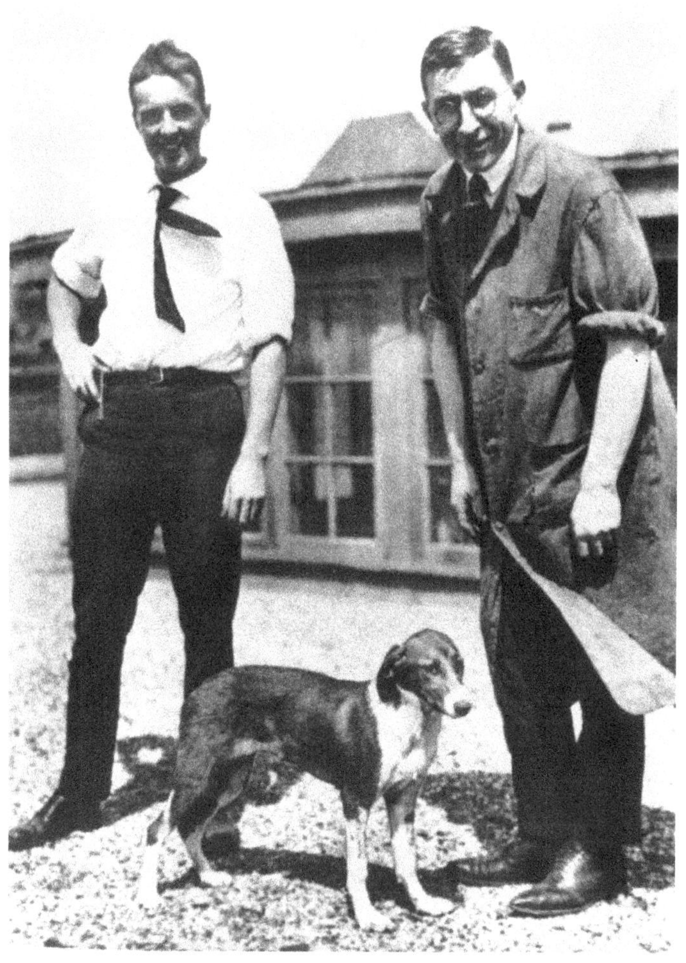

History

Frederick Banting, born on November 14, 1891, in Alliston, Ontario, is an orthopedic surgeon with a keen interest in diabetes. His pivotal moment came on October 31, 1920, when he conceptualized a novel approach to isolating the pancreas's internal secretion, hypothesizing that it could treat diabetes.

Despite his lack of experience in diabetes treatment and research, Banting's idea was rooted in the belief that the internal secretion, destroyed by the digestive enzymes produced by the pancreas, could be isolated if the flow of these enzymes was stopped.

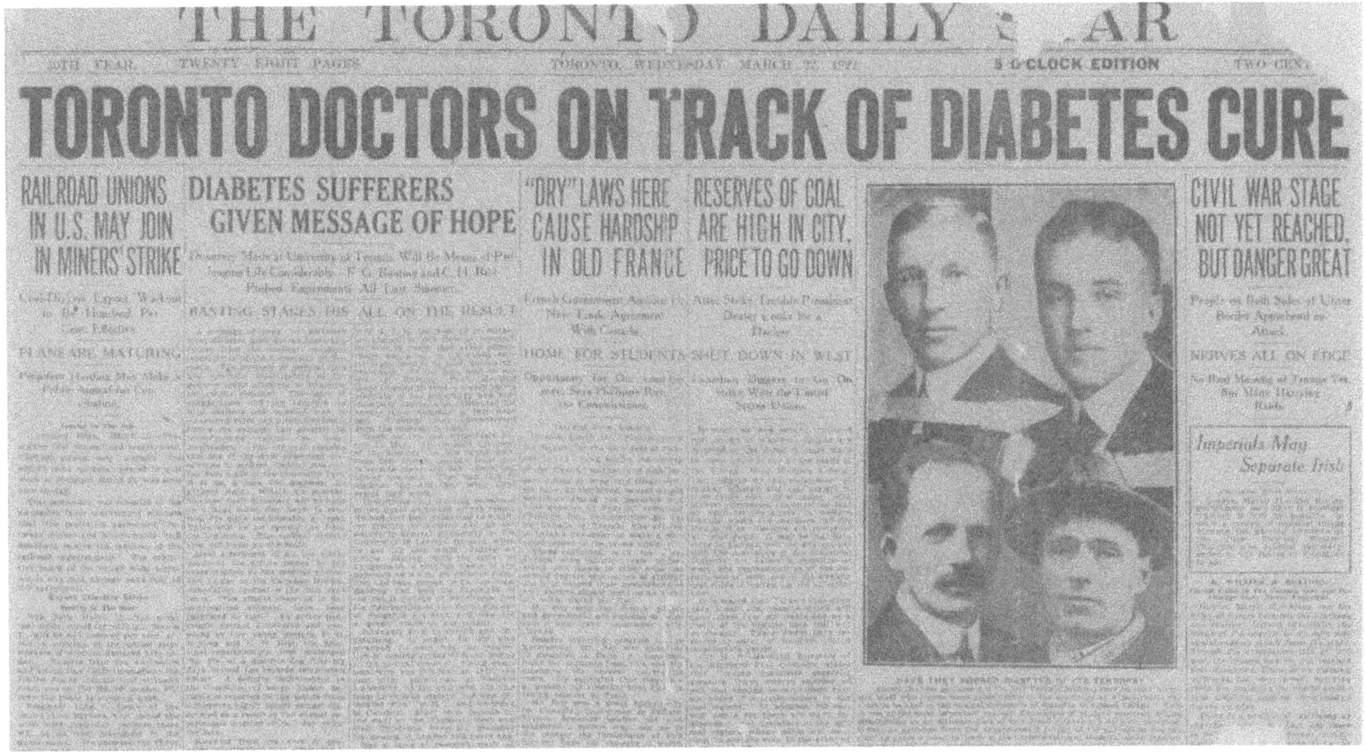

John J.R. Macleod, a professor at the University of Toronto and an expert in carbohydrate metabolism, initially met Banting's proposal with skepticism. However, recognizing the potential of Banting's hypothesis, Macleod provided him with laboratory space, research animals, and the assistance of Charles Best, a medical student, in the summer of 1921.

The research conducted at the University of Toronto was fraught with challenges. Banting and Best's experiments with dogs, aiming to ligate the pancreatic ducts and isolate the internal secretion, faced technical and methodological hurdles. Despite these obstacles, they achieved a breakthrough in July 1921, successfully reducing a diabetic dog's blood sugar levels with pancreatic extract injections. This initial success was followed by further experimentation and refinement of their extraction methods, with biochemist James Bertram Collip joining the team to improve the consistency and effectiveness of the pancreatic extracts.

The culmination of their efforts was the successful treatment of Leonard Thompson, a 14-year-old boy with diabetes, in January 1922, marking the first successful clinical use of insulin. This achievement was not only a testament to the team's determination and innovation but also a turning point in the treatment of diabetes, offering hope to millions worldwide.

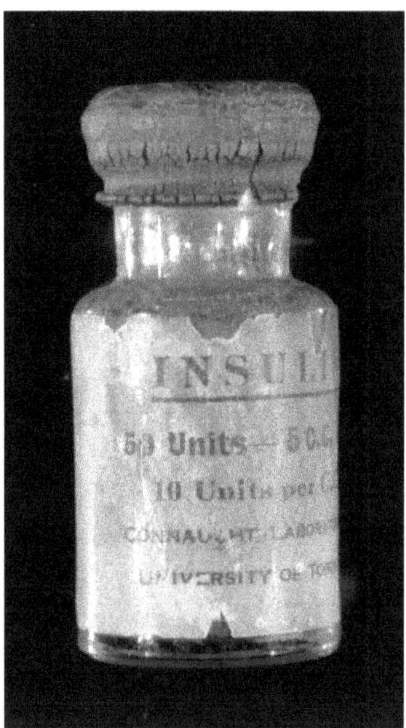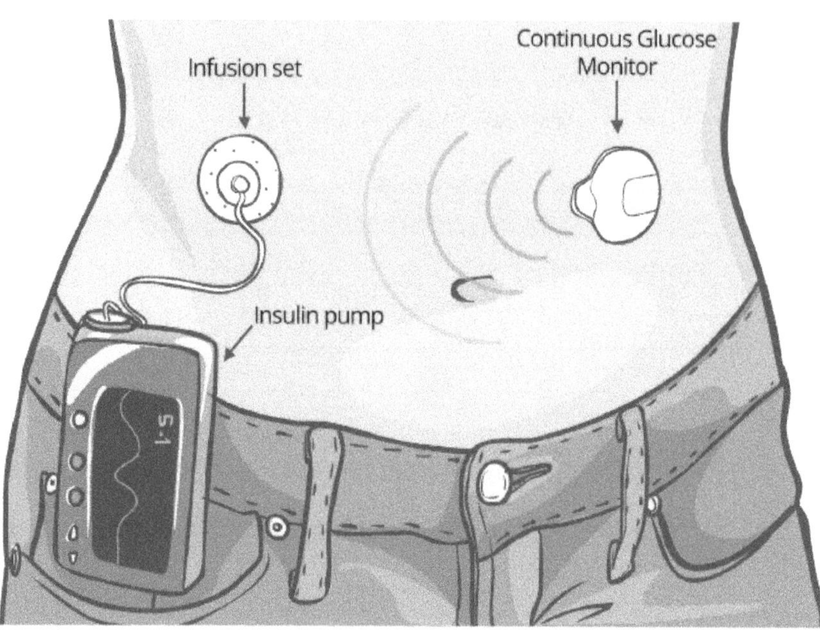

The evolution : The original insulin and the automated pump with a glucose sensor

Snippets

The discovery of insulin represents a pivotal moment in medical history, marking a transition from a period where Type I diabetes was essentially a death sentence to one where patients could lead full and healthy lives. The narrative of this discovery is deeply entwined with the work of Frederick Banting, Charles Best, John J.R. Macleod, and James Bertram Collip at the University of Toronto.

Before the advent of insulin therapy, individuals with Type I diabetes had very limited options for the management of their condition, primarily relying on starvation diets that at best could only extend life for a short period. The development and successful human trial of insulin dramatically changed this, offering not just hope but a tangible solution to those suffering from diabetes.

The discovery process itself was fraught with challenges, including difficult pancreatic surgeries on dogs during the extreme heat of the Toronto summer in 1921, and the meticulous and often frustrating task of measuring the effects of their experimental treatments accurately. Despite these obstacles, Banting and Best, under the guidance of Macleod, persevered. Their experiments led to the crucial finding that extracts from the degenerated pancreas of duct-ligated dogs could significantly reduce blood sugar levels in diabetic dogs.

The journey was marked by scientific disagreements and the need for critical refinement of their approach. Macleod's skepticism and insistence on rigorous methodology pushed the team to refine their extraction and purification techniques, ultimately leading to the production of a more consistent and effective insulin preparation. This process was significantly advanced by the addition of Collip, a skilled biochemist, who improved the extract's consistency and effectiveness

A major controversy erupted when the Nobel prize was announced.

When Banting and Macleod won the Nobel Prize for discovering insulin, it caused tension between them. Banting was upset that Macleod got the prize instead of Best. Banting made sure Best got credit for the work. He shared his prize money with Best. Macleod also shared his prize money with Collip. Later, the Nobel Committee agreed that Best should have received part of the prize.

Current Implications

Insulin therapy remains a cornerstone of diabetes care, offering life-saving treatment for millions worldwide. The development and refinement of insulin types, including rapid-acting, long-acting, and mixed formulations, cater to the varying needs of patients, allowing for personalized treatment plans. These advancements have significantly improved the quality of life for those with diabetes, enabling tighter blood glucose control and reduced risk of complications.

Insulin therapy is tailored to individual needs, with treatment strategies ranging from augmentation, where insulin is used alongside oral antidiabetic drugs to improve glucose control, to full replacement in cases where endogenous insulin production is minimal or absent. The management of insulin involves detailed regimens that include basal (long-acting) insulin to manage fasting glucose levels and bolus (short-acting) insulin to cover carbohydrate intake during meals.

The combination of insulin with oral medications, particularly insulin sensitizers like metformin, illustrates the ongoing evolution of diabetes treatment strategies. This combination therapy is often preferred for its potential to enhance glycemic control while minimizing adverse effects, highlighting the importance of a comprehensive approach to diabetes management that incorporates both pharmacological and lifestyle interventions.

Impact and Products

Synthetic Human Insulin Production

Introduced in the 1970s, utilizing recombinant DNA technology. This was a significant breakthrough, offering a more consistent and reliable source of insulin than animal-derived insulins.

Development of Insulin Analogs

Engineered to have altered absorption profiles, allowing for faster onset or longer duration of action to more closely mimic natural insulin release from the pancreas. Examples include rapid-acting and long-acting insulins.

Insulin Delivery Innovations

Introduction of insulin pens for easier dosing, insulin pumps for continuous insulin delivery, and needle-free injection systems.

Continuous Glucose Monitoring (CGM) Systems

Allow real-time tracking of glucose levels, providing users and healthcare providers with detailed glucose data to inform treatment decisions.

Closed-loop Systems/Artificial Pancreas

Combine insulin pumps and CGM to automatically adjust insulin delivery based on glucose readings, significantly improving glycemic control and reducing the burden on individuals.

Advances in Diabetes Care

Including telemedicine for remote diabetes management, mobile apps for tracking food intake and medication, and predictive algorithms to prevent hypoglycemia.

Biotechnological Research

Ongoing research into beta-cell transplantation, stem cell therapies, and the development of oral insulin formulations to provide new treatment avenues.

Global Accessibility and Affordability Initiatives

Efforts to improve access to insulin and diabetes care in low – and middle-income countries through partnerships, generic manufacturing, and policy advocacy.

WILLEM EINTHOVEN (1924)

The mercurial Dutch, whose colossal discovery ECG, taught us the electrical language of heart

Willem Einthoven was awarded the Nobel Prize in Medicine in 1924 for his pioneering work in developing the electrocardiogram (ECG), a device essential for the diagnosis of heart diseases. His groundbreaking research unveiled the electrical properties of the heart, marking a significant advancement in medical science and cardiac care.

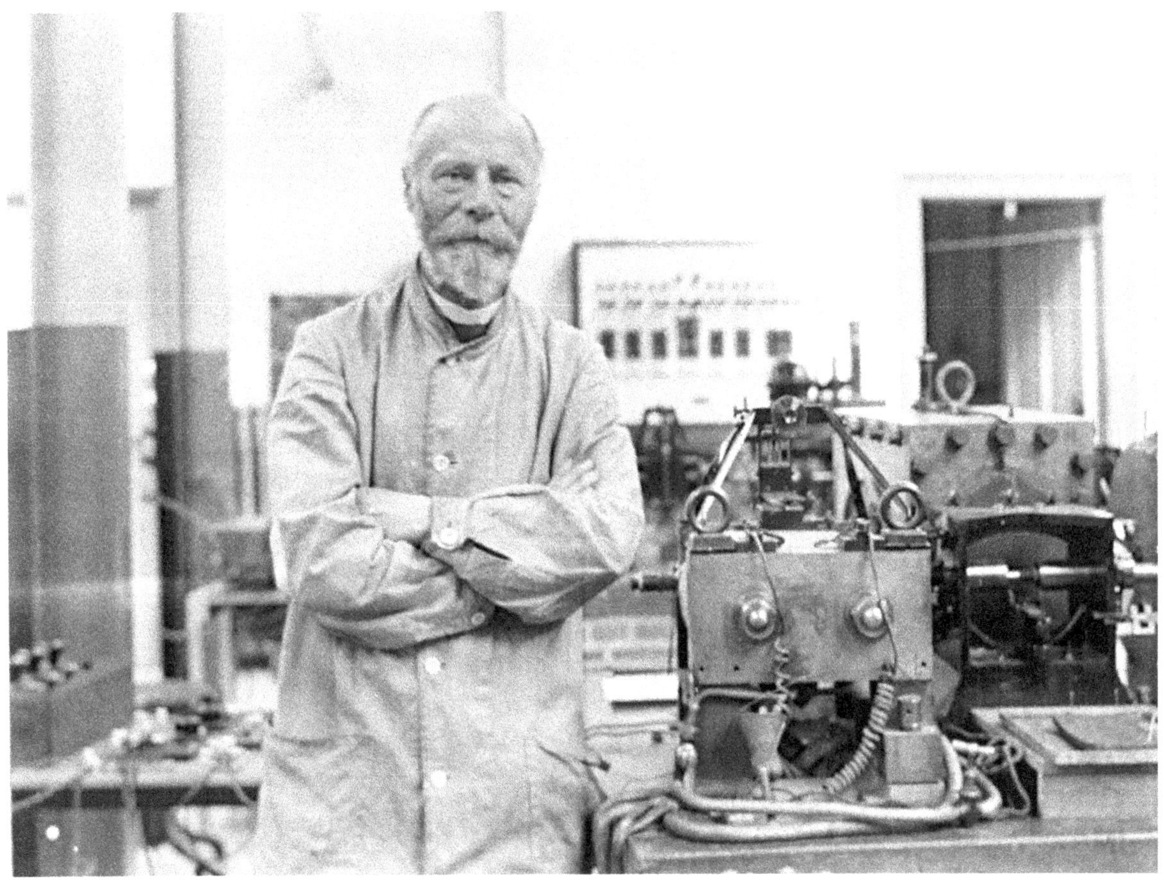

The brilliance of this man & understanding of cardiac electricity prodigious

History

Willem Einthoven, born on May 21, 1860, in Semarang, Java, in what was then the Dutch East Indies, stands as a monumental figure in the realm of medical science, especially known for his pioneering development of electrocardiography (ECG). After obtaining his medical degree from the University of Utrecht, Einthoven embarked on a career that would lead him to invent the string galvanometer in 1903, a device essential for the modern practice of recording the heart's electrical activity.

Einthoven's journey was characterized by his innovative spirit and relentless pursuit of understanding the electrical phenomena associated with the human heart. His invention of the string galvanometer was not just a moment of brilliance but the result of meticulous research and experimentation that transformed the way heart diseases are diagnosed and treated. This contribution has had a profound and lasting impact on the medical field, enabling precise diagnoses and opening new pathways for the therapeutic intervention of cardiac conditions.

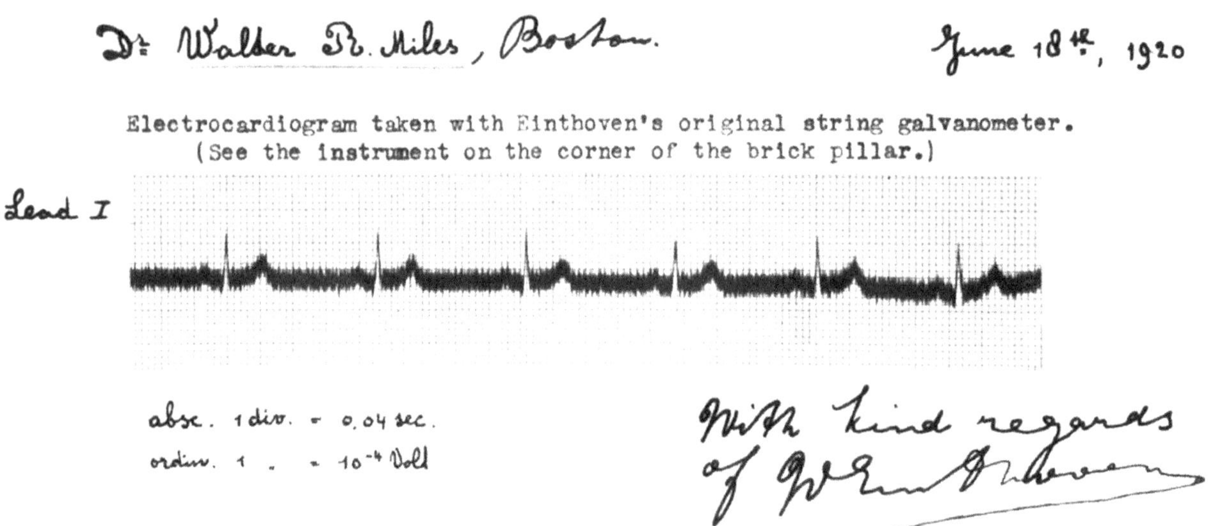

Snippets

Einthoven's career was marked by significant achievements and contributions to medical science. He became a professor at the University of Leiden in 1886, where he dedicated his research to exploring the electrical activity of the heart. The challenge at the time was the inability to accurately measure the heart's electrical currents without direct contact with the organ. Einthoven addressed this challenge by developing the string galvanometer in 1901, a device capable of measuring the electrical activity of the heart through the skin and bones of the chest.

The string galvanometer was a sophisticated instrument that used a thin filament of conductive wire positioned between strong electromagnets. Electrical currents from the heart would cause the wire to move, with these movements being recorded as a continuous curve on photographic paper. Despite its initial size and complexity, requiring water cooling and multiple operators, this invention laid the groundwork for modern electrocardiography by significantly enhancing the sensitivity compared to previous methods.

Einthoven's dedication to his work had a lasting impact on cardiology. He introduced the standardization of the ECG, assigning the letters P, Q, R, S, and T to the various deflections seen in an ECG reading, a convention that remains in use today. His concept of "Einthoven's triangle," an imaginary triangle formed on the chest to explain the lead placements for ECG readings, is also a testament to his influence on the field.

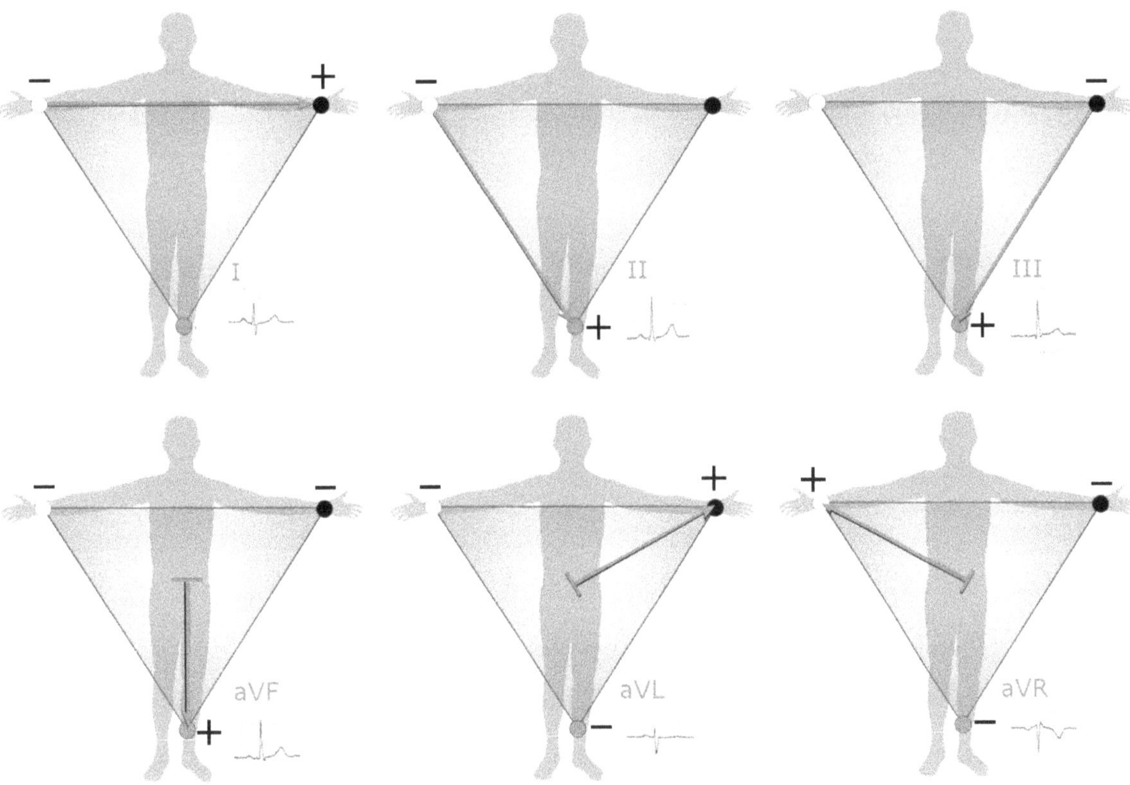

Einthoven triangle is the first step to understand ECG for medical students even today,

Beyond his invention of the ECG, Einthoven continued to contribute to medical science, later turning his attention to acoustics and the study of heart sounds in collaboration with Dr. P. Battaerd. His legacy extends beyond his lifetime, with his work continuing to be a cornerstone in the diagnosis and understanding of cardiovascular disorders.

Einthoven's contributions were recognized not only by the Nobel Prize but also through various honors and remembrances, including a Google Doodle on his 159th birthday. His burial site in the graveyard of the Reformed "Green Church" in Oegstgeest, Netherlands, remains a place where admirers can pay their respects. A town in the Netherlands is named after him.

Early Researchers

The Bohemian physiologist Johannes Purkinje, for instance, identified the fibers that bear his name in 1839, which are crucial for conducting the heart's electrical signals. His findings on the specialized tissue responsible for the heart's rhythmic contractions underscored the significance of the electrical properties within the heart.

In 1907, the combined efforts of Martin Flack and Sir Arthur Keith led to the discovery of the sinoatrial (SA) node, which acts as the heart's natural pacemaker, initiating the electrical impulses that govern the heartbeat. This discovery was pivotal, as it identified the primary source of the heart's rhythmic electrical activity.

The atrioventricular (AV) bundle, discovered by Wilhelm His Jr. in 1893, and the bundle branches identified shortly thereafter, were also critical in mapping the heart's electrical conduction pathway. The discovery of these structures provided insights into the heart's complex electrical system, enabling further advancements in cardiac diagnostics and treatment.

The work of Karl Albert Aschoff and Sunao Tawara in describing the AV node, as well as Ivan Mahaim's research on the connections in the bundle of His, contributed significantly to the detailed understanding of the heart's electrical conduction system.

Jean George Bachmann's experiments on canines in 1916 demonstrated the importance of the atrial connection in cardiac conduction, highlighting the intricate relationship between the heart's structural components and its electrical activity.

While Einthoven won the Nobel Prize for inventing the string galvanometer, two others, Dr. James Waller who worked with the capillary electrometer, and Dr. Thomas Lewis who saw its value at the bedside earlier, also deserved recognition.

Current Implications

The integration of artificial intelligence (AI) with ECG technology has marked a pivotal advancement in cardiovascular disease management. AI-enhanced ECGs, particularly through the development of convolutional neural networks (CNNs), are enabling more accurate and comprehensive interpretations of cardiac signals, pushing the boundaries of traditional cardiac monitoring and diagnosis.

The current implications of the electrocardiogram (ECG) in cardiac care underscore its indispensable role in diagnosing and monitoring heart conditions, reflecting a significant evolution from Einthoven's original invention to the sophisticated systems in use today. The integration of artificial intelligence (AI) with ECG technology has marked a pivotal advancement in cardiovascular disease management. AI-enhanced ECGs, particularly through the development of convolutional neural networks (CNNs), are enabling more accurate and comprehensive interpretations of cardiac signals, pushing the boundaries of traditional cardiac monitoring and diagnosis.

AI-driven algorithms have significantly improved the ability to interpret ECG data, enabling the detection of subtle patterns that may not be visible to the human eye. This has led to the development of models capable of diagnosing a wide range of cardiac abnormalities with high accuracy.

CNNs have been applied to large datasets of ECG records to identify various types of abnormalities, demonstrating the potential of AI to augment or even surpass the diagnostic capabilities of practicing cardiologists in some cases.

The application of AI to ECG interpretation aims to achieve a level of comprehensive, human-like interpretation capability that has been a goal since the advent of the digital ECG. Early efforts in computer-generated ECG interpretation could recognize basic points and measurements, but modern AI technologies have advanced to recognize complex patterns within extensive datasets.

Impact and Products

Foundation of Modern Cardiac Diagnostics: Einthoven's invention of the ECG has become a cornerstone of cardiovascular medicine, enabling the detection and analysis of heart rhythms, diagnosing heart diseases, and guiding treatment decisions.

Portable ECG Monitors: Technological advancements have led to the development of portable and wearable ECG monitors. These devices allow for continuous monitoring of heart activity, enabling early detection of arrhythmias and other cardiac issues in real-time, even outside clinical settings.

Telemetry Systems: The principles laid down by Einthoven have been expanded upon with the advent of telemetry systems in hospitals. These systems allow for the wireless monitoring of cardiac patients, providing continuous data transmission to healthcare providers for real-time analysis and intervention.

Smartphone Integration: Modern ECG technology has been integrated with smartphones and smartwatches, making it accessible to a broader audience. This integration promotes proactive health monitoring and can alert users to potential cardiac issues requiring further medical evaluation.

Advanced Diagnostic Tools: The legacy of Einthoven's ECG has paved the way for more sophisticated diagnostic tools, such as the combination of electrocardiography and electroencephalography (EEG) to simultaneously monitor heart and brain activity. This dual approach enhances the diagnosis and treatment of conditions affecting both the heart and the brain.

Screening and Preventive Medicine: ECG technology is instrumental in screening for heart conditions in at-risk populations, such as those with a family history of heart disease or high blood pressure. This preventive approach helps in early detection and management of potential heart issues before they become life-threatening.

Willem Einthoven's invention of the ECG has made a huge impact on heart care. It led to new technologies that keep getting better, helping diagnose, monitor, and treat heart issues, and advancing global health

JOHANNES FIBIGER (1926)

Tentative steps towards the origin story of cancer, still good enough for a Nobel

Johannes Fibiger, a Danish pathologist and physician, was awarded the Nobel Prize in Medicine in 1926 for his research on cancer. Fibiger's work, initially celebrated for its pioneering approach to inducing cancer in laboratory animals, later faced significant scrutiny, yet it marked a crucial phase in cancer research and the study of carcinogens.

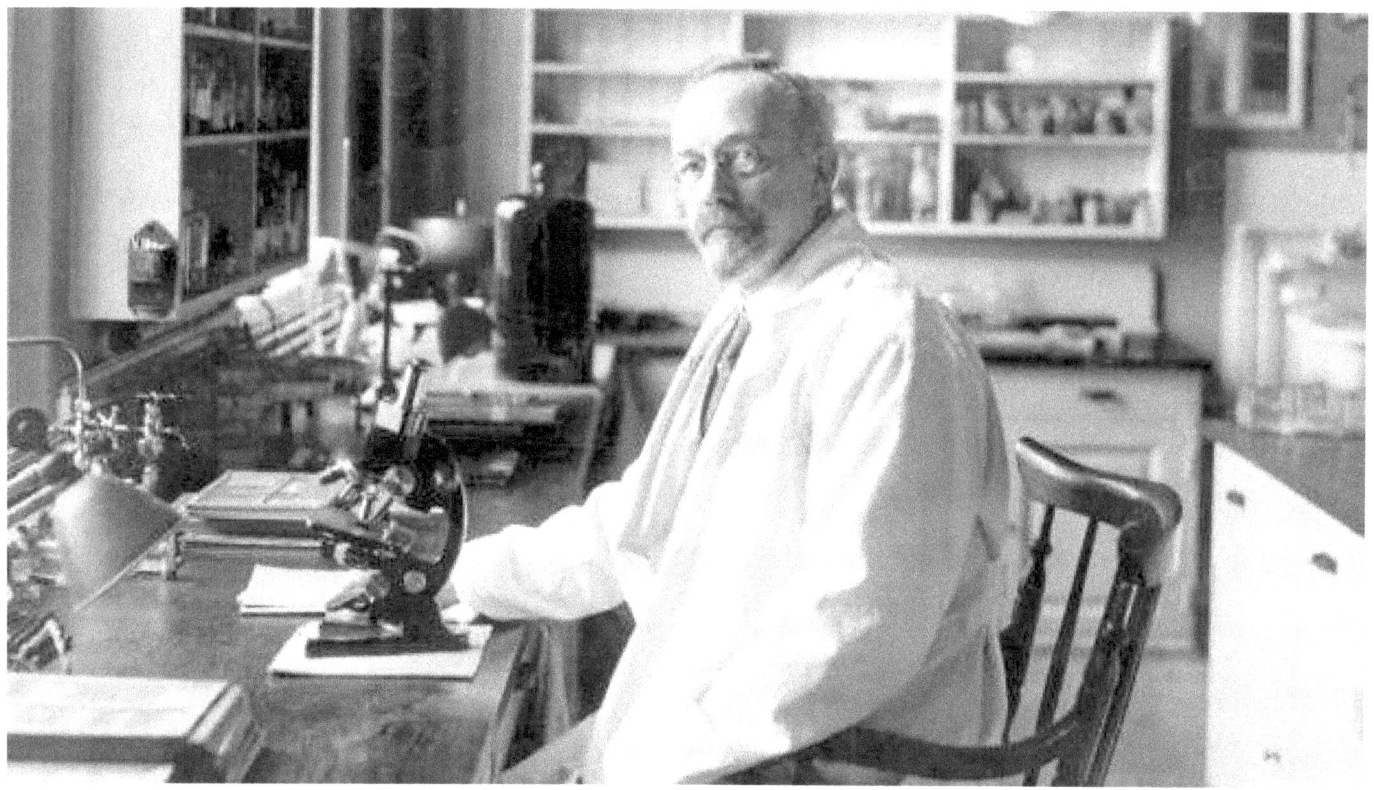

History

Born in Silkeborg, Denmark, in 1867, Fibiger's medical journey began with his graduation from the University of Copenhagen. His academic and professional endeavors were driven by a keen interest in pathology and bacteriology. Fibiger's Nobel-awarded work involved his discovery that a specific type of worm, which he thought induced cancerous tumors in rats and mice, could be a potential cause of cancer. He announced his findings in 1913, sparking international acclaim and furthering the scientific community's understanding of cancer development.

Snippets

Fibiger's research was groundbreaking for several reasons. He was among the first to experimentally produce what he believed were cancerous tumors in the laboratory, a feat that positioned him as a pioneer in cancer research. Despite later criticisms and the refutation of his findings—particularly the assertion that the observed tumors were not cancerous and were not caused by the parasites as he had thought—his work laid the groundwork for future research into the causes and mechanisms of cancer.

Current Implications

While Johannes Fibiger's specific hypothesis about parasitic worms causing cancer was disproven, his approach and methodology opened new avenues for cancer research. His efforts underscored the importance of experimental models in understanding cancer and its etiology. Subsequent research has built upon and moved beyond Fibiger's initial findings, leading to significant advancements in our understanding of cancer, including the roles of genetic predisposition, environmental factors, and indeed, viruses in cancer development.

Impact and Products

Fibiger's legacy in cancer research is a testament to the evolution of scientific inquiry. Although his specific conclusions were eventually contested, the spirit of his work contributed to the broader field of oncology, inspiring further studies on chemical carcinogens and the environmental causes of cancer. His initial success and later controversies remind us of the complex, iterative nature of scientific discovery. Notably, his work indirectly encouraged the exploration of cancer viruses and the environmental and genetic factors contributing to cancer, areas that have since led to groundbreaking discoveries and innovations in cancer treatment and prevention.

JULIUS WAGNER-JAUREGG (1927)

Pyrotherapy, a not so crazy innovation, when malaria was used as a weapon against syphilis

In 1927, Julius Wagner-Jauregg was recognized with the Nobel Prize in Medicine for his innovative use of malaria inoculation in treating dementia paralytica, a late stage of syphilis affecting the nervous system.

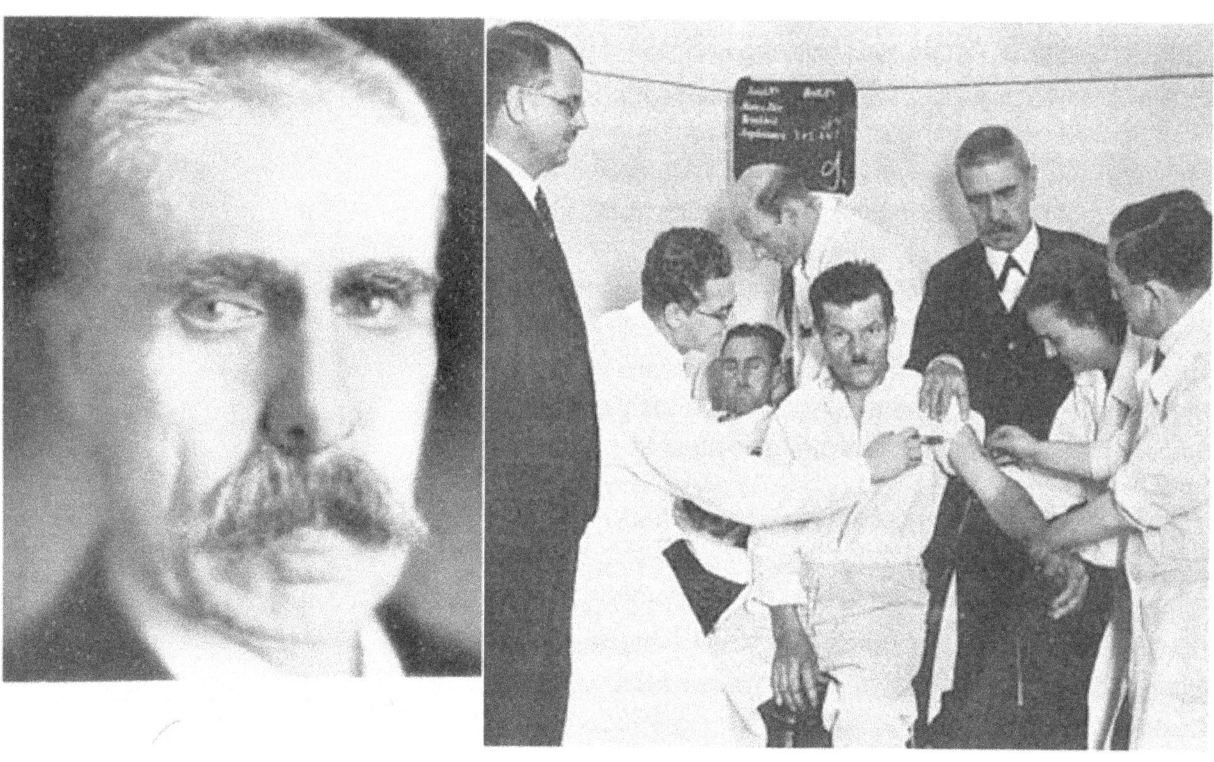

History

Julius Wagner-Jauregg was born on March 7, 1857, in Wels, Austria. Throughout his career in Austria, he was a leading figure in psychiatry and neurology, dedicating his work to understanding and treating mental illnesses. After completing his medical studies, Wagner-Jauregg held positions at psychiatric clinics and later at the University of Vienna, where he explored the biological bases of mental disorders.

Snippets

Wagner-Jauregg's groundbreaking contribution was his development of malaria therapy for neurosyphilis patients. By deliberately infecting patients with malaria, he could induce fever that would kill the syphilis bacteria, significantly improving or curing the condition. This method, known as pyrotherapy, marked a pivotal moment in the treatment of psychiatric illnesses, showing that biological interventions could have profound therapeutic effects.

Current Implications

While malaria therapy is no longer in use due to its risks and the development of antibiotics, Wagner-Jauregg's approach laid the groundwork for the biological treatment of mental illnesses, influencing contemporary psychiatric treatments.

Impact and Products

The success of malaria therapy in treating neurosyphilis revolutionized approaches to psychiatric disease, leading to the establishment of fever therapy as a legitimate and effective treatment method for certain disorders. Wagner-Jauregg's work has inspired ongoing research into the use of immunological and biological treatments in psychiatry, impacting the evolution of treatments for psychiatric disorders significantly.

CHARLES NICOLLE (1928)

Breakthrough in microbiology: Lice was found to be the vector for the giant killer Typhus

In 1928, Charles Jules Henri Nicolle, a distinguished French bacteriologist, was honored with the Nobel Prize in Medicine for his groundbreaking work on typhus. His discovery that lice were the vector for transmitting this deadly disease marked a significant advancement in medical science, contributing to the control of typhus epidemics and saving countless lives.

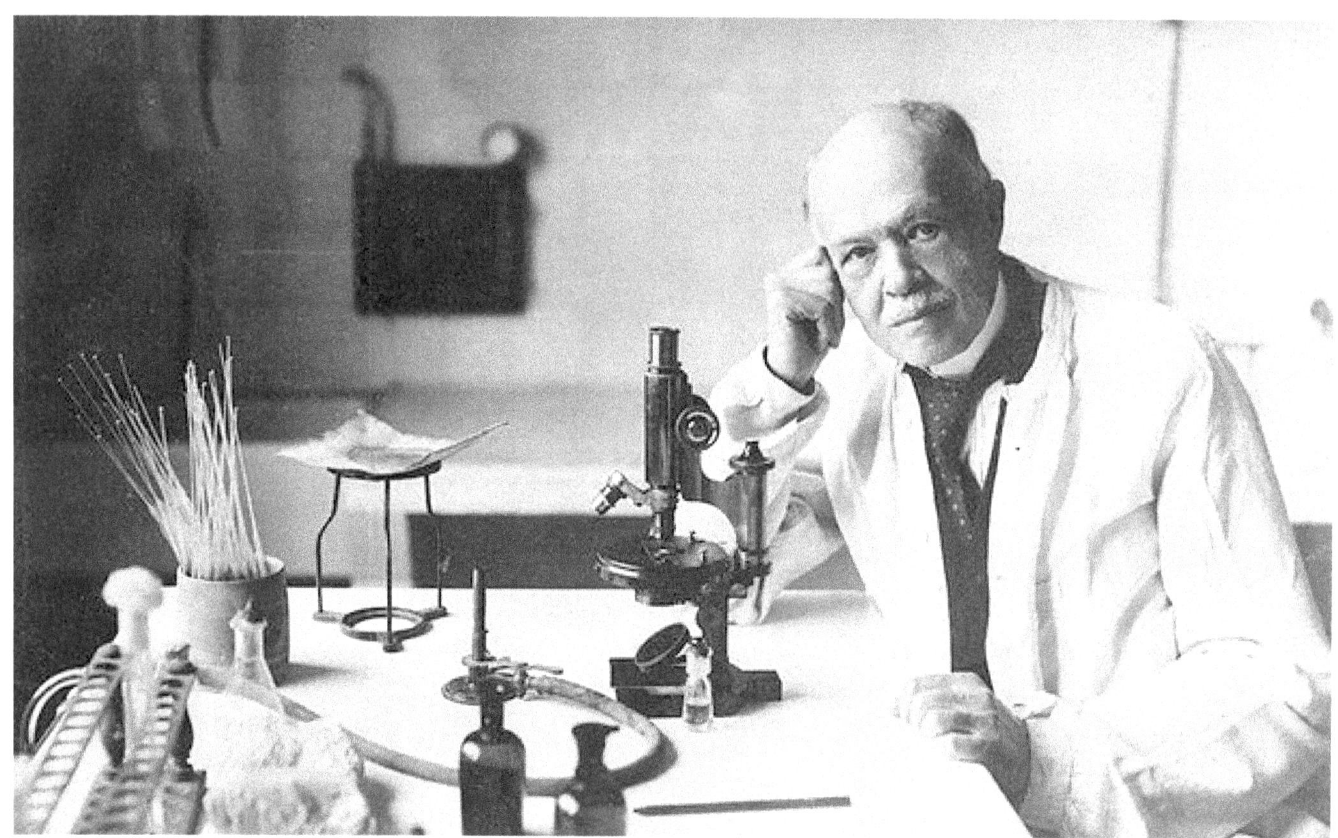

History

Born on September 21, 1866, in Rouen, France, Nicolle's early career was shaped by his profound interest in infectious diseases. His work at the Institute Pasteur in Tunis, Tunisia, provided him with the unique opportunity to study infectious diseases prevalent in North Africa and the Mediterranean Basin. Nicolle's keen observations and innovative experiments led to the discovery that lice acted as the vector for typhus transmission, a revelation that fundamentally changed the understanding of the disease's spread.

Snippets

Nicolle's discovery stemmed from his observation that typhus patients ceased to be infectious after undergoing a hot bath and changing clothes, leading him to hypothesize the role of lice in the disease's transmission. In 1909, he confirmed his theory by transferring typhus from infected to uninfected apes through lice, a finding that highlighted the importance of cleanliness and hygiene in controlling typhus outbreaks.

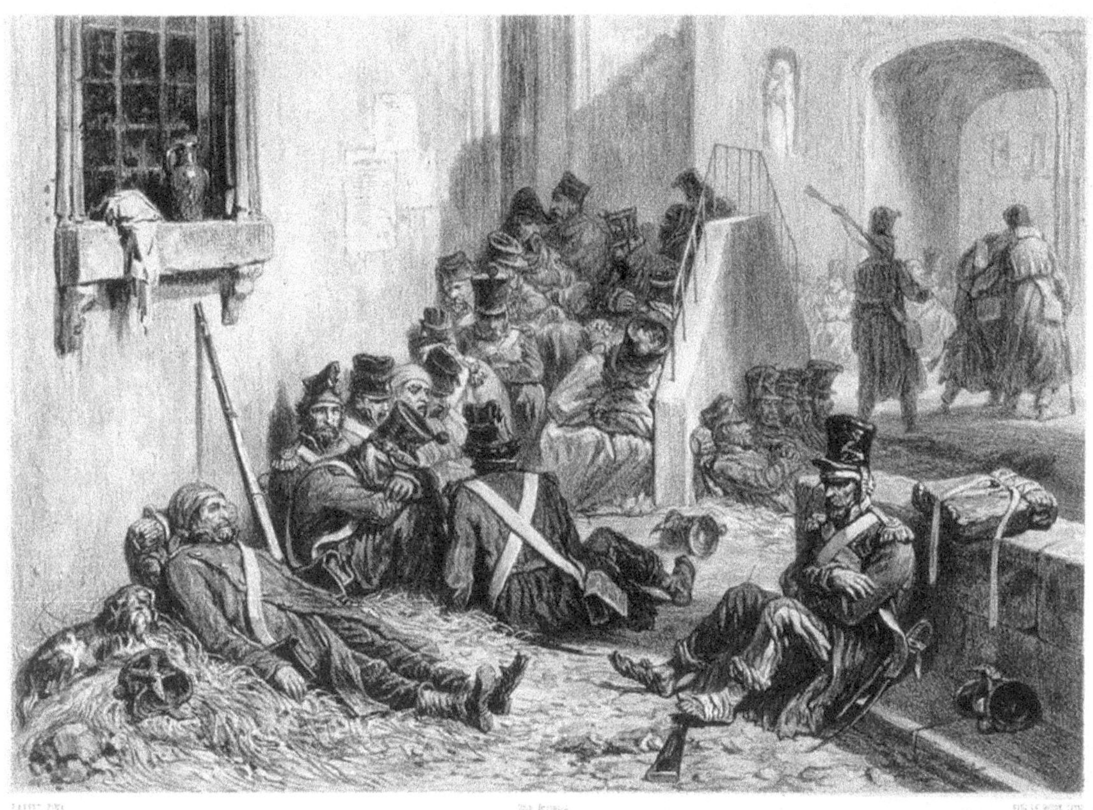

Soldiers at Mainz with typhus

Current Implications

Today, Nicolle's work on typhus and his broader contributions to infectious disease research continues to influence public health strategies and vaccine development. His approach to scientific inquiry, emphasizing observation, hypothesis testing, and the application of findings to improve health outcomes, remains a cornerstone of medical research.

Impact and Products

Beyond his scientific achievements, Nicolle's legacy includes his contributions to vaccine development and his efforts to combat other diseases, such as Malta fever and tick fever. Despite facing challenges in developing a practical vaccine for typhus, Nicolle's innovative use of sodium fluoride in vaccine development paved the way for future advancements in the field.

CHRISTIAAN EIJKMAN AND SIR FREDERICK HOPKINS (1929)

Vitamin discovery, a vital leap in decoding biochemical secrets in human nutrition

Christiaan Eijkman and Sir Frederick Hopkins, awarded the Nobel Prize in Medicine in 1929, are pivotal figures in the history of nutritional science. Their groundbreaking work laid the foundation for understanding the vital role of vitamins in human health.

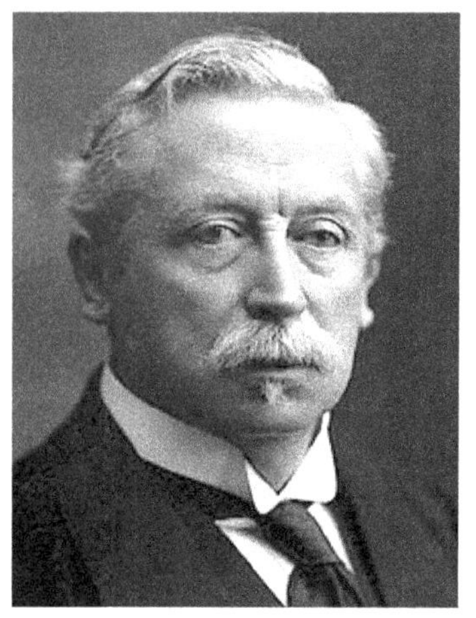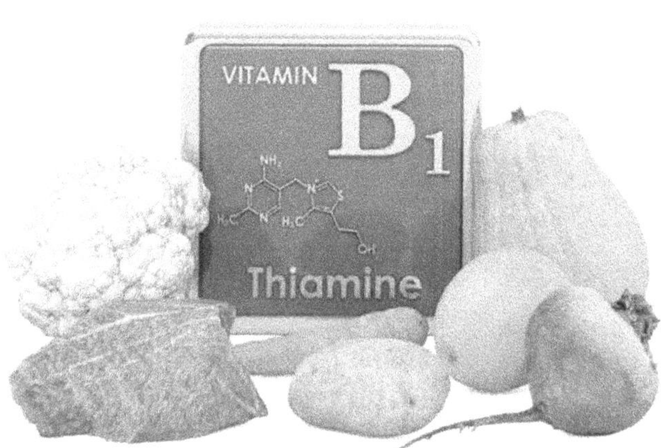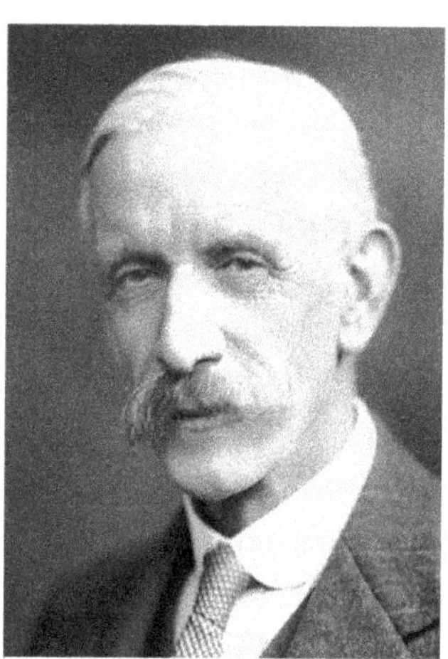

History

Christiaan Eijkman

Born on August 11, 1858, in Nijkerk, Netherlands, Christiaan Eijkman would become a pivotal figure in the field of nutrition. His early interest in medicine led him to pursue his studies at the University of Amsterdam, where he graduated with a degree in medicine. Eijkman's career took a significant turn when he joined the military and was subsequently stationed as a medical officer in the Dutch East Indies (now Indonesia).

It was in the Dutch East Indies that Eijkman's path to his Nobel Prize-winning discovery began. Tasked with investigating the cause of beriberi, a disease that afflicted thousands in the region, Eijkman's work took a pivotal turn in 1886. Beriberi, characterized by nerve degeneration, weakness, and heart failure, was a common and often fatal disease among the local population and Dutch colonial soldiers.

Sir Frederick Hopkins

Sir Frederick Gowland Hopkins, born on June 20, 1861, in Eastbourne, England, emerged as another foundational figure in the study of vitamins. Hopkins' academic journey led him to the University of

London, where he studied medicine, and later to the University of Cambridge, where he would make his most significant scientific contributions.

Hopkins is best known for his proposition of "accessory food factors" – substances that were critical for the maintenance of health but were neither macronutrients nor minerals. In a series of experiments conducted in the early 20th century, Hopkins demonstrated that animals fed a diet solely consisting of purified macronutrients failed to thrive unless the diet was supplemented with minute quantities of milk.

Snippets

Eijkman's Discovery

Christiaan Eijkman's breakthrough came from an unexpected turn in his research when he noticed a peculiar similarity between the symptoms of beriberi in humans and the conditions observed in chickens being used for nutritional experiments. Initially, these chickens were fed a diet of polished rice—the same kind of rice that was a staple in the diet of those populations among whom beriberi was rampant. These chickens developed symptoms akin to human beriberi, including muscle weakness and nerve degeneration.

The turning point in Eijkman's research occurred quite by accident. Due to a change in the personnel handling the chicken's diet, the chickens started receiving unpolished rice, which included the outer husk. Remarkably, the chickens that had shown symptoms of beriberi began to recover swiftly after the switch in their diet. This observation was the eureka moment for Eijkman. He hypothesized that the outer layer of rice, discarded during the polishing process, contained a vital nutrient that was essential for preventing beriberi. This nutrient, unknown to Eijkman at the time, was what we now know as vitamin B1 or thiamine.

Hopkins' Work

Sir Frederick Hopkins' contributions to nutritional science were grounded in meticulous experimentation and an unwavering belief in the existence of "accessory factors" in food, which were crucial for health but not yet identified or understood. Hopkins conducted a series of experiments on animals, demonstrating that a diet solely consisting of purified proteins, fats, carbohydrates, and minerals was insufficient for growth and survival.

This led Hopkins to propose the existence of essential dietary factors, which he initially termed "accessory food factors" and are now known as vitamins. His work provided compelling evidence that these substances were necessary for the body to function correctly and that their absence could lead to specific diseases.

Early Researchers

Gerrit Grijns (1865-1944): A Dutch physician and colleague of Christiaan Eijkman, Grijns continued Eijkman's work on beriberi and was the first to explicitly suggest the concept of "vital substances" missing from the diet of those suffering from beriberi. Grijns' insights were crucial in framing the hypothesis that led to the discovery of vitamins, yet his contributions are often overshadowed by Eijkman's Nobel Prize recognition.

Casimir Funk (1884-1967): A Polish biochemist, Funk is credited with coining the term "vitamine" in 1912, later shortened to "vitamin." He hypothesized that certain diseases were caused by the absence of specific substances in the diet, a theory that was groundbreaking at the time. Despite his significant contribution to the conceptual foundation of vitamin research, Funk's work did not receive the same level of acclaim as that of Hopkins or Eijkman.

Axel Holst (1860-1931) and Theodor Frølich (1870-1947): Norwegian scientists who conducted pivotal research on scurvy. Through their experiments with guinea pigs, they demonstrated that scurvy could be induced and cured with specific dietary changes, leading to the understanding that certain diseases were caused by dietary deficiencies. Their work laid the foundation for the discovery of vitamin C, yet their names are often absent from mainstream narratives of nutritional science history.

Current Implications

Fortification of Foods

Prevention of Nutritional Deficiencies: One of the most direct implications of Eijkman's and Hopkins' discoveries is the widespread fortification of foods with essential vitamins and minerals. This initiative has been instrumental in combating nutritional deficiencies around the globe. For example, the fortification of salt with iodine to prevent goiter, flour with folic acid to reduce the incidence of neural tube defects, and milk with vitamin D to combat rickets are all practices that stem from an understanding of the vital role nutrients play in health.

Global Health Initiatives: The knowledge that certain diseases could be prevented by dietary components led to international health initiatives aimed at eliminating or reducing the prevalence of vitamin deficiency diseases. Programs targeting vitamin A deficiency, for example, have significantly reduced mortality rates among children in developing countries

Emphasis on Balanced Diets

Nutritional Guidelines: The work of Eijkman and Hopkins has underpinned the development of nutritional guidelines that emphasize the importance of a balanced diet rich in vitamins and minerals. Dietary recommendations now routinely include a focus on consuming a variety of foods to ensure an adequate intake of all essential nutrients, reflecting the understanding that a diverse diet is key to preventing nutritional deficiencies and promoting overall health.

Public Health Policies: Governments and health organizations worldwide have implemented policies to promote nutritional education and awareness, recognizing the critical role of diet in preventing chronic diseases such as heart disease, diabetes, and cancer. The emphasis on eating fruits, vegetables, whole grains, and lean proteins can be traced back to the foundational work of Eijkman and Hopkins, highlighting the importance of micronutrients for health.

Impact on Food Security and Agriculture

Biofortification: Beyond the fortification of processed foods, there is an increasing focus on biofortification—the breeding of crop varieties with higher contents of vitamins and minerals. This agricultural strategy aims to improve the nutritional quality of food crops to address micronutrient malnutrition, particularly in regions where people rely heavily on staple crops for their diet.

Sustainable Diets: The recognition of the importance of vitamins and other micronutrients in diet has also contributed to the promotion of sustainable diets that are not only healthful but also environmentally sustainable. There is a growing understanding that food systems must not only provide nutritional security but also preserve natural resources and biodiversity.

Impact and Products

Influence on the Nutritional Supplements Industry

The research by Eijkman and Hopkins has directly influenced the nutritional supplements industry, which has grown into a multi-billion dollar sector. Their work demonstrated the critical role of vitamins and micronutrients in maintaining health, leading to the development of a wide range of dietary supplements aimed at preventing nutritional deficiencies and improving overall health.

Development of Dietary Guidelines

Their discoveries have also been instrumental in the formulation of dietary guidelines that emphasize the importance of vitamin intake. For instance, the Dietary Guidelines for Americans, 2020-2025, developed by the U.S. Department of Agriculture and the U.S. Department of Health and Human Services, offers advice on what to eat and drink to meet nutrient needs, promote health, and prevent chronic disease.

Ongoing Research into Micronutrients

Modern scientific inquiries have expanded beyond their initial discoveries to explore the nuanced roles of vitamins and minerals in preventing chronic diseases, such as cardiovascular diseases, cancer, and diabetes.

Christiaan Eijkman and Sir Frederick Gowland Hopkins' research on vitamins and nutrition has had a lasting impact, shaping the supplements industry, dietary guidelines, and ongoing micronutrient research for health and disease prevention.

KARL LANDSTEINER (1930)

Discovery of blood groups : A momentous moment in medical science

Karl Landsteiner was awarded the Nobel Prize in Medicine in 1930 for his discovery of human blood groups. His work laid the foundation for safe blood transfusions, transforming medical practice and saving countless lives. Landsteiner's identification of the A, B, AB, and O blood groups was a groundbreaking achievement that enabled the development of blood typing and cross matching techniques critical for transfusion medicine.

History

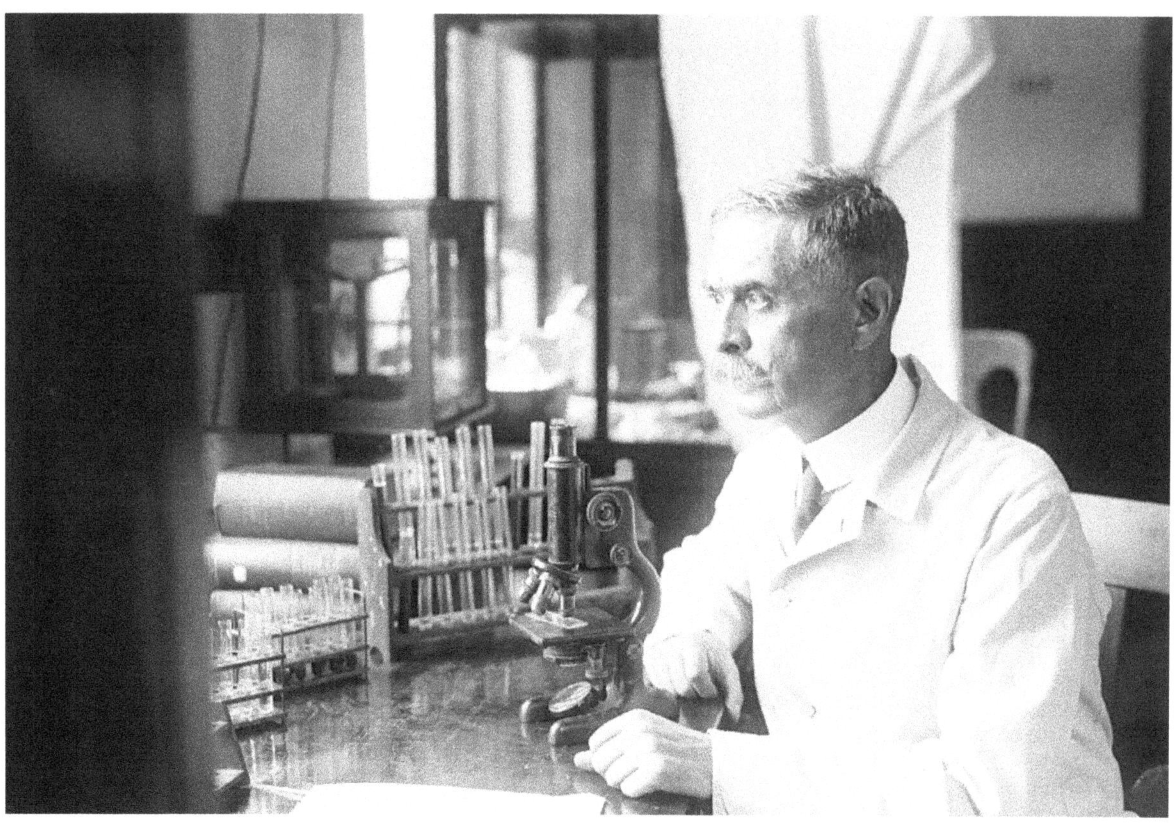

Born in Vienna, Austria, on June 14, 1868, Landsteiner was immersed in academia from an early age, following the death of his father when he was just six years old. His early education was heavily influenced by his devoted mother, Fanny Hess. Landsteiner pursued his medical studies at the University of Vienna, graduating in 1891, and began his foray into biochemical research during his time as a student, publishing a paper on the influence of diet on the composition of blood ash.

From 1898 to 1908, Landsteiner served as an assistant in the University Department of Pathological Anatomy in Vienna, under the leadership of Professor A. Weichselbaum. It was during this period that Landsteiner made significant contributions to the study of morbid physiology and immunology, including the discovery of new facts about the immunology of syphilis and the Wassermann reaction, as well as the immunological factors he named haptens.

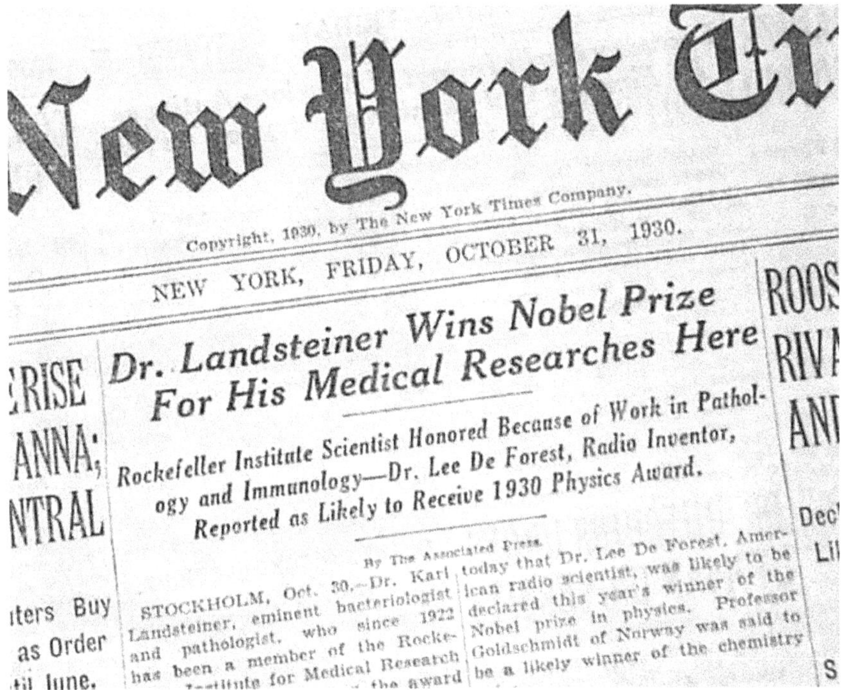

In 1919, Landsteiner moved to The Hague, and in 1922, he relocated to the United States to work at the Rockefeller Institute for Medical Research in New York. He married Helen Wlasto in 1916, with whom he had a son, Dr. E. Landsteiner. Landsteiner continued his research until his death on June 26, 1943, following a heart attack in his laboratory, a poignant end to the life of a scientist who was truly dedicated to his work until his final moments.

Snippets

Discovery of ABO Blood Groups: Karl Landsteiner's identification of the A, B, AB, and O blood groups in 1900 revolutionized the practice of blood transfusion. Before this discovery, transfusions were highly risky and frequently fatal due to incompatible blood types.

Blood Compatibility and Safe Transfusions: Landsteiner's work made it clear that blood compatibility was crucial for safe transfusions. This understanding led to the development of blood typing and cross-matching practices, significantly reducing the risk of adverse reactions and making transfusions safer.

ABO Phenotypes and Antibodies: The identification of ABO phenotypes and the understanding that individuals form antibodies against the ABO blood group antigens not present on their own red blood cells laid the foundation for modern transfusion medicine. This knowledge is pivotal in preventing immune reactions during blood transfusions.

	Group A	Group B	Group AB	Group O
Red blood cell type	A	B	AB	O
Antibodies in plasma	Anti-B	Anti-A	None	Anti-A and Anti-B
Antigens in red blood cell	A antigen	B antigen	A and B antigens	None

Universal Donors and Recipients: The discovery of the O blood type as a universal donor and AB as a universal recipient has been critical in emergency transfusions and when a patient's blood type is unknown, thereby saving countless lives.

Early researchers

The journey towards understanding blood transfusions began with experiments that spanned hundreds of years, with many early attempts resulting in adverse reactions or the death of the patient due to incompatible blood types. Early researchers noted that some transfusions were successful while others were not, hinting at an underlying compatibility issue, but without understanding the immunological basis behind these reactions.

Significant contributions came from the field of serum therapy, where scientists like Emil von Behring and Shibasaburo Kitasato made strides in understanding the role of antibodies in the blood. Their work, although not directly related to blood transfusion, enriched the scientific background necessary for later breakthroughs in immunology and transfusion medicine.

Attempts to store and preserve blood for later use, even though primitive by today's standards, were essential steps towards developing modern blood banking and transfusion services. Observations of hemolysis in early transfusion experiments highlighted the risks associated with incompatible transfusions, even if the precise reasons for these reactions—later identified as the ABO blood group antigens and antibodies—remained elusive.

Current Implications

Foundation of Modern Transfusion Medicine

Landsteiner's identification of the major blood groups (A, B, AB, and O) laid the groundwork for the safe practice of blood transfusion. This discovery is fundamental to transfusion medicine, enabling the matching of blood types between donors and recipients, thus preventing adverse reactions during transfusions.

Development of Blood Typing and Crossmatching Techniques

Landsteiner's work led to the development of precise blood typing and crossmatching techniques. These methods are critical for ensuring compatibility between donor and recipient blood, significantly reducing the risks of transfusion reactions. Today, these techniques are standard practice in hospitals and blood banks worldwide, ensuring patient safety during blood transfusions

Understanding and Managing Rh Factor Complications

The discovery of the Rh factor by Landsteiner and Alexander S. Wiener in 1937 further refined the safety of blood transfusions by addressing the complications related to Rh incompatibility. This discovery has crucial implications for managing Rh-negative mothers' pregnancies, preventing hemolytic disease of the newborn (HDN).

Impact on Autoimmune Diseases and Immunology

Landsteiner's contributions extended beyond transfusion medicine into the broader field of immunology. His work on the mechanisms of immunity and the nature of antibodies paved the way for understanding autoimmune diseases, where the body's immune system attacks its own tissues. This understanding has led to the development of diagnostics and treatments for autoimmune conditions.

Impact and Products

Complex Surgical Procedures: The ability to safely transfuse blood has enabled the advancement and complexity of surgical procedures. Surgeons can now perform operations that require significant blood replacement, knowing that matched blood types can be transfused with minimal risk of reaction.

Organ Transplantation: Landsteiner's work has also been instrumental in the field of organ transplantation. Understanding blood groups and the immune system's response to foreign antigens has helped in matching donors and recipients, reducing the risk of organ rejection.

Treatment of Trauma Patients: Trauma care has been significantly improved with the ability to quickly and safely transfuse blood to victims of accidents and injuries, helping to prevent shock and support recovery.

Understanding Immune Reactions: Beyond transfusion, Landsteiner's discovery has advanced the understanding of the immune system's functioning, particularly how it reacts to foreign substances.

This has implications for immunology, including the development of vaccines and treatments for autoimmune diseases.

Global Practices of Blood Donation and Transfusion: The principles established by Landsteiner underpin the global practices of blood donation, storage, and transfusion. Blood typing and crossmatching are standard procedures before any blood transfusion, ensuring compatibility and minimizing risks.

His work continues to influence current medical practices and research, demonstrating the enduring value of his contributions to improving human health and saving lives.

Wherever a blood transfusion happens today, wherever a worried mother's child is saved, Karl Landsteiner is there in spirit. These were the last words of Hermann Chiari, his colleague, during the unveiling of the Landsteiner memorial at the University of Vienna in 1961.

His groundbreaking role in isolating the Polio virus showed the way for the creation of a vaccine later on. Not many are aware that he was posthumously inducted into the Polio Hall of Fame at Warm Springs, Georgia, a dedication made in 1958.

OTTO HEINRICH WARBURG (1931)

The prodigious German, who proved that every cell in the body respires
with its mitochondria

Otto Heinrich Warburg was awarded the Nobel Prize in Medicine in 1931 for his pioneering research on cellular respiration. Specifically, his work identified the nature and mode of action of the respiratory enzyme, fundamentally altering our understanding of cell metabolism and laying the groundwork for future research in cellular respiration and metabolism.

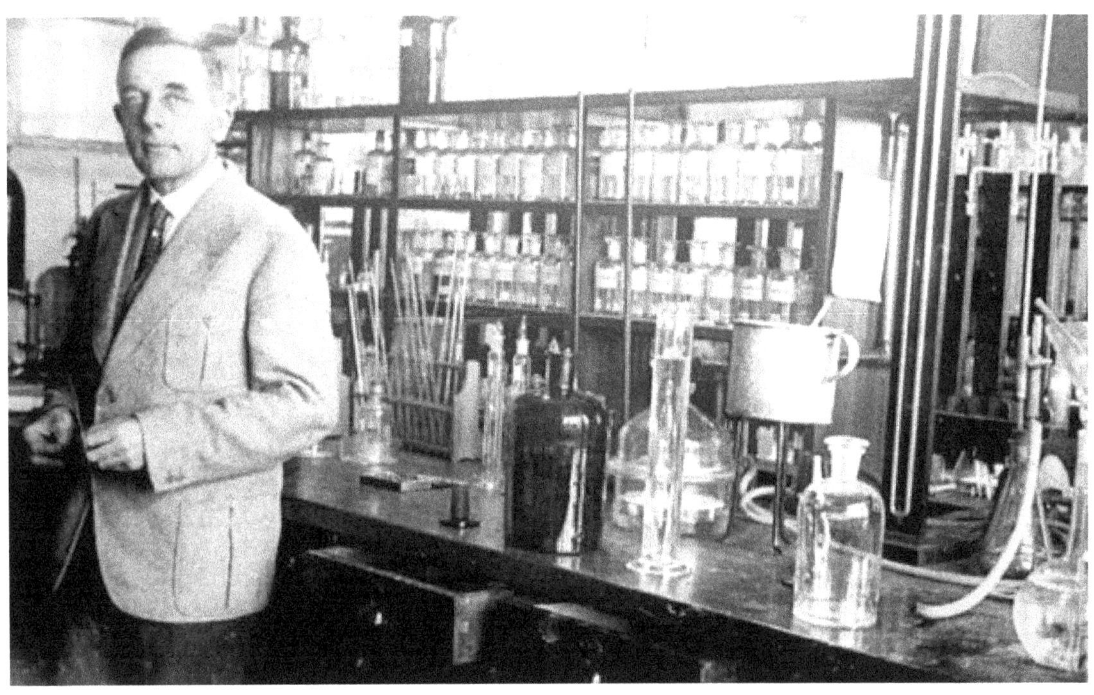

History

Otto Heinrich Warburg's life and career were as distinguished as they were influential, beginning with his birth on October 8, 1883, in Freiburg, Germany, into a family with a rich heritage of scholars and professionals. His father, Emil Warburg, was a prominent physicist, which undoubtedly influenced Otto's scientific path. Warburg's academic journey was comprehensive; after studying chemistry under Emil Fischer at the University of Berlin and earning a Doctorate in Chemistry in 1906, he pursued medicine at Heidelberg University, obtaining a Doctorate in Medicine in 1911.

Warburg's work at the Naples Marine Biological Station between 1908 and 1914 marked the beginning of his lifelong dedication to understanding the fundamental processes of life, particularly cellular respiration.

His military service during World War I, where he was awarded the Iron Cross, provided him with a unique perspective on life outside academia, enriching his approach to scientific inquiry. During this time, Albert Einstein asked Warburg to go back to teaching for the benefit of science, showing how respected Warburg was in the scientific world.

Despite never marrying, Warburg had a passion for equestrian sports, maintaining personal interests alongside his groundbreaking scientific work until his death on August 1, 1970.

Snippets

Discovery of Aerobic Glycolysis: Warburg observed that tumor cells exhibit an increased uptake of glucose and produce lactic acid from this glucose even in the presence of oxygen. This is in contrast to normal cells, which primarily rely on oxidative phosphorylation for energy production when oxygen is available. This phenomenon, termed the Warburg effect, indicates that cancer cells prefer fermentation to aerobic respiration for energy production, even in oxygen-rich environments.

Debate on Mitochondrial Functionality: While Warburg initially hypothesized that cancer cells resort to fermentation due to mitochondrial damage, this was later contested. Studies showed that tumor cells' mitochondria are functional, and these cells utilize both aerobic glycolysis and oxidative phosphorylation. The choice for aerobic glycolysis is believed to support rapid proliferation, providing not just energy (ATP) but also metabolic intermediates for biomass accumulation necessary for cell growth.

Clinical Significance of the Warburg Effect: The Warburg effect has profound implications in cancer diagnosis and treatment. For instance, PET imaging exploits the high glucose uptake of cancer cells to detect tumors and monitor treatment response. Furthermore, research into gene expression profiles related to glycolysis could help in prognostication, with glycolytic phenotypes often correlating with poorer survival outcomes in cancers like lung adenocarcinoma and triple-negative breast cancer.

Metabolic and Genetic Reprogramming: The metabolic shift seen in cancer cells, known as the Warburg effect, is now understood to be influenced by various oncogenes and tumor suppressor genes. This reprogramming enables cancer cells to sustain high rates of proliferation and resist cell death, contributing to tumor growth and metastasis. Key players in this process include HIF-1α, which promotes glycolysis, and oncogenes like MYC and Ras, as well as the tumor suppressor TP53, all of which modulate the balance between glycolysis and oxidative phosphorylation in favor of rapid energy production.

Heterogeneity in Tumor Metabolism: The Warburg effect is not uniform across all cancer types or even within a single tumor, reflecting the metabolic flexibility of cancer cells. This heterogeneity is driven by various factors, including the activation of different oncogenic pathways. Understanding these variations is crucial for developing targeted therapies that can exploit the unique metabolic vulnerabilities of cancer cells.

Early Researchers

Before Otto Warburg's significant contributions, pioneers like Eduard Buchner demonstrated that alcoholic fermentation occurs in cell-free extracts, laying the groundwork for understanding biochemical reactions outside living cells. Additionally, the work of scientists like Louis Pasteur on fermentation and the role of microorganisms, as well as the discoveries related to enzymes' roles in chemical reactions, provided essential knowledge that paved the way for Warburg's groundbreaking research in cellular metabolism. These early discoveries in biochemistry and physiology were crucial for Warburg's later work on cellular respiration and metabolism, illustrating the collaborative nature of scientific progress.

Current Implications

Foundation of Cancer Metabolism Understanding: Warburg's identification of altered glucose metabolism in cancer cells, known as the "Warburg Effect," laid the foundation for the field of cancer metabolism, shifting the focus toward understanding how metabolic alterations drive cancer progression.

Advancements in Diagnostic Techniques: His discoveries led to the development of PET imaging, exploiting cancer cells' increased glucose uptake. This technique has become indispensable in oncology for tumor detection and monitoring treatment response.

Influence on Therapeutic Strategies: The Warburg Effect has inspired strategies targeting cancer cell metabolism, aiming to disrupt their energy supply and inhibit tumor growth, opening new avenues for cancer treatment.

Implications Beyond Oncology: Warburg's work has implications beyond cancer, influencing research into metabolic disorders and providing insights into the metabolic aspects of various diseases.

Stimulating Ongoing Research: Warburg's findings continue to inspire and challenge researchers, driving advancements in understanding the complex role of metabolism in health and disease.

Impact and Products

Pioneering Biochemical Research: Otto Warburg's groundbreaking discovery of the Warburg effect laid the foundational stone for modern biochemical research, particularly in understanding the metabolic processes of cancer cells. His work has illuminated the pathways of cellular respiration and metabolism, marking a significant advancement in biochemistry.

Revolutionizing Cancer Treatment: Warburg's insights into cellular metabolism have been crucial in developing targeted cancer therapies. By exploiting the unique metabolic needs of cancer cells, researchers are devising novel treatments aimed at starving cancer cells of their energy supply, thereby inhibiting their growth.

Enhancing Diagnostic Technologies: The Warburg effect's characterization has led to improvements in cancer diagnosis, notably through the use of PET scans. This technique takes advantage of cancer cells' increased glucose consumption, allowing for more precise tumor detection and monitoring of treatment efficacy.

Influencing Various Scientific Fields: The implications of Warburg's research extend beyond cancer, impacting physiology, medicine, and even aging research. Understanding cellular metabolism's role in disease has opened new research avenues, aiming to uncover treatments for various metabolic disorders.

Fostering Ongoing Research and Innovation: Today, Warburg's legacy continues to inspire research into the complexities of cellular metabolism. Scientists worldwide are exploring metabolic pathways, seeking new interventions for diseases where altered metabolism is a key factor, demonstrating the enduring value of his contributions to science and medicine.

CHARLES SHERRINGTON AND EDGAR ADRIAN (1932)

Critical experiments in neural communications

In 1932, Sir Charles Scott Sherrington and Edgar Douglas Adrian were jointly awarded the Nobel Prize in Medicine for their pioneering discoveries regarding the functions of neurons.

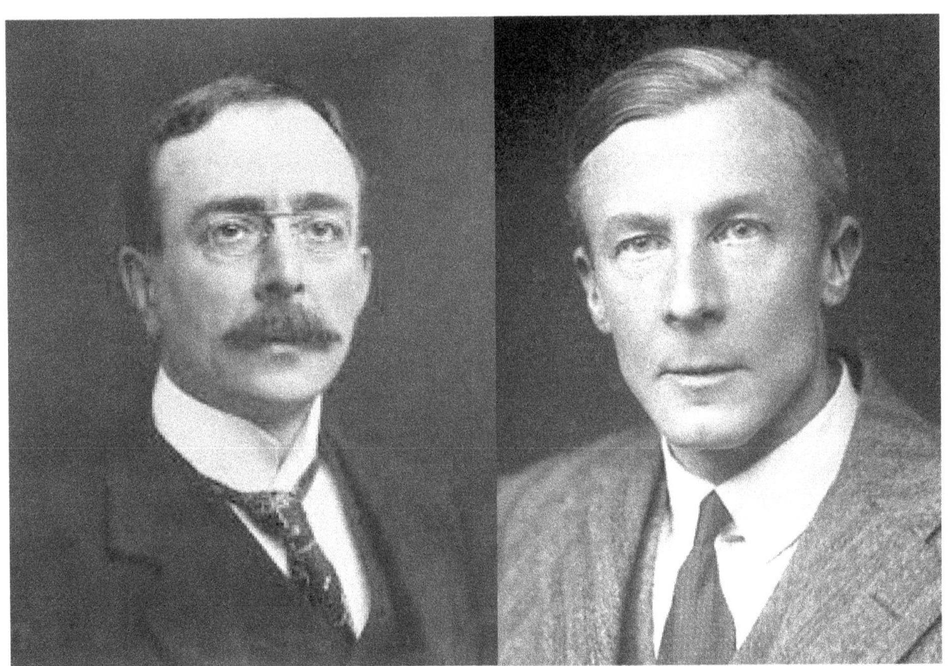

History

Sir Charles Scott Sherrington, born on November 27, 1857, in London, United Kingdom, contributed extensively to the understanding of the nervous system. His research in the 1890s demonstrated how reflexes—unconscious muscular movements triggered by stimuli—involve complex interactions within the spinal cord and brain to process and respond to nerve impulses. Sherrington's work provided insights into the integrative action of the nervous system, exploring how different reflexes are coordinated through the spinal cord and brain.

Edgar Douglas Adrian, born on November 30, 1889, also in London, focused on how nerve cells signal physiological processes. His development of methods to measure electrical signals in the nervous system led to the discovery that these signals have a consistent size, showing that intensity of stimuli is represented by the frequency and number of nerve signals rather than their individual strength.

Current Implications

Their discoveries have profound implications for neuroscience, offering a basis for understanding a wide range of neurological functions and disorders. By establishing the all-or-nothing law of neural response and elucidating the roles of excitatory and inhibitory signals in neural communication, Sherrington and Adrian set the stage for decades of research into how the brain processes information.

Impact and Products

Sherrington's and Adrian's work together forms the cornerstone of neurophysiology, influencing subsequent research in synaptic transmission, neural signaling pathways, and the overall understanding of the nervous system's structure and function. Their insights into synaptic plasticity, the dynamics of neurotransmission, and the molecular mechanisms underpinning these processes continue to inform current research, driving forward advancements in diagnosing and treating neurological conditions.

Their discoveries remain crucial to neuroscience, underpinning ongoing studies into brain function and dysfunction, and contributing to the development of treatments for neurological diseases.

THOMAS MORGAN (1933)

The founder & leader in the theory of Chromosomal Inheritance

Thomas Hunt Morgan was awarded the Nobel Prize in Medicine in 1933 for his discoveries concerning the role played by the chromosome in heredity, establishing the chromosome theory of heredity through his work with Drosophila melanogaster, the fruit fly.

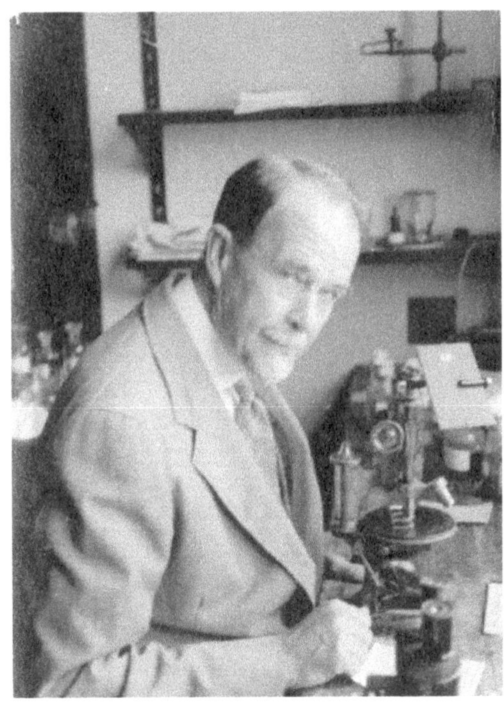

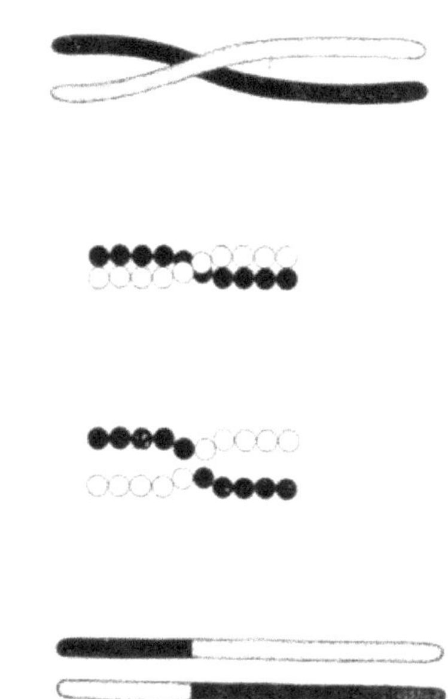

Fig. 64. Scheme to illustrate a method of crossing over of the chromosomes.

History

Morgan was born on September 25, 1866, in Lexington, Kentucky, USA, into a family with significant historical connections, including ties to Confederate General John Hunt Morgan and Francis Scott Key, the author of the "Star Spangled Banner." He displayed a keen interest in natural history from a young age. Morgan graduated from the State College of Kentucky (now the University of Kentucky) in 1886 with a B.S. degree in zoology and went on to earn his Ph.D. from Johns Hopkins University in 1890. Morgan's work at Columbia University's Fly Room was pivotal in demonstrating that genes are carried on chromosomes and are the mechanical basis of heredity, which laid the foundation for modern genetics.

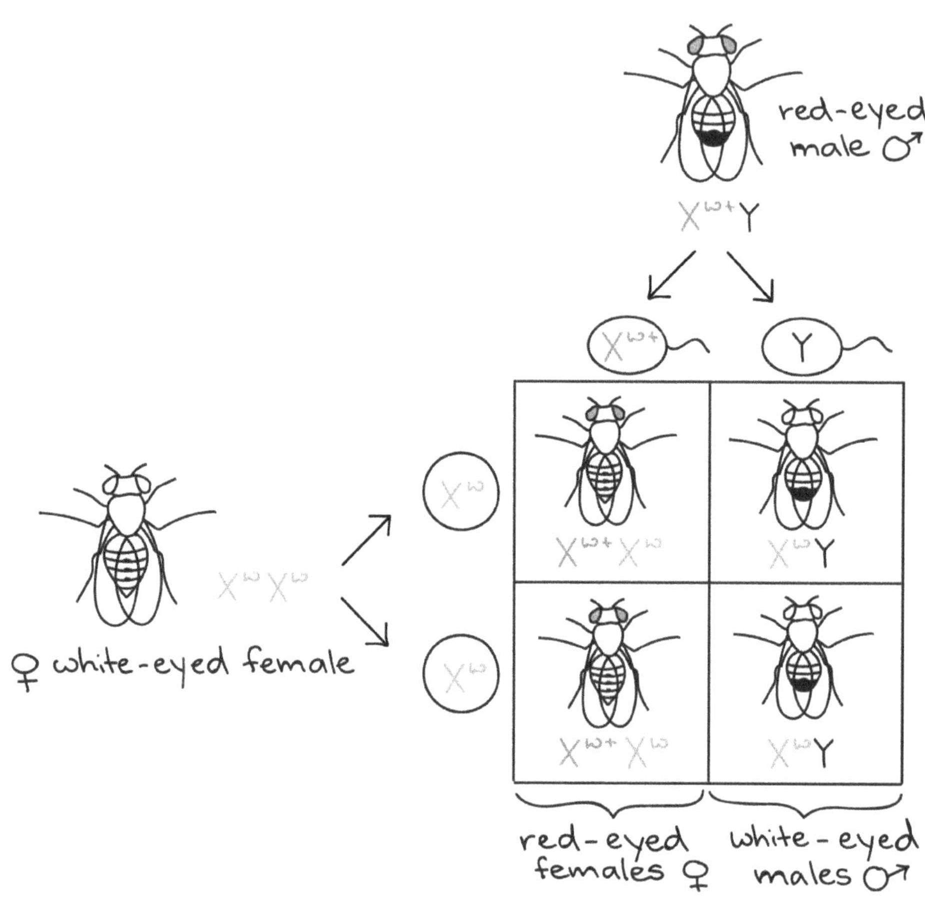

Morgan's fruit fly experiments

Morgan's professional journey took him from Johns Hopkins to Bryn Mawr and finally to Columbia University, where he would conduct his groundbreaking work in genetics. At Columbia, in the famous "Fly Room," Morgan and his students used Drosophila melanogaster to unlock the secrets of heredity and chromosome function.

Snippets

Model Organism Selection: Morgan chose Drosophila melanogaster, a type of fruit fly, for his genetic studies due to its simple care requirements, short life cycle, and high reproductive rate, making it an ideal model organism for genetic research.

Discovery of Sex-Linked Inheritance: One of Morgan's significant early findings was the discovery of a white-eyed mutant in Drosophila, which led to the first demonstration of sex-linked inheritance, showing that some traits are carried on specific chromosomes (the X chromosome in this case).

Chromosome Theory of Inheritance: Morgan's work provided crucial evidence for the chromosome theory of inheritance, which posits that genes are located on chromosomes, and these chromosomes are the basis for hereditary transmission of traits from parents to offspring.

Genetic Linkage and Recombination: Through breeding experiments with fruit flies, Morgan and his team discovered genetic linkage and recombination, demonstrating that genes on the same chromosome tend to be inherited together but can be separated through recombination, or "crossing over," during meiosis.

Gene Mapping: Morgan's research led to the creation of the first genetic maps, which showed the relative positions of genes on chromosomes. These maps were constructed based on the frequencies of recombination between different gene pairs, laying the groundwork for modern genetics and genomics.

Mutation Studies: Morgan's lab observed spontaneous mutations in their Drosophila populations, which were instrumental in understanding the role of mutations in genetic variation and evolution. This work highlighted the dynamic nature of the genome and its importance in adaptive processes.

Foundation of Modern Genetics: Morgan's findings challenged and expanded upon the principles of Mendelian genetics, integrating them into a chromosomal framework. This integration formed the foundation of modern genetics, influencing future research in biology, medicine, and other fields.

Early Researchers

Francis Galton, a polymath, pioneered the study of heredity and was among the first to use statistical methods to analyze genetic traits. He introduced regression and correlation concepts to study hereditary characteristics, contributing to the emergence of genetics as a scientific discipline. His work on biometrics and eugenics, though controversial today, played a significant role in shaping genetic studies.

Further, Hugo de Vries, Carl Correns, and Erich Tschermak independently rediscovered Gregor Mendel's pea plant experiments at the turn of the 20th century. Their simultaneous rediscovery in 1900 reaffirmed Mendel's findings, reigniting interest in heredity studies. Additionally, Walter Sutton and Theodor Boveri formulated the chromosome theory of inheritance, proposing chromosomes as gene carriers, laying the foundation for modern genetics. This theory aligned cytology with Mendel's heredity rules, marking a crucial advancement in genetics. Simultaneously, Lucien Cuénot, working with mice, provided early evidence supporting Mendel's theory in animals, expanding the scope of Mendelian genetics beyond plants.

Current Impication

Genetic Research and Genomics: Morgan's demonstration of the chromosomal basis of inheritance paved the way for the fields of molecular biology and genomics. Today, we can sequence entire genomes, identifying the genetic basis of diseases, understanding evolutionary relationships, and enhancing our knowledge of genetic diversity among populations.

Medicine and Gene Therapy: Insights from Morgan's work are directly applied in medical genetics, where understanding the genetic basis of diseases has led to better diagnosis, treatment, and the development of gene therapy. Gene therapy seeks to correct or replace faulty genes responsible for disease development, offering potential cures for previously untreatable conditions.

Education and Research: Morgan's methodological approach and use of model organisms have become standard practices in genetic research and education. Drosophila melanogaster remains a widely used model organism in genetics and developmental biology, providing invaluable insights into human biology and disease.

Ethical, Legal, and Social Implications (ELSI): The advancements spurred by Morgan's research have also led to the emergence of ethical, legal, and social questions regarding genetic information, privacy, genetic testing, and genetic modification. The field of bioethics continues to evolve in response to these challenges, addressing concerns about genetic discrimination, consent, and the implications of genetic engineering.

Impacts and Products

Advances in Genetic Research: Morgan's work has directly contributed to our ability to conduct advanced genetic research, leading to the development of technologies such as CRISPR-Cas9 for genome editing. This allows for precise manipulation of DNA in organisms, opening up possibilities for scientific research, agriculture, and medicine.

Gene Therapy and Precision Medicine: Building on Morgan's discoveries, gene therapy has emerged as a revolutionary approach to treat and potentially cure genetic disorders by correcting defective genes. Precision medicine, which tailors medical treatment to the individual characteristics of each patient based on their genetic profile, is another direct outcome of understanding genetic inheritance and variability.

Agricultural Improvements: The principles of heredity discovered by Morgan have been applied to develop genetically modified crops that are more resistant to pests, diseases, and environmental stresses. These advancements have led to increased agricultural productivity and food security in various parts of the world.

Model Organisms in Research: Morgan's use of Drosophila melanogaster as a model organism has established a precedent for using model organisms in biological research. This practice has led to significant discoveries in genetics, developmental biology, neurology, and many other fields, contributing to our understanding of complex biological processes.

Bioinformatics and Computational Biology: The understanding of genetic linkage and chromosomal inheritance has propelled the fields of bioinformatics and computational biology, where computer technologies are used to manage, analyze, and understand biological data, including genetic sequences. These fields are crucial for interpreting the vast amounts of data generated by genomic research.

Biodiversity and Conservation Genetics: Insights from genetic research have applications in biodiversity conservation, helping to understand the genetic diversity within and between species, which is crucial for conservation planning and efforts. This has led to the development of conservation strategies that preserve genetic diversity and reduce the risk of extinction.

GEORGE WHIPPLE, GEORGE MINOT, WILLIAM MURPHY
(1934)

The pivotal discovery of Vitamin B-12, liver extracts, & the dramatic cure for Anemia

In 1934, George Hoyt Whipple, George Richards Minot, and William Parry Murphy were jointly awarded the Nobel Prize in Medicine "for their discoveries concerning liver therapy in cases of anemia".

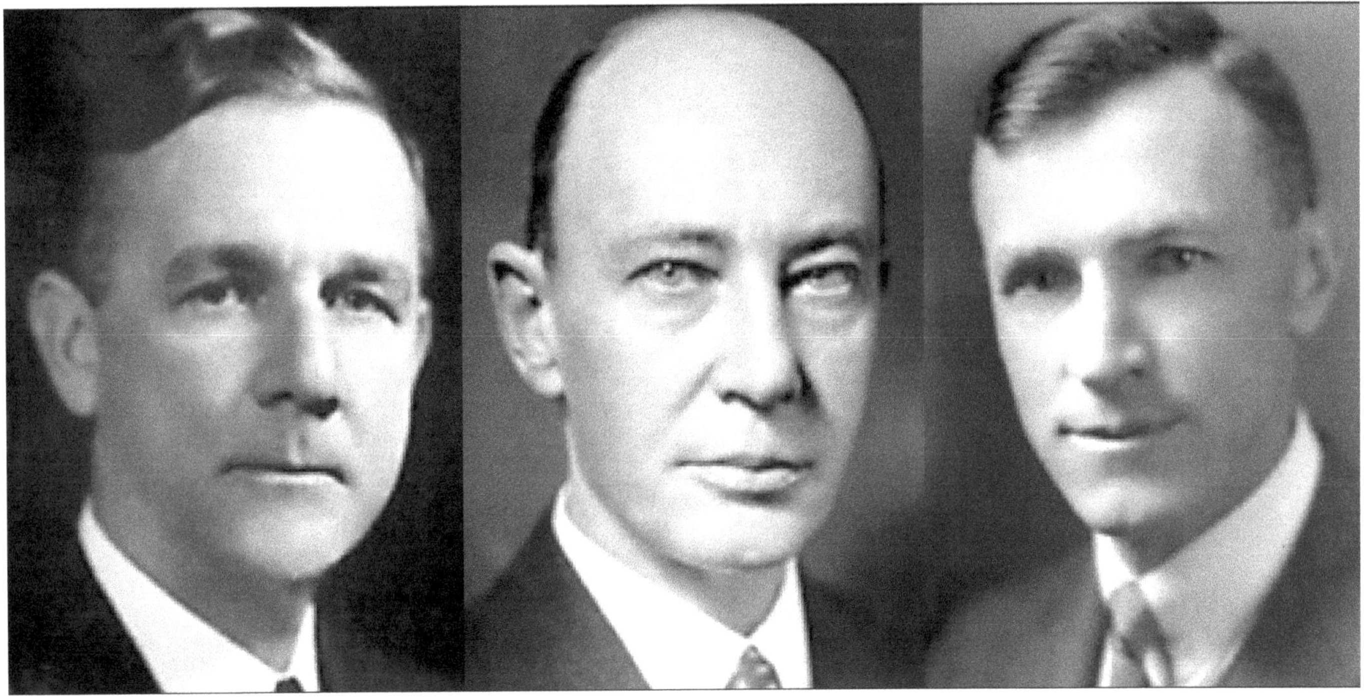

History

George Hoyt Whipple, born in 1878, was an American physician, pathologist, and biomedical researcher whose initial studies on the regeneration of blood and the effects of diet on blood production set the stage for liver therapy in anemia. His work demonstrated that ingesting liver led to rapid recovery in dogs with anemia from blood loss, suggesting a potential therapeutic approach for similar conditions in humans.

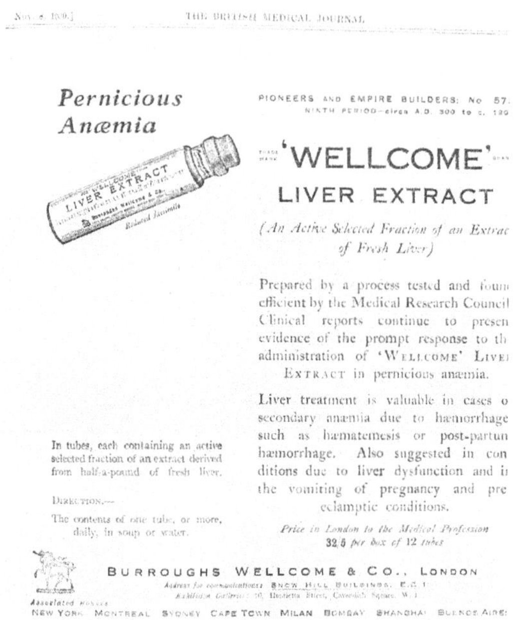

George Richards Minot, born in 1885, and William Parry Murphy, born in 1892, were also American physicians who made significant contributions to this research. Minot and Murphy collaborated on extending Whipple's findings, proving that a diet of liver could treat patients with pernicious anemia, a condition then considered fatal. Before their work, the nature and treatment of anemia were poorly understood, with few effective treatments available.

Their discovery was pivotal, illustrating the critical role of diet and specific nutrients in treating diseases. This work not only provided an effective treatment for pernicious anemia but also opened new avenues for research into nutritional deficiencies and their impact on health.

Snippets

Foundation of Liver Therapy: Whipple's experiments with dogs showed that feeding liver to anemic animals significantly improved their condition, leading to the hypothesis that liver could have therapeutic effects in human anemia.

Pivotal Publication: In 1926, Minot and Murphy published their landmark paper demonstrating the effectiveness of liver in treating pernicious anemia, fundamentally changing the management of the disease and saving countless lives.

Personal Triumph Over Adversity: Minot's personal battle with diabetes and the newly discovered insulin treatment not only saved his life but also allowed him to continue his research, contributing significantly to the discovery of the liver therapy for pernicious anemia.

Broadening Medical Understanding: Their work significantly advanced the understanding of anemia's nutritional basis, leading to the exploration of vitamins and other dietary treatments for various health conditions.

Early Researchers

Among these pivotal figures was William Castle, a physician whose work on the "intrinsic factor" concept was fundamental to understanding pernicious anemia. Castle's research proposed that the stomach secreted a substance necessary for vitamin B12 absorption, a theory that would later prove instrumental in comprehending the disease's pathophysiology. This intrinsic factor, coupled with the extrinsic factor found in liver therapy, outlined the complex nature of anemia treatment and its reliance on both dietary intake and physiological processes for the absorption of essential nutrients.

Another key figure was Frederick Banting, whose discovery of insulin not only revolutionized the treatment of diabetes but also indirectly influenced the work on pernicious anemia. Banting's breakthrough enabled George Minot to manage his own diabetes, thus allowing him to continue his research endeavors, including the critical studies on liver therapy.

Current Implications

Advances in Anemia Treatment: Today, the treatment of pernicious anemia has evolved from dietary liver therapy to more efficient methods, such as vitamin B12 injections or supplements. This shift was made possible by the foundational understanding that anemia could be treated through dietary intervention, a concept pioneered by Whipple, Minot, and Murphy.

Nutritional Science: Their work underscored the critical role of specific nutrients in health and disease management, catalyzing the field of nutritional science. Modern nutritional research continues to uncover how vitamins, minerals, and other dietary components affect various aspects of health, disease prevention, and treatment.

Holistic Approach to Medicine: The success of liver therapy highlighted the importance of considering dietary factors in medical treatment, encouraging a more holistic approach to patient care. This perspective is evident in contemporary practices that integrate nutrition and lifestyle modifications alongside conventional treatments for a wide range of conditions.

Research and Development: The trio's work has inspired ongoing research into the mechanisms by which nutrients and diets influence blood production and overall health. This includes exploring new treatments for various forms of anemia and other diseases with nutritional components.

Public Health and Policy: Understanding the link between diet and disease has informed public health initiatives and policy decisions aimed at preventing nutritional deficiencies in populations. Efforts to fortify foods with essential vitamins and minerals are direct outcomes of recognizing the impact of nutrition on diseases like anemia.

Impact and Products

Vitamin B12 Therapy: The foundational liver therapy has been replaced by direct vitamin B12 supplementation, most commonly through intramuscular injections. This method quickly replenishes the body's B12 stores, critical for the production of healthy red blood cells and neurological function.

Oral and Sublingual Supplements: For ongoing management, high-dose oral B12 supplements or sublingual forms (dissolving under the tongue) are available. These methods cater to individuals with less severe B12 absorption issues or for maintenance therapy after initial B12 levels have been restored.

Nasal Gel or Spray: B12 is also available in the form of a nasal gel or spray, providing an alternative route of administration for those who may not prefer injections or have difficulties with oral supplements.

Comprehensive Diagnosis Techniques: Diagnosis of pernicious anemia involves a combination of blood tests, including checks for B12 levels, the presence of antibodies to intrinsic factor (indicating an autoimmune response that inhibits B12 absorption), and a complete blood count to assess the impact on red blood cells.

Long-term Treatment Requirement: For many individuals with pernicious anemia, B12 supplementation becomes a lifelong necessity to manage the condition and prevent recurrence of symptoms. The specific treatment regimen may vary based on the severity of the deficiency and the patient's response to initial treatments.

HANS SPEMANN (1935)

A thought leader and a embryo researcher who made the organ transplantation a reality

Hans Spemann was awarded the Nobel Prize in Medicine in 1935 for his discovery of the organizer effect in embryonic development. This recognition was based on his pioneering work using micro-surgical techniques to manipulate amphibian embryos, leading to fundamental insights into how cells and tissues organize during the development of an organism.

History

Spemann, born on June 27, 1869, in Stuttgart, Germany, was deeply influenced by his work at the University of Würzburg under scientists like Theodor Boveri, Julius Sachs, and Wilhelm Röntgen.

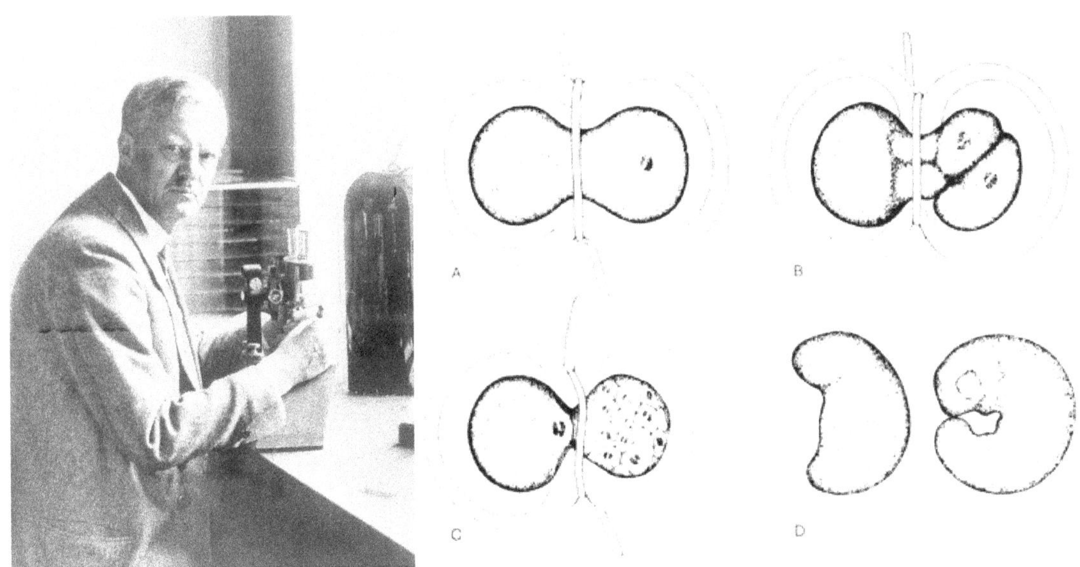

Speman's constriction experiments on single egg

His academic career commenced with studies in medicine at the University of Heidelberg, but it was his transfer to the University of Würzburg that truly marked the beginning of his scientific quest. At Würzburg, he was profoundly influenced by Theodor Boveri, Julius Sachs, and Wilhelm Röntgen, prominent scientists whose work would shape his future contributions to biology.

Spemann's groundbreaking research began in earnest while he was a professor at the University of Rostock, and later at the Kaiser Wilhelm Institute of Biology in Berlin-Dahlem. Here, through meticulous micro-surgical techniques, Spemann embarked on experiments that would redefine our understanding of embryonic development. By manipulating the cells of amphibian embryos, he demonstrated the organizer effect, where specific groups of cells, when transplanted to a host embryo, could dictate the developmental pathway of the host's cells, guiding the formation of various organs and tissues.

Snippets

Discovery of the Organizer: Spemann's groundbreaking experiment with Hilde Mangold demonstrated the "organizer" concept, where transplanted tissue induced the development of a secondary embryonic axis in host embryos, illustrating the directed development of embryonic cells.

Micro-surgical Techniques: Spemann's mastery of micro-surgical techniques, notably using a strand of baby hair as a noose to manipulate embryonic cells, showcased his innovative approach to experimental embryology and is considered foundational in the field of micro-surgery.

The Concept of Induction: His work elucidated the process of embryonic induction, where certain cells influence the developmental pathway of neighboring cells, laying the groundwork for understanding how complex organisms develop from a single fertilized egg.

Somatic Cell Nuclear Transfer Experiment: In 1928, Spemann performed the first somatic cell nuclear transfer using amphibian embryos, a pioneering step towards cloning, which highlighted the potential for cellular differentiation and reprogramming.

Early Influencers

Wilhelm Roux, a German embryologist who is often considered one of the founding fathers of experimental embryology. Roux's innovative use of microsurgical techniques to manipulate frog embryos established the methodological foundation upon which Spemann would later build. Roux's "mosaic theory" of development, though later revised, sparked considerable debate and research into how cells acquire their fates during development.

Another important contributor was August Weismann, whose germ plasm theory proposed that hereditary information is transmitted via a special substance, the germ plasm, contained only in the reproductive cells. This theory influenced Spemann's thinking about the cellular mechanisms underlying embryonic development.

Ethel Browne Harvey is yet another significant figure, known for her discovery that the unfertilized egg of the sea urchin can be triggered to develop into a larva without sperm, through chemical means. This finding hinted at the chemical cues that might guide embryonic development, a concept that resonates with Spemann's work on induction.

Current Implications

Stem Cell Research: Spemann's discovery of the organizer effect has significantly influenced stem cell research, guiding scientists in understanding how cells determine their fate and the potential for these cells to be manipulated for therapeutic purposes.

Regenerative Medicine: Insights from Spemann's work contribute to the field of regenerative medicine, particularly in developing strategies for tissue and organ regeneration, offering hope for repairing or replacing damaged parts of the human body.

Developmental Disorders: Understanding the organizer effect and the principles of embryonic induction helps in diagnosing and potentially treating developmental disorders, as many congenital abnormalities arise from disruptions in normal developmental processes.

Cancer Research: The study of how cells communicate and influence each other's development, a concept stemming from Spemann's organizer effect, is crucial in cancer research, helping to uncover how cancer cells evade normal growth controls and how they might be targeted for treatment.

Gene Therapy and CRISPR: Spemann's legacy informs the development of gene therapy techniques, including CRISPR-Cas9, by providing a deeper understanding of developmental biology and genetics, thus enabling precise edits to DNA to correct genetic defects.

Evolutionary Developmental Biology (Evo-Devo): The organizer concept has also impacted evolutionary developmental biology, a field that explores how the evolution of developmental processes contributes to the diversity of life, helping to elucidate the genetic and developmental mechanisms that drive evolution.

Biotechnological Applications: Knowledge of embryonic development and cell differentiation, inspired by Spemann's findings, is applied in biotechnology for creating artificial organs and tissues, which can be used for research, drug testing, and transplantation.

Impact and Products

Enhancement of Microsurgical Techniques: Spemann's pioneering use of microsurgery has been refined and expanded, leading to advanced microsurgical instruments and techniques. These advancements have broad applications, including intricate operations in ophthalmology, neurosurgery, and reconstructive surgery, thereby improving surgical outcomes and patient recovery.

Development of Cloning Technologies: Spemann's early experiments on somatic cell nuclear transfer laid the groundwork for cloning technologies. This has led to the development of therapeutic cloning and the production of genetically identical animals, contributing to medical research, conservation efforts, and agricultural practices.

Educational and Research Models: The organizer concept introduced by Spemann has become a fundamental model in developmental biology education and research. It has facilitated the development of various experimental models in amphibians and other organisms, enabling detailed studies of developmental processes and gene function.

Bioinformatics Tools for Developmental Biology: Insights from Spemann's work have fueled the creation of bioinformatics tools that model developmental processes. These tools help researchers understand the complex signaling pathways and genetic interactions that guide embryonic development, fostering discoveries in gene regulation and cellular differentiation.

Innovations in Regenerative Medicine: Understanding embryonic development and cell signaling pathways, influenced by Spemann's organizer effect, is crucial for regenerative medicine. This includes the engineering of tissues and organs from stem cells, offering potential treatments for diseases and injuries by harnessing the body's innate ability to heal and regenerate.

Pharmaceutical Development for Developmental Disorders: Spemann's research has also informed the development of pharmaceuticals targeting developmental disorders. By understanding the molecular basis of these conditions, new drugs and therapies are being designed to correct or mitigate the effects of developmental anomalies at the molecular level.

HENRY DALE AND OTTO LOEWI (1936)

Their work on the biochemical basis of Neurotransmission is monumental

Henry Dale and Otto Loewi were awarded the Nobel Prize in Medicine in 1936 for their discoveries relating to the chemical transmission of nerve impulses. Their groundbreaking work established the foundation of neurochemistry and significantly advanced our understanding of how neurons communicate.

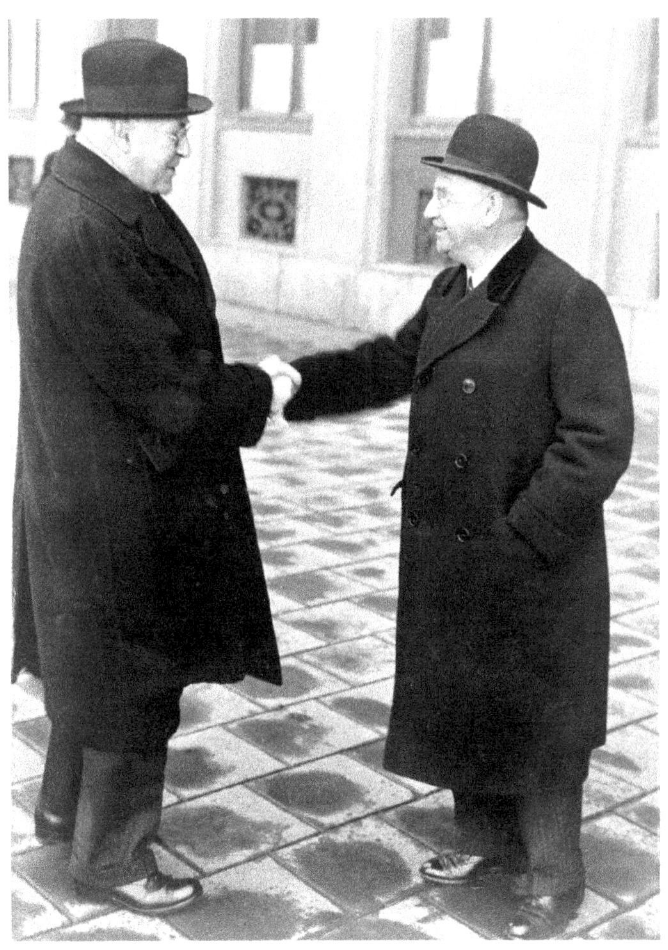

History

Henry Hallett Dale began his journey in London, where he was born in 1875. After attending Leys School in Cambridge and Trinity College, where he specialized in physiology and zoology, Dale's path led him through various prestigious research positions. His work under notable scientists like J.N. Langley and Ernest Starling significantly influenced his scientific outlook. It was at University College London where Dale met his lifelong friend Otto Loewi, marking the beginning of a collaboration that would eventually contribute to their joint Nobel Prize. Dale's tenure at the Wellcome Physiological Research Laboratories and later at the National Institute for Medical Research in London saw his investigation into the pharmacology of ergot alkaloids and the physiological actions of various biologically active substances, including acetylcholine, a key neurotransmitter in the nervous system.

The diagram below shows a classic experiment by Sir Henry Dale, a Nobel prize-winning British pharmacologist. It shows changes in blood pressure in an anaesthetized cat following intravenous injections of acetylcholine and atropine at various doses.

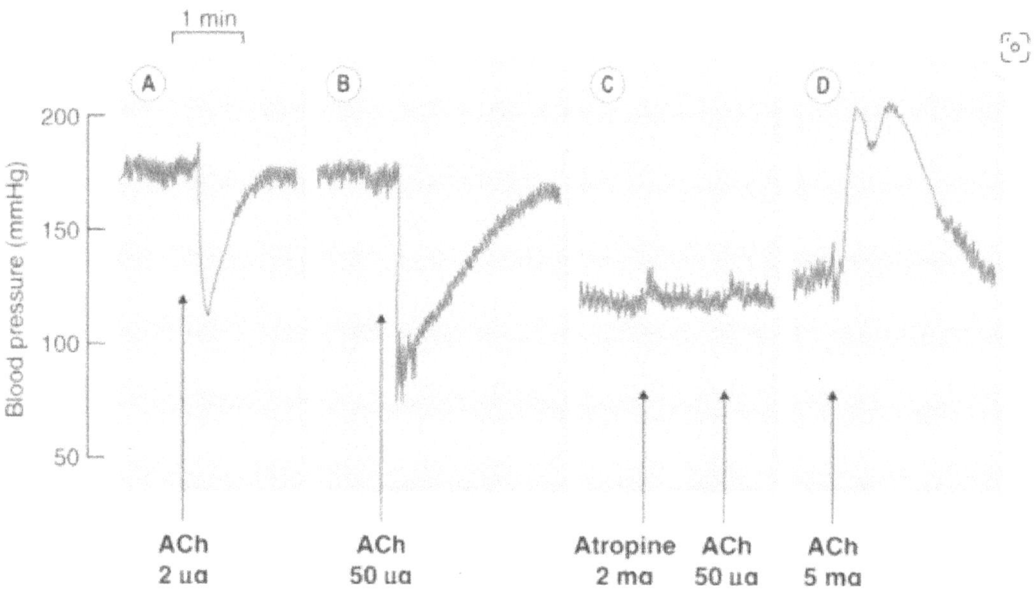

Otto Loewi's story, on the other hand, traces back to Frankfurt, Germany, where he was born in 1873. His initial intention to pursue a clinical career shifted dramatically after witnessing the limitations of medical treatments for diseases like tuberculosis and pneumonia. This realization steered him towards research in basic medical science, particularly pharmacology. Loewi's career blossomed under the mentorship of Hans Horst Meyer, first at the University of Marburg and then in Vienna. His research spanned metabolism, the vegetative nervous system, and notably, the mechanisms of neurotransmission. Loewi's famous experiment in 1921, which demonstrated the chemical basis of nerve impulse transmission through his work with frog hearts, firmly established him as a pioneer in neurochemistry.

Snippets

Dale's Acetylcholine Research: Identified acetylcholine as a neurotransmitter in 1914, establishing its central role in neurotransmission and the nervous system's function.

Loewi's Chemical Neurotransmission Discovery: Demonstrated neurotransmission via chemical messengers through his iconic frog heart experiment in 1921, identifying acetylcholine as the first neurotransmitter.

Collaborative Foundations: Although working independently, Dale and Loewi's discoveries were deeply interconnected, illustrating the complementary nature of scientific research across disciplines and geographies.

Controversy and Confirmation: Engaged in scientific debate over synaptic signaling being chemical vs. electrical. Dale and others' stance on chemical signaling was eventually confirmed, shaping our understanding of synaptic function.

Neurotransmitter Classification: Dale originated the scheme to classify neurons based on their neurotransmitters, a method that significantly advanced the study of neural networks and brain function.

Early Researchers

Paul Ehrlich stands out for his contributions to immunology and his innovative work in staining techniques, which allowed for the visualization of neural circuits and laid the groundwork for understanding neural communication. His concept of the "magic bullet" for targeting specific pathogens without harming the host organism hints at the specificity that would later be discovered in neurotransmitter action.

Another significant figure is John Newport Langley, whose concept of the autonomic nervous system and the idea of "receptive substances" provided a theoretical framework that would later support the idea of chemical neurotransmission. Langley's work, although not directly related to neurotransmitters, paved the way for the understanding of how chemicals could affect neural activity.

Sir Charles Sherrington's studies on reflex arcs and synaptic transmission also deserve mention. His work on the integrative action of the nervous system introduced the concept of synapses as the junctions between neurons, even though he believed synaptic transmission was purely electrical.

Current Implications

Neurological and Psychiatric Disorder Treatment: Understanding chemical neurotransmission has directly influenced the development of treatments for neurological and psychiatric disorders. Medications that modulate neurotransmitter levels, such as antidepressants, antipsychotics, and anxiolytics, are now fundamental in managing conditions like depression, schizophrenia, and anxiety disorders.

Pharmacological Research and Development: The identification of neurotransmitters and their receptors has been crucial in pharmacology, enabling the development of drugs that specifically target these molecules to treat a wide range of diseases, from pain management to neurodegenerative disorders like Parkinson's and Alzheimer's diseases.

Neuroscience Research: Dale and Loewi's work laid the foundation for the field of neuroscience, particularly in understanding how neurons communicate and process information. This has implications for research into brain function, cognition, and memory, contributing to advances in artificial intelligence and neural networks by providing biological insights into information processing.

Addiction and Substance Abuse: Insights into neurotransmission have informed approaches to treating addiction and substance abuse. Understanding how drugs of abuse alter neurotransmitter levels has led to better strategies for intervention and rehabilitation, focusing on restoring the balance in brain chemistry.

Pain Management: The study of neurotransmitters involved in pain perception has led to the development of new analgesics that target specific pathways in the nervous system, offering more effective and targeted pain relief options for chronic pain conditions.

Impact and Products

Antidepressants and Antipsychotics: These medications, which adjust the levels of neurotransmitters in the brain, have improved the quality of life for millions of people worldwide. Selective serotonin reuptake inhibitors (SSRIs), for example, specifically target serotonin systems to treat depression and anxiety disorders.

Treatments for Parkinson's Disease: Medications like Levodopa work by increasing dopamine levels in the brain, counteracting the dopamine deficiency that characterizes Parkinson's disease. This approach was made possible by an understanding of neurotransmitter roles and functions.

Alzheimer's Disease Medications: Drugs such as donepezil and rivastigmine are designed to increase acetylcholine concentrations in the brain, aiming to offset the loss of cholinergic neurons seen in Alzheimer's disease. These treatments are rooted in the foundational knowledge of neurotransmitter roles in memory and cognition.

Analgesics: The development of targeted analgesics, such as those acting on the endocannabinoid system or specific neurotransmitter receptors involved in pain transmission, offers more effective pain management options with fewer side effects.

Nicotine Replacement Therapies (NRTs): Understanding the role of acetylcholine in addiction has led to the development of NRTs, helping individuals overcome nicotine dependency by mimicking the neurotransmitter's effects to reduce withdrawal symptoms.

Migraine Treatments: Triptans, used to alleviate migraine symptoms, function by stimulating serotonin receptors to reduce inflammation and constrict blood vessels, demonstrating the application of neurotransmitter research in treating vascular headaches.

Their impact endures in scientific history and drives the ongoing advancements in new drugs and treatments that benefit society.

ALBERT SZENT-GYÖRGYI (1937)

The man who discovered the Vitamin C amidst the ravages of the world war

In 1937, Albert Szent-Györgyi was awarded the Nobel Prize in Medicine for his seminal discoveries in biological combustion processes, particularly emphasizing the role of vitamin C and the catalysis of fumaric acid.

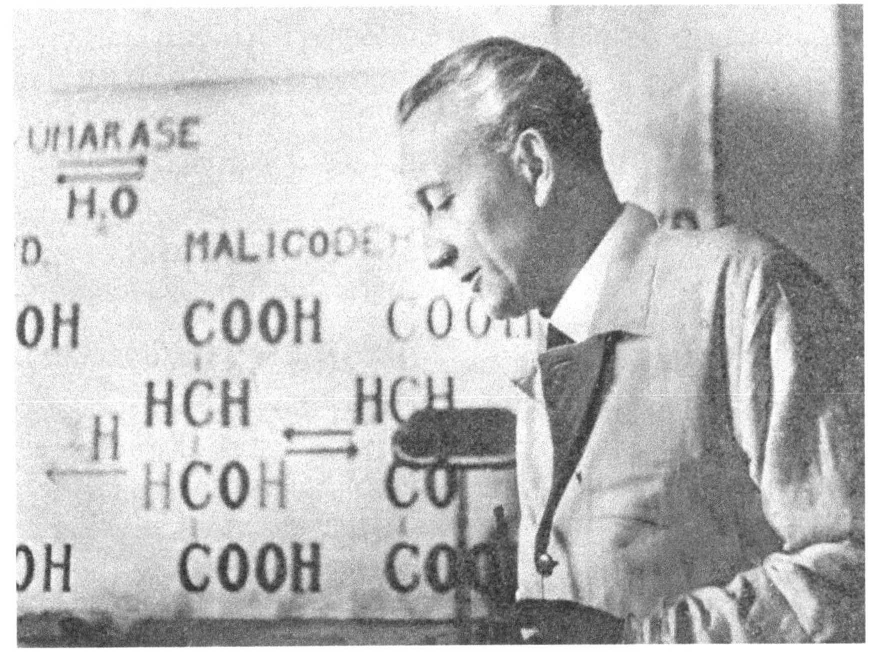

History

Albert Szent-Györgyi was born on September 16, 1893, in Budapest, then part of the Austro-Hungarian Empire. He hailed from a family with a rich scientific heritage, which undoubtedly influenced his future pursuits. Despite the interruption of his studies due to World War I, Szent-Györgyi earned his medical degree in 1917. His early academic career took him across Europe, contributing to his diverse scientific background.

Snippets

Szent-Györgyi's groundbreaking work in the early 20th century led to the isolation of vitamin C, initially termed "hexuronic acid." His research illuminated the vital role of vitamin C in preventing scurvy, a discovery that stemmed from centuries of observation regarding the disease's prevention through citrus fruits but without a scientific explanation until Szent-Györgyi's experiments. This work laid the groundwork for understanding the biological effects of vitamins and their role in human health.

Current Implications

Today, Szent-Györgyi's research on vitamin C continues to influence nutrition science, medicine, and our understanding of antioxidants. His studies on cellular respiration also contributed to the foundation of biochemistry, impacting how we understand energy transfer within cells.

Impact and Products

Albert Szent-Györgyi's contributions extend far beyond his discovery of vitamin C, marking significant advancements in our understanding of biological processes. His work on muscle contraction led to identifying actin and myosin, proteins essential for this mechanism.

His work significantly advanced our understanding of cellular metabolism and the biochemical basis of vitamin C's importance in health and disease prevention.

CORNEILLE HEYMANS (1938)

Discovery of secret bio-chemical sensors in the aortic arch that modulated respiration

In 1938, Corneille Heymans, a distinguished Belgian physiologist, was honored with the Nobel Prize in Medicine for unveiling the mechanisms by which respiration is regulated through the sinus and aortic mechanisms.

History

Corneille Heymans was born on March 28, 1892, in Ghent, Belgium. Immersed in an environment of scientific inquiry from a young age, he pursued medical studies at the University of Ghent. His education, briefly interrupted by his service in World War I, culminated in a medical degree in 1920.

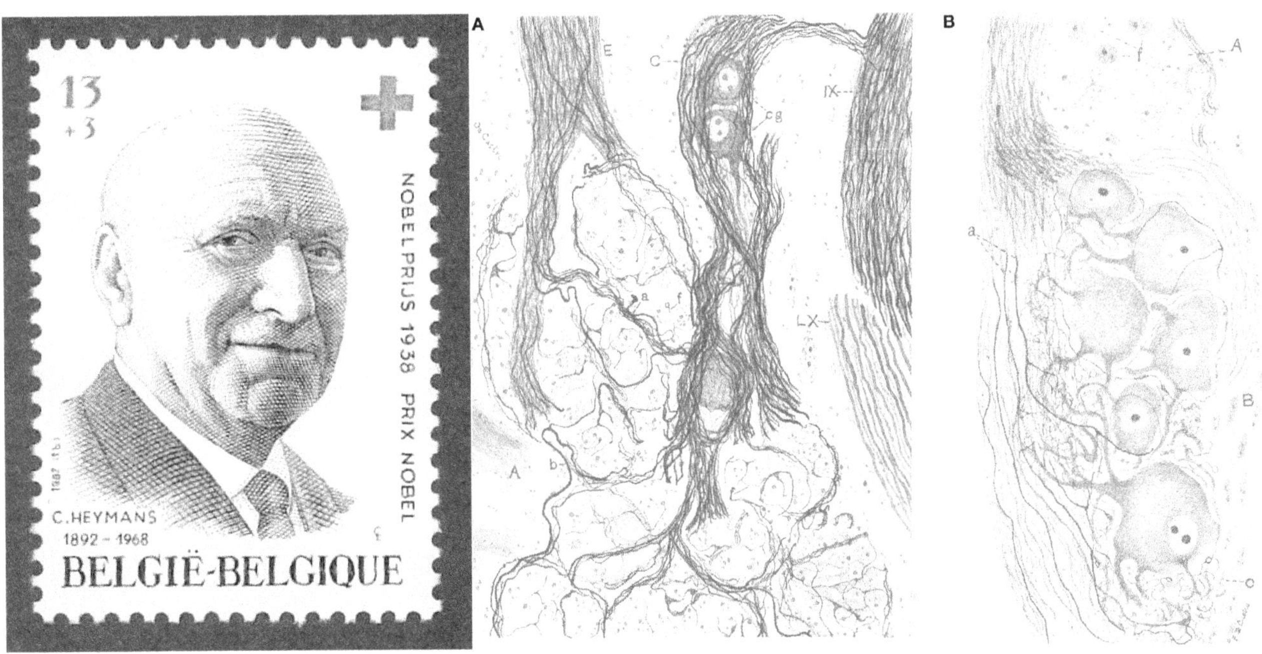

Heymans histological study on carotid and aortic bodies

Heymans' post-war years were spent enriching his scientific expertise across Europe and the USA, collaborating with eminent scientists of his era. In 1922, he embarked on his lifelong academic and research career at the University of Ghent, succeeding his father, Jean François Heymans, as Professor of Pharmacology in 1930 and continuing the family's pioneering research in respiratory and circulatory physiology.

Snippets

Heymans' groundbreaking research focused on understanding how the body's respiratory rate is influenced by chemical stimuli detected by receptors in the carotid body and sinus. His meticulous experiments, primarily conducted on animals, demonstrated the crucial role these receptors play in monitoring and adjusting the respiratory process based on the blood's oxygen and carbon dioxide levels.

Current Implications

Today, Heymans' discoveries remain foundational in medical and physiological education, influencing how respiratory and cardiovascular systems are understood and treated. His work on chemoreceptors continues to inform clinical approaches to managing conditions like sleep apnea, hypertension, and heart failure, underscoring the enduring relevance of his research.

Impact and Products

Heymans' legacy is immortalized in over 800 scientific publications and numerous awards, reflecting his broad impact on medical science. His leadership at the J.F. Heymans Institute of Pharmacodynamics and Therapeutics facilitated a vibrant research environment that attracted international scholars and furthered studies in various pharmacological and physiological disciplines.

His work not only advanced the fundamental understanding of respiratory regulation but also laid the groundwork for future research in cardiovascular physiology.

GERHARD DOMAGK (1939)

The German who scripted the success story of first antibiotic Prontosil in human domain

In 1939, Gerhard Domagk, a German bacteriologist and pathologist, received the Nobel Prize in Medicine for his discovery of the antibacterial effects of Prontosil, marking a monumental advancement in medical science by introducing the first commercially available antibiotic.

History

Born on October 30, 1895, in Lagow, Brandenburg, Germany (now Poland), Domagk's journey into medicine was shaped by his experiences in World War I, where he served as a medic. Witnessing firsthand the devastation caused by bacterial infections on the battlefield, Domagk was determined to find a solution to combat these deadly microorganisms.

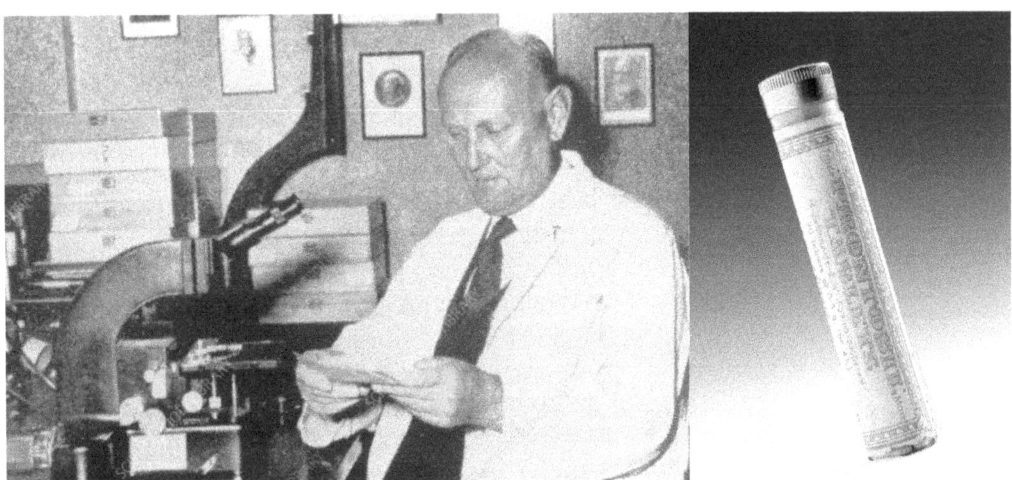

After the war, he pursued his medical studies, eventually joining the German chemical company IG Farben. Here, he led a team that discovered Prontosil, the first of the sulfonamide drugs, which proved effective against a wide range of bacterial infections.

Snippets

Domagk's research at IG Farben was focused on testing chemical compounds for their antimicrobial properties. Among these, Prontosil stood out for its effectiveness against streptococcal infections in mice and later in humans, including Domagk's own daughter, who was successfully treated for a severe infection with the drug. This breakthrough opened the door to the development of sulfa drugs, laying the groundwork for modern antibiotics.

Current Implications

Domagk's work on Prontosil and the subsequent development of sulfa drugs revolutionized the treatment of bacterial infections, significantly reducing the mortality rate from such diseases before the advent of penicillin and other antibiotics. Although the focus in antibiotic therapy has shifted over the years, the discovery of Prontosil remains a landmark event in the history of medicine, illustrating the potential of chemical compounds in combating infectious diseases.

Impact and Products

Domagk's legacy includes his contributions to the field of chemotherapy and his later research efforts aimed at finding treatments for tuberculosis, contributing to the discovery of isoniazid, one of the most effective drugs against the disease. His pioneering work has not only saved countless lives but also paved the way for future generations of scientists to explore the therapeutic potential of synthetic drugs.

Domagk's story is a testament to the power of scientific inquiry and perseverance in the face of adversity, illustrating how dedicated research can lead to breakthroughs that changed the course of medical history.

HENRIK DAM AND EDWARD DOISY (1943)

*The transatlantic discovery of Vitamin K which led to the development of
oral anticoagulants*

Henrik Dam, from Denmark, and Edward Doisy, from the United States, were jointly awarded the Nobel Prize in Medicine in 1943. Their research into vitamin K and its role in blood coagulation significantly advanced our understanding of hematology and nutrition.

History

Henrik Dam, born on February 21, 1895, in Copenhagen, Denmark, embarked on a career that would fundamentally change our understanding of nutrition and its relationship to health. He graduated from the University of Copenhagen, where he initially studied biochemistry, his academic pursuits laying the groundwork for his later groundbreaking discoveries in the field of vitamins.

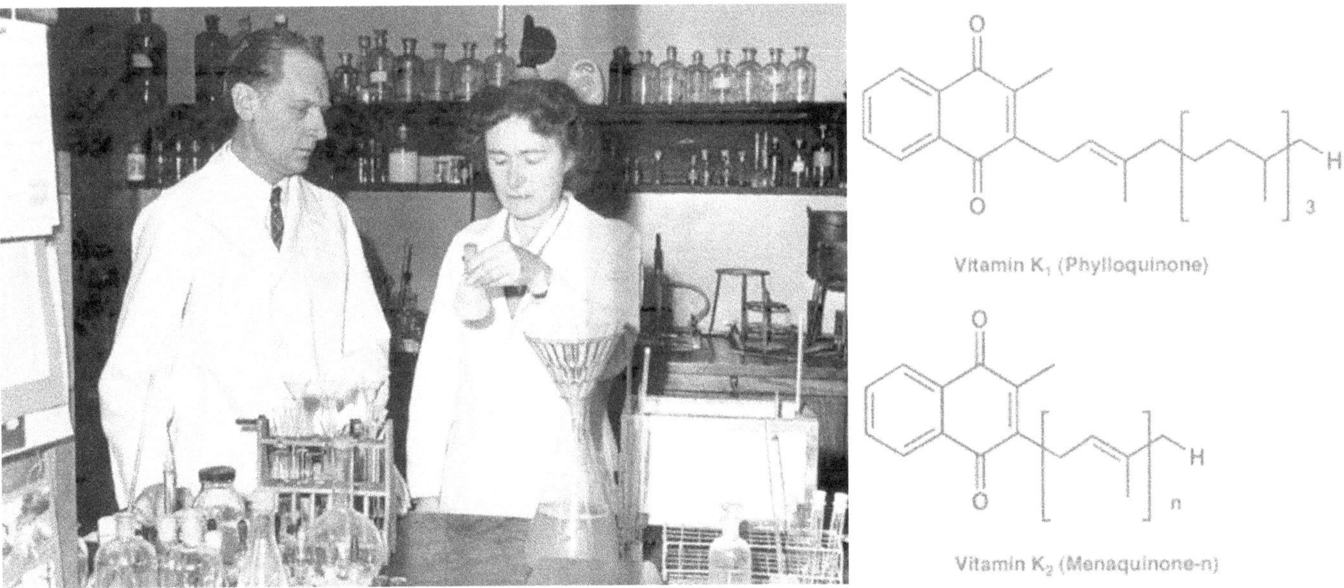

Edward Adelbert Doisy, on the other hand, was born on November 13, 1893, in Hume, Illinois, USA. He pursued his higher education at Harvard University, where he developed a keen interest in biochemistry and medical research. This educational background set the stage for his future achievements in isolating and understanding the chemical nature of vitamin K, for which he would share the Nobel Prize with Dam.

Dam's research into cholesterol metabolism and the effects of diet on health led him to the discovery of an essential factor in blood coagulation, which he named vitamin K for "Koagulation," the Danish word for coagulation. This discovery was pivotal, identifying a direct link between diet and the prevention of bleeding diseases.

Doisy's work complemented Dam's discovery by elucidating the chemical structure of vitamin K, making it possible to synthesize the vitamin and further explore its therapeutic potential. His efforts in isolating and characterizing vitamin K marked a significant milestone in the fields of biochemistry and medicine, directly impacting the treatment and prevention of coagulation disorders.

Early Influencers

Paul Ehrlich, a German scientist known for his work in immunology and chemotherapy, who laid the foundational principles for staining tissues and cells, enabling future scientists to visualize and understand cellular components and reactions better.

Albert Szent-Györgyi, who discovered vitamin C, is another unsung hero in the vitamin research field. His work on vitamins and their role in cellular functions paved the way for further research into essential nutrients, including vitamin K.

Finally, the work of scientists like Fritz Pregl and Richard Kuhn, who made significant contributions to the analytical and synthetic chemistry of vitamins, respectively, provided the tools and knowledge necessary for the isolation and structural elucidation of vitamin K by Dam and Doisy.

Current Implications

Prevention and Treatment of Hemorrhagic Disease in Newborns: Vitamin K is now routinely administered to newborns to prevent hemorrhagic disease, a potentially life-threatening condition. This practice underscores the critical role of vitamin K in blood clotting and newborn care.

Management of Coagulation Disorders: Knowledge of vitamin K's role in coagulation has improved the treatment of patients with certain blood clotting disorders. It has also informed the use of anticoagulants like warfarin, which work by inhibiting vitamin K-dependent clotting factors, in conditions such as atrial fibrillation and deep vein thrombosis.

Surgical and Medical Procedures: Understanding the mechanisms of vitamin K has led to better management of bleeding risks associated with surgical and medical procedures. Patients on anticoagulation therapy may require careful adjustment of their medication and monitoring of vitamin K intake to maintain optimal coagulation status.

Nutritional Supplementation and Diet: The importance of vitamin K extends into dietary recommendations and nutritional supplementation, especially in populations at risk of deficiency, such as individuals with certain digestive disorders that affect nutrient absorption.

Bone Health: Beyond coagulation, research has uncovered a role for vitamin K in bone metabolism, suggesting that adequate vitamin K intake is important for bone health and may help prevent osteoporosis. This has implications for dietary guidelines and supplements targeting bone health.

Cardiovascular Health: Emerging research indicates that vitamin K may play a role in cardiovascular health by preventing arterial calcification. While this area of research is still developing, it highlights the potential broader health implications of vitamin K beyond coagulation.

Impacts and Products

Vitamin K Supplements: One of the direct products stemming from their discovery is the range of vitamin K supplements available on the market. These supplements are crucial for individuals who are at risk of vitamin K deficiency due to dietary restrictions or absorption issues.

Neonatal Care Products: Vitamin K injections for newborns are a standard practice worldwide to prevent vitamin K deficiency bleeding (VKDB), a serious condition that can lead to brain damage or death. This preventive measure is a direct application of Dam and Doisy's research.

Anticoagulation Therapy: The understanding of vitamin K's role in blood coagulation has been instrumental in the development of anticoagulant drugs such as warfarin. Warfarin works by inhibiting the vitamin K cycle, a mechanism directly linked to the clotting process discovered by Dam and Doisy. These medications are vital for patients with an elevated risk of forming blood clots.

Osteoporosis Treatments: Emerging evidence of vitamin K's role in bone health has led to the formulation of combined calcium and vitamin K supplements aimed at improving bone density and reducing fracture risk, especially among the elderly.

Topical Creams and Serums: Vitamin K is also used in a variety of dermatological products, including creams and serums designed to reduce bruising, improve skin healing, and diminish the appearance of spider veins and dark circles under the eyes.

Dietary Guidelines and Fortified Foods: The discovery has influenced dietary guidelines, advocating for the inclusion of vitamin K-rich foods such as leafy greens, broccoli, and Brussels sprouts. Additionally, some food products are fortified with vitamin K to enhance their nutritional value.

Research and Diagnostic Kits: The understanding of vitamin K's mechanism has spurred the development of research tools and diagnostic kits for studying coagulation disorders and monitoring anticoagulation therapy effectiveness, contributing to advanced research and patient care in hematology.

JOSEPH ERLANGER AND HERBERT GASSER (1944)

Unraveled path breaking facts in both Neural anatomy and physiology

Joseph Erlanger and Herbert Spencer Gasser were awarded the Nobel Prize in Medicine in 1944 for their pioneering discoveries concerning the highly differentiated functions of single nerve fibers. Their work provided fundamental insights into the electrical signals of nerve fibers, marking a significant advancement in neurophysiology.

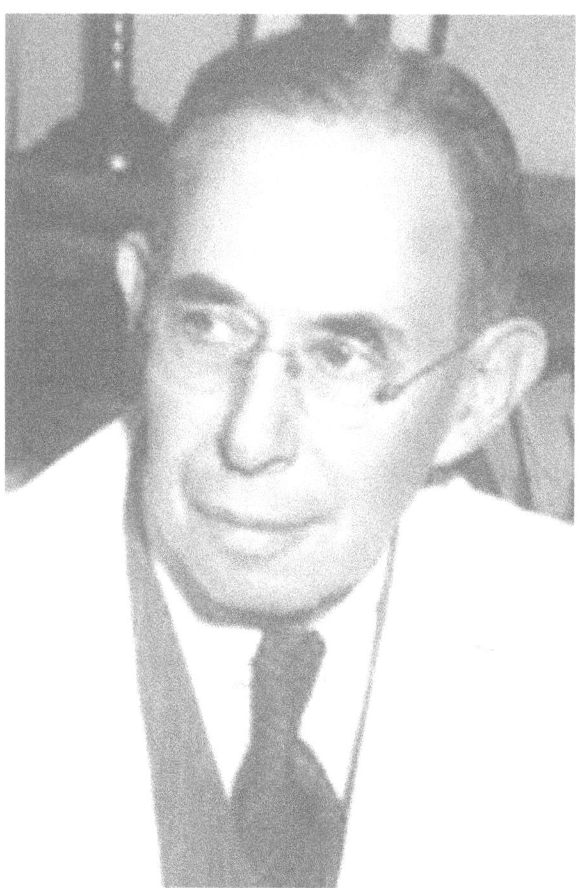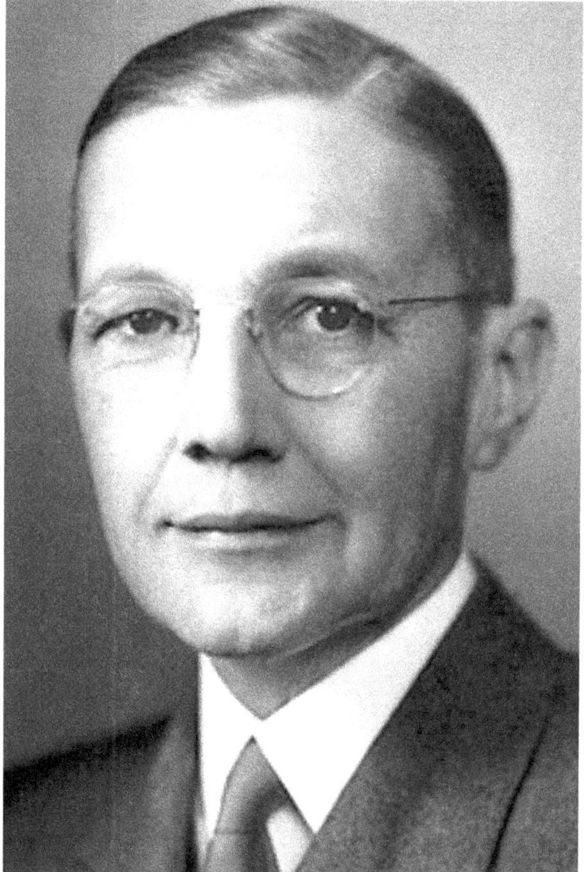

History

Joseph Erlanger was born on January 5, 1874, in San Francisco, California. He pursued his undergraduate studies in chemistry at the University of California, Berkeley, and later attended Johns Hopkins University School of Medicine, where he earned his medical degree. Erlanger's academic and professional career was distinguished by his contributions to understanding the cardiovascular system and electrophysiology.

Herbert Spencer Gasser, born on July 5, 1888, in Platteville, Wisconsin, followed a similar path of academic excellence. He graduated from the University of Wisconsin, where he initially embarked on his journey into physiology. Gasser's work eventually led him to collaborate with Erlanger, marking the beginning of a partnership that would significantly impact neurophysiology. After completing his Ph.D., Gasser joined Erlanger at Washington University in St. Louis, where their groundbreaking experiments on nerve function took place.

Together, Erlanger and Gasser embarked on a series of experiments that would unveil the complexities of nerve fiber functionality. By modifying a Western Electric oscilloscope, they made it possible to observe the electrical signals of nerve fibers in unprecedented detail. Their research demonstrated that nerve fibers exhibited differentiated functions, a discovery that challenged existing notions about nerve signals and laid the groundwork for modern neurophysiology.

Snippets

Innovative Techniques: They modified a Western Electric oscilloscope for low-voltage operations, enabling the detailed observation of action potentials in nerve fibers—a major breakthrough in measuring neural activity.

Discovery of Nerve Fiber Functions: Their research demonstrated that neurons exhibited varied forms and functions, with the velocity of action potentials being directly proportional to the diameter of the nerve fiber. This insight was crucial in understanding the complexity of neural communication.

Educational and Professional Backgrounds: Erlanger pursued chemistry and medicine at the University of California and Johns Hopkins University, while Gasser completed his Ph.D. at the University of Wisconsin before their paths converged at Washington University in St. Louis.

Early Researchers

Sir Charles Scott Sherrington is another key figure whose concept of the synapse and work on reflex arcs greatly influenced the understanding of how neurons communicate. His studies on the integration of sensory and motor responses laid the groundwork for exploring neural function at a physiological level.

Another notable pioneer is Edgar Adrian, who, along with Sherrington, was awarded the Nobel Prize in Medicine in 1932 for their work on the functions of neurons. Adrian's efforts in quantifying neural activity and his discovery of the all-or-nothing principle of nerve conduction were pivotal advancements that set the stage for Erlanger and Gasser's later work.

Additionally, scientists like Julius Bernstein, who proposed the membrane theory of electrical potentials in neurons, and Luigi Galvani and Emil du Bois-Reymond, who conducted early experiments on bioelectricity, were instrumental in developing the theoretical and experimental framework necessary for understanding nerve impulses.

Current Implications

Neurological Diagnostics: The understanding of action potentials and nerve function differentiation is fundamental in modern neurological diagnostics. Techniques such as electromyography (EMG) and nerve conduction studies, which assess the health of muscles and the nerve cells that control them, are directly built upon Erlanger and Gasser's findings. These diagnostic tools are essential for identifying diseases of the nerve and muscle.

Treatment of Neurological Disorders: Insights into nerve fiber functionality have informed therapeutic strategies for a range of neurological disorders. For example, understanding the properties of different nerve fibers aids in the development of more effective treatments for neuropathic pain, a condition resulting from nerve damage.

Development of Anesthetics: The differentiation of nerve fibers has implications for the development and application of local anesthetics. By targeting specific nerve fibers, anesthetics can be more effectively used to block pain without affecting other types of nerve function, such as motor control.

Neurosurgical Techniques: Knowledge of the varied functions of nerve fibers has refined neurosurgical techniques, allowing surgeons to better preserve nerve function during operations. This is particularly crucial in surgeries involving the brain and spinal cord, where precise understanding of nerve fiber functions can minimize damage and improve outcomes.

Brain-Machine Interfaces: The principles discovered by Erlanger and Gasser also underpin the development of brain-machine interfaces (BMIs), which rely on decoding neural signals for controlling prosthetic limbs or restoring sensory feedback. Understanding how different nerve fibers transmit information is key to creating more effective and naturalistic BMIs.

Research on Neuroplasticity: Their work laid the groundwork for studies on neuroplasticity, the brain's ability to reorganize itself by forming new neural connections. This research is vital for developing rehabilitation methods for stroke and injury recovery, showing how flexible and adaptable the nervous system can be in response to damage.

Impact And Products

Advanced Neurodiagnostic Devices: Building on the principles uncovered by Erlanger and Gasser, there has been the development of sophisticated neurodiagnostic devices. These include high-resolution oscilloscopes and advanced EEG machines capable of detecting and analyzing the intricate activities of different nerve fibers within the nervous system.

Precision Neurotherapeutics: Their research has led to the creation of targeted therapeutic interventions, such as selective nerve blocks and precision medicine approaches for treating neuropathic pain. By understanding the specific functions of different nerve fibers, treatments can be tailored to more effectively target pathological processes without affecting healthy nerve function.

Enhanced Surgical Equipment: Innovations in neurosurgical tools and techniques, including nerve monitoring systems used during surgery, owe much to the foundational knowledge of nerve function differentiation. These tools help surgeons to avoid damaging critical nerve pathways, thereby improving surgical outcomes and patient recovery times.

Educational Models and Simulations: The detailed study of nerve impulses and their differentiation has also been translated into educational models and software simulations. These tools are used in medical and biological education to teach students about neural physiology, enhancing their understanding through interactive learning experiences.

Pharmaceutical Development: Erlanger and Gasser's discoveries have informed the pharmaceutical industry, particularly in the development of drugs that modulate nerve activity. New classes of medications that specifically target certain types of nerve fibers for the treatment of epilepsy, anxiety, and other conditions have been developed based on an understanding of nerve fiber functions.

Rehabilitation Technologies: The differentiation of nerve fibers has influenced the design of rehabilitation technologies, including electrical stimulation devices for recovery after nerve injury. These devices aim to selectively stimulate specific nerve fibers to promote healing and restore function, leveraging insights into the varied roles of different types of nerve fibers.

ALEXANDER FLEMING, ERNST CHAIN, HOWARD FLOREY (1945)

The three stellar stars presented the Godly gift of Penicillin to mankind

Alexander Fleming, Ernst Boris Chain, and Howard Florey were jointly awarded the Nobel Prize in Medicine in 1945 for their discovery of penicillin and its development into a life-saving antibiotic. This groundbreaking work ushered in the era of antibiotics, revolutionizing the treatment of bacterial infections.

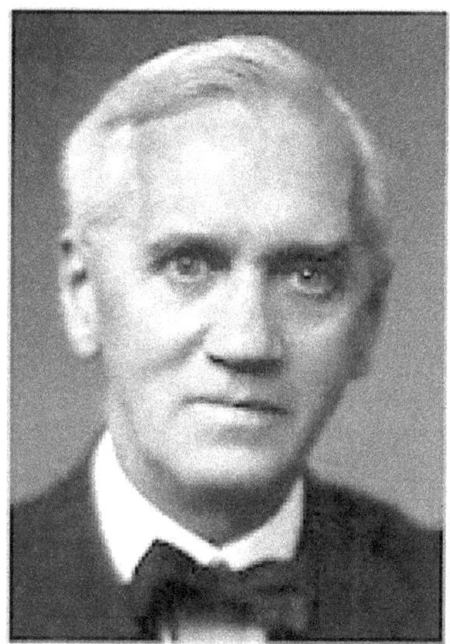

Sir Alexander Fleming
(1881-1955)

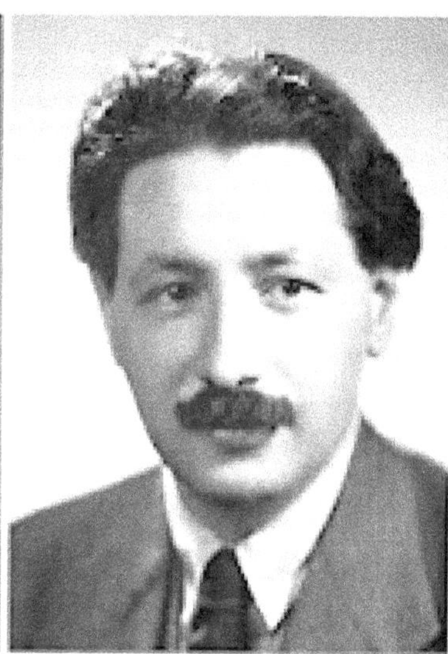

Ernst Boris Chain
(1906-1979)

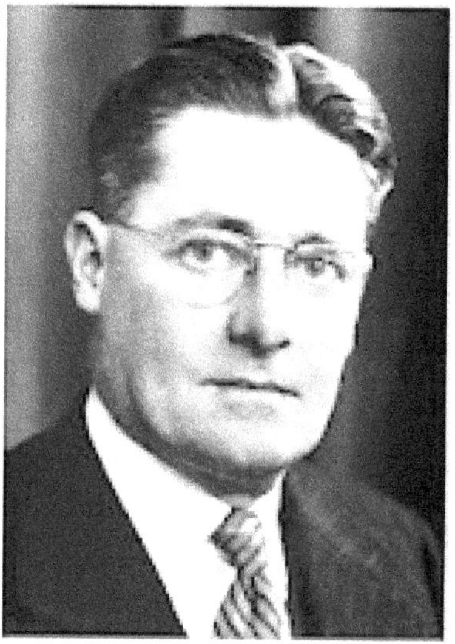

Sir Howard Walter Florey
(1898-1968)

History

Alexander Fleming was born on August 6, 1881, in Ayrshire, Scotland. Initially planning to become a surgeon, Fleming's direction changed after inheriting some money, leading him to study medicine at St. Mary's Hospital Medical School, London, where he later embarked on a career in research. Fleming's accidental discovery of penicillin in 1928 occurred when a mold contaminated a petri dish in his laboratory, inhibiting bacterial growth.

Ernst Boris Chain was born on June 19, 1906, in Berlin, Germany. He fled Nazi Germany due to his Jewish heritage, eventually joining the University of Oxford. There, alongside Howard Florey, Chain was instrumental in isolating and purifying penicillin, making it viable for clinical use.

Howard Florey, born on September 24, 1898, in Adelaide, Australia, was a pathologist whose work at Oxford University with Chain led to the first clinical trials of penicillin. Their successful development of penicillin as a drug represented a monumental achievement in medical history.

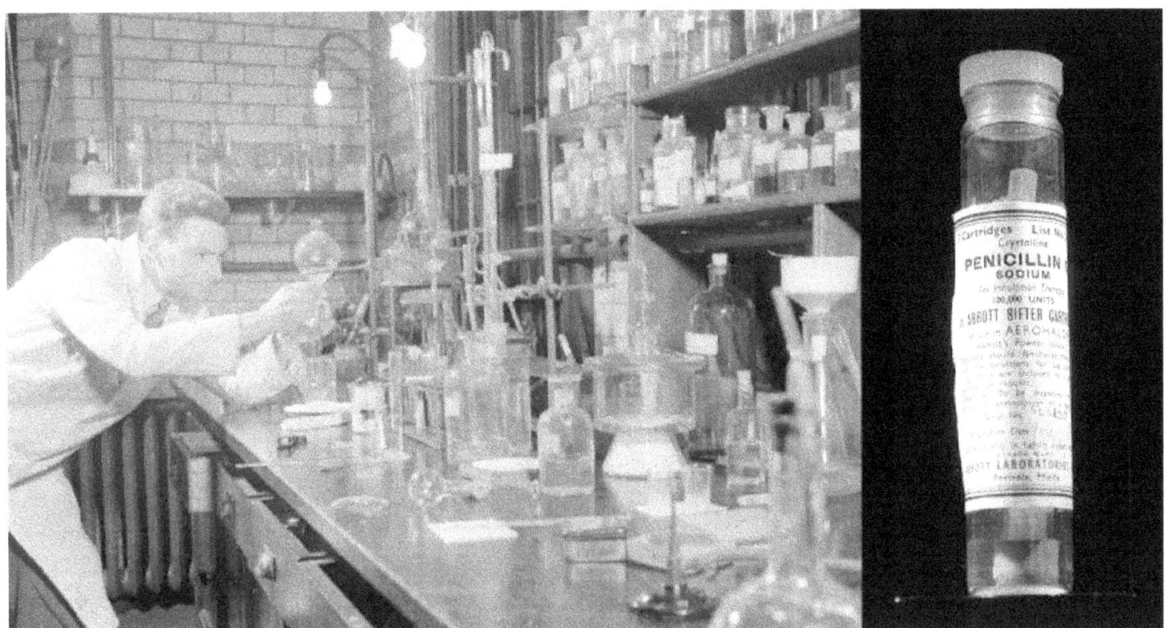

Snippets

Penicillin's Accidental Discovery: Alexander Fleming noticed a mold (Penicillium notatum) that killed bacteria in his Staphylococcus culture plates, marking the first step toward the antibiotic revolution.

Penicillin Purification and Clinical Use: Ernst Boris Chain and Howard Florey successfully isolated and purified penicillin, transforming it into a viable therapeutic agent used extensively during World War II to treat wounded soldiers.

Global Impact on Medicine: Their work not only ushered in the age of antibiotics, dramatically reducing deaths from bacterial infections but also set the stage for the development of other antibiotics, fundamentally changing medical practices.

Continued Relevance: The discovery of penicillin remains one of the most significant achievements in medical history, highlighting the importance of research, observation, and interdisciplinary collaboration in advancing healthcare.

Early Researchers

Selman Waksman is another notable contributor whose work led to the discovery of streptomycin, the first antibiotic effective against tuberculosis. Waksman's efforts in soil microbiology and the identification of antibiotics further expanded the arsenal of drugs available for combating bacterial infections, following in the footsteps paved by penicillin.

Gerhard Domagk, a German pathologist and bacteriologist, made significant contributions with his discovery of sulfonamides, the first class of antibiotics. While not directly related to penicillin, Domagk's work on sulfonamides represented a parallel path in the search for substances that could kill bacteria, underscoring the broader quest for antimicrobial agents during the early 20th century.

Current Implication

Foundation for Modern Antibiotic Therapy: Penicillin's success paved the way for the discovery and development of other antibiotics, creating a cornerstone for modern antibiotic therapy. This revolutionized the treatment of bacterial infections, significantly reducing mortality rates from previously fatal conditions like sepsis, pneumonia, and bacterial meningitis.

Surgical Advances: The availability of penicillin and later antibiotics has dramatically reduced the risk of post-surgical infections, enabling more complex and invasive surgical procedures to be performed safely. This has had a transformative impact on fields such as transplant surgery, cardiac surgery, and orthopedics.

Treatment of Sexually Transmitted Infections (STIs): Penicillin and its derivatives have been crucial in the treatment of STIs such as syphilis and gonorrhea, helping to control these infections and reduce their spread.

Antibiotic Resistance: While the development of penicillin has saved countless lives, it has also led to the emergence of antibiotic resistance due to overuse and misuse of antibiotics. This ongoing challenge underscores the need for responsible antibiotic use, continuous surveillance, and the development of new antimicrobial agents.

Continued Research and Development: The story of penicillin inspires ongoing research in the field of antimicrobial resistance (AMR) and the search for novel antibiotics to combat resistant strains. It highlights the importance of interdisciplinary research in developing new therapeutic strategies to address emerging health threats.

Impact And Products

Broad Spectrum of Antibiotics: The success of penicillin inspired the discovery and production of a wide range of antibiotics, each targeting different bacteria. This diversity has allowed for more tailored treatments of bacterial infections, improving patient outcomes.

Antibiotic Production Techniques: The processes developed for the production of penicillin set the standard for antibiotic manufacturing, leading to advancements in fermentation technology and pharmaceutical production that have been crucial for scaling up the availability of various drugs.

Vaccination Programs: While not a direct product of penicillin, the methodology and understanding of infectious diseases that came from its development have bolstered vaccination programs by highlighting the importance of preventing bacterial infections.

Antibiotic Resistance Solutions: The emergence of antibiotic-resistant bacteria due to the widespread use of penicillin and other antibiotics has spurred innovation in developing new antimicrobial agents and strategies to combat resistance, including the exploration of bacteriophage therapy and novel drug molecules.

Medical and Laboratory Supplies: Penicillin's discovery led to the development of standardized laboratory techniques for testing antibiotic sensitivity, which are now commonplace in clinical microbiology labs. These techniques are essential for diagnosing infections and guiding appropriate antibiotic treatment.

Public Health Initiatives: Penicillin's success has underscored the importance of antibiotics in public health, leading to initiatives aimed at educating the public and healthcare professionals on the prudent use of antibiotics to mitigate the rise of resistance.

HERMANN MULLER (1946)

The man who visualized an X factor in the X – rays and defined radiation injury to genes

In 1946, Hermann Muller, an American geneticist renowned for his contributions to the field of genetics, was awarded the Nobel Prize in Medicine. His groundbreaking discovery that X-rays could induce genetic mutations revolutionized our understanding of genetics and heredity.

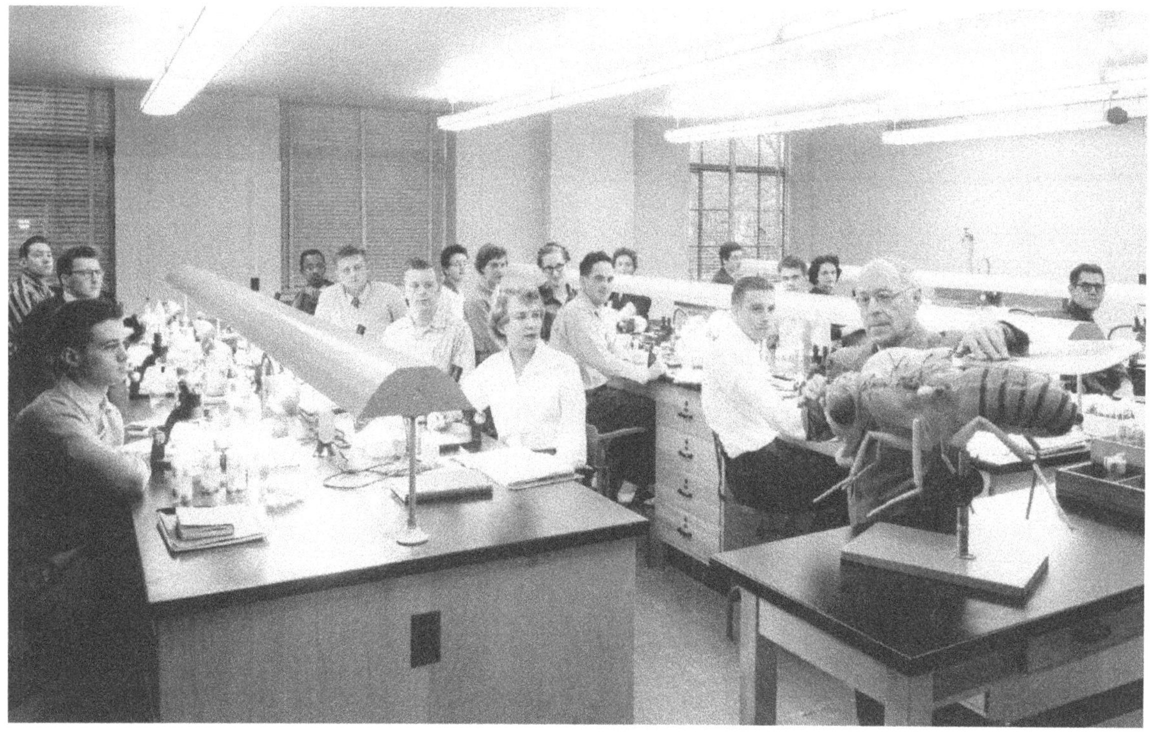

History

Born on December 21, 1890, in New York City, Muller's academic path led him to Columbia University, where he was mentored by some of the early pioneers in genetics. This environment nurtured his growing interest in genetic research, particularly using Drosophila as a model organism.

Snippets

Muller's pivotal research showed that exposure to X-rays could significantly increase the mutation rate in fruit flies. This was the first clear demonstration that environmental factors could cause genetic mutations, providing invaluable insight into the mechanisms of mutation and laying the groundwork for the field of radiation genetics.

Current Implications

The implications of Muller's work extend far beyond his initial discovery. His research into the effects of radiation on genetics has informed safety standards for radiation exposure and contributed to our understanding of the risks associated with radiation. Muller's findings have played a crucial role in cancer research, aiding in the development of treatments and prevention strategies.

Impact and Products

Muller's contributions to genetics and his pioneering work in radiation genetics have had a lasting impact on multiple scientific disciplines. His research has not only enhanced our understanding of genetic mutations and their causes but also paved the way for advances in genetic engineering, cancer treatment, and radiation safety protocols. Today, Muller is remembered as a pioneer whose work continues to influence the fields of genetics and medicine.

CARL CORI, GERTY CORI, BERNARDO HOUSSAY (1947)

The Coris' and their famous (family) cycle that got deep into Glycogen metabolism

In 1947, the Nobel Prize in Medicine was awarded to Carl and Gerty Cori, a pioneering husband-and-wife scientific duo, and Bernardo Houssay. The Coris were recognized "for their discovery of the course of the catalytic conversion of glycogen," and Houssay "for his discovery of the part played by the hormone of the anterior pituitary lobe in the metabolism of sugar." These discoveries provided significant insights into carbohydrate metabolism and its hormonal regulation, fundamental for understanding metabolic diseases such as diabetes.

History

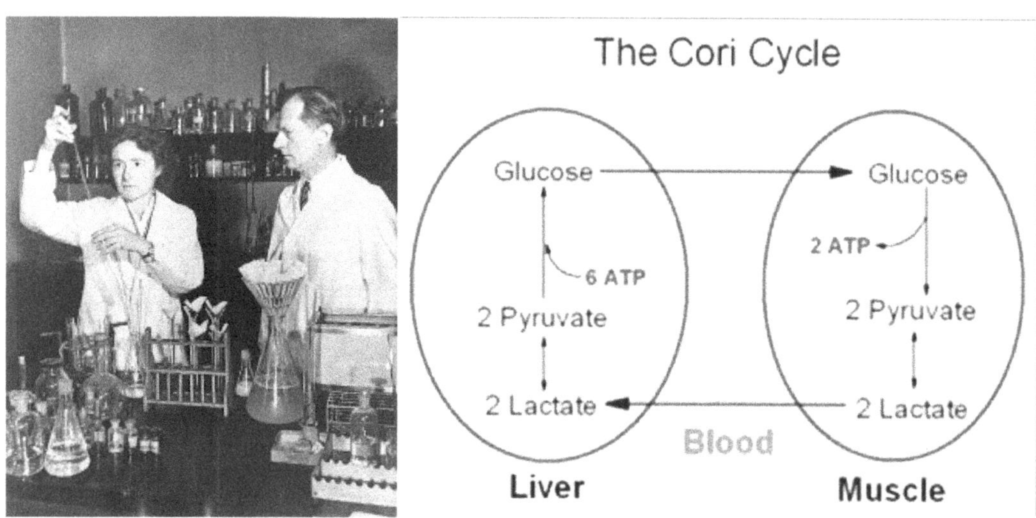

Carl Ferdinand Cori and Gerty Theresa Cori, both born in Prague (then part of the Austro-Hungarian Empire) in 1896, embarked on a journey that would revolutionize the understanding of biochemistry and metabolic processes. After meeting at the German University of Prague, where they both studied medicine, they married in 1920, the same year they received their medical degrees. The Coris moved to the United States in 1922, starting their work at the State Institute for the Study of Malignant Diseases in Buffalo, New York, and later joining the faculty of Washington University in St. Louis in 1931. Their collaborative research led to the discovery of the enzyme that facilitates the conversion of glycogen into glucose, as well as the process that came to be known as the Cori cycle, explaining the metabolic pathway of glucose production and utilization in the liver and muscles.

Bernardo Houssay, born in Buenos Aires, Argentina, in 1887, had a prolific career in physiology that spanned several decades. After earning his medical degree from the University of Buenos Aires at the young age of 23, Houssay went on to become a professor of physiology at the same university, eventually founding the Institute of Biology and Experimental Medicine in Buenos Aires. His research on the role of pituitary hormones in regulating blood sugar levels in diabetic dogs laid the groundwork for understanding the hormonal control of glucose metabolism, a key factor in the treatment of diabetes.

Snippets

The Cori Cycle: The Coris elucidated the Cori cycle, demonstrating how glycogen is converted into glucose in the liver, then used by muscles for energy, with lactate produced by muscles transported back to the liver to synthesize glycogen again, a critical insight into energy metabolism

Houssay's Hormonal Research: Bernardo Houssay's experiments on dogs showcased how pituitary hormones influence blood sugar levels, providing a foundational understanding of the hormonal regulation of glucose metabolism, pivotal for diabetes research.

A Transatlantic Collaboration: The Coris, originally from Prague, and Houssay, from Buenos Aires, Argentina, exemplify the international collaboration and diverse perspectives that contribute to scientific advancement, underscoring the global nature of research and discovery.

Legacy in Metabolic Disease: Their combined research has had a profound impact on understanding and treating metabolic diseases, especially diabetes, by highlighting the intricate balance between carbohydrate metabolism and hormonal regulation.

Early Influencers

One notable pioneer is Sir Frederick Gowland Hopkins, awarded the Nobel Prize in 1929 for his discovery of vitamins, demonstrating the importance of micronutrients in health and disease, including their role in metabolic processes. His work highlighted the critical role of diet in metabolism, setting the stage for the Coris' later discoveries in glycogen and glucose metabolism

Another significant contributor was Gustav Embden, known for his work on the glycolytic pathway, the Embden-Meyerhof pathway, which detailed the process of glucose breakdown within the cell. This pathway is integral to understanding the biochemical basis of the Cori cycle and the metabolic fluxes that occur during exercise and in various pathological conditions.

Oscar Minkowski and Joseph von Mering were instrumental in establishing the role of the pancreas in diabetes after observing that dogs developed diabetes following pancreatectomy. This discovery was crucial for later research into insulin and the hormonal regulation of blood sugar, areas where Houssay made significant contributions.

Current Implications

Diabetes Research and Treatment: The Coris' elucidation of the glycogenolysis process and Houssay's work on the role of pituitary hormones in glucose regulation have significantly impacted the understanding of diabetes. This has contributed to the development of targeted treatments that improve glucose control and insulin sensitivity in diabetic patients.

Sports Medicine and Nutrition: Knowledge of the Cori cycle has influenced recommendations for athlete nutrition and recovery strategies, emphasizing the role of carbohydrates in energy metabolism during and after intense physical activity. This understanding helps in optimizing performance and recovery in sports settings.

Metabolic Syndrome and Obesity: The research into carbohydrate metabolism has shed light on the pathophysiology of metabolic syndrome and obesity. Insights into how the body processes and stores carbohydrates contribute to developing dietary guidelines and treatments aimed at preventing and managing these conditions.

Endocrinology: Houssay's discoveries regarding hormonal influence on glucose metabolism have deepened the understanding of various endocrine disorders beyond diabetes, including conditions affecting the pituitary and adrenal glands. This has led to better diagnostic and therapeutic approaches in endocrinology.

Pharmacological Advances: The foundational work of the Coris and Houssay has paved the way for the development of new pharmacological agents that modulate metabolic pathways for therapeutic purposes, offering new treatments for metabolic diseases.

Impact And Products

Advancements in Insulin Therapy: Their work laid the groundwork for the refinement of insulin therapy techniques and formulations, providing more effective and tailored treatment options for individuals with diabetes. This includes the development of long-acting insulins and insulin analogs designed to mimic natural insulin secretion more closely.

New Diagnostic Tests: Understanding the biochemical pathways involved in carbohydrate metabolism has led to the creation of sophisticated diagnostic tests for metabolic disorders. These tests can more accurately assess liver function, insulin resistance, and other aspects of glucose metabolism, aiding in early detection and management of diseases.

Metabolic Modulators: The insights gained from their research have spurred the development of drugs that target specific enzymes in the metabolic pathways they elucidated. These metabolic modulators offer potential treatments for metabolic disorders by adjusting the flow through metabolic pathways, such as those involved in glycogen breakdown and synthesis.

Educational Tools: The Cori cycle and the hormonal regulation of glucose metabolism have become fundamental concepts in medical and biological education. The development of educational models, animations, and simulations based on their discoveries has enhanced the learning experience for students across the globe, fostering a deeper understanding of human physiology.

Nutritional Supplements and Strategies: The practical application of their metabolic research has influenced the formulation of nutritional supplements and dietary strategies aimed at optimizing glycogen storage and utilization, benefiting athletes, individuals with metabolic disorders, and the general population seeking to improve their metabolic health.

Research Methodologies: Lastly, the techniques pioneered by the Coris and Houssay have evolved into standard research methodologies in biochemistry and physiology, enabling ongoing discoveries in metabolic diseases and beyond. These methodologies continue to facilitate breakthroughs in understanding the complex interplay between hormones, enzymes, and nutrients in the body.

PAUL HERMANN MÜLLER (1948)

The DDT scientist who went all out to cleanse the world from insects borne diseases

In 1948, Paul Hermann Müller, a Swiss chemist, was awarded the Nobel Prize in Medicine for his discovery of DDT's high efficiency as a contact poison against various arthropods.

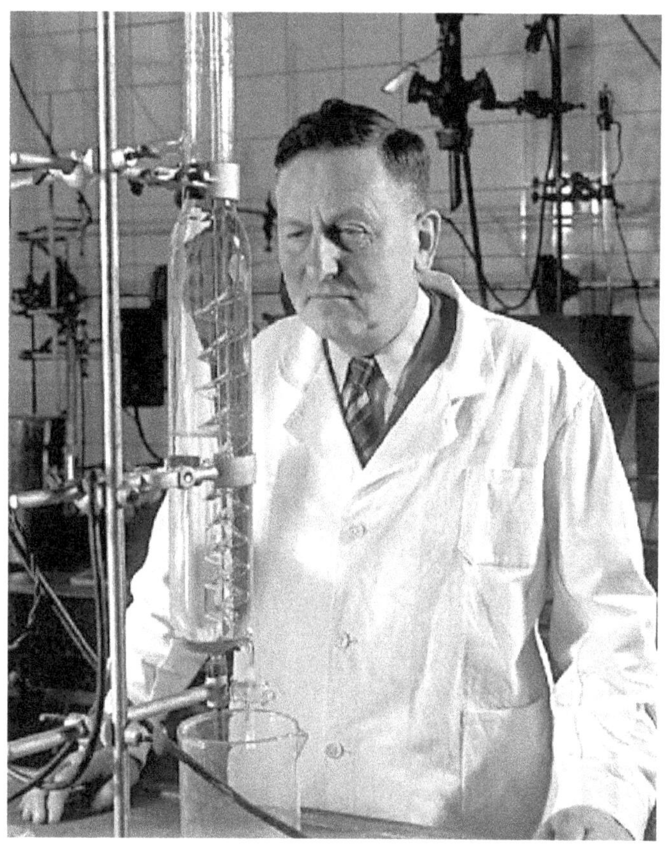

History

Born on January 12, 1899, in Olten, Switzerland, Müller's early career was marked by his work as a laboratory assistant and later as an assistant chemist. He pursued his education at Basle University, obtaining a doctorate in 1925. Müller's career at J.R. Geigy A.G. began in the same year, leading to his role as Deputy Director of Scientific Research on Substances for Plant Protection by 1946.

Snippets

Müller's journey to discovering DDT was driven by the need for effective, yet safe, insecticides. Previous solutions were either too expensive, ineffective, or dangerously toxic to both pests and humans. After years of research and hundreds of trials, Müller identified DDT in 1939, recognizing its potential as a powerful insecticide that was both long-lasting and safe for mammals. This discovery was a result of his dedication to synthesizing a chemical that could combat insect pests without harming plants or warm-blooded animals.

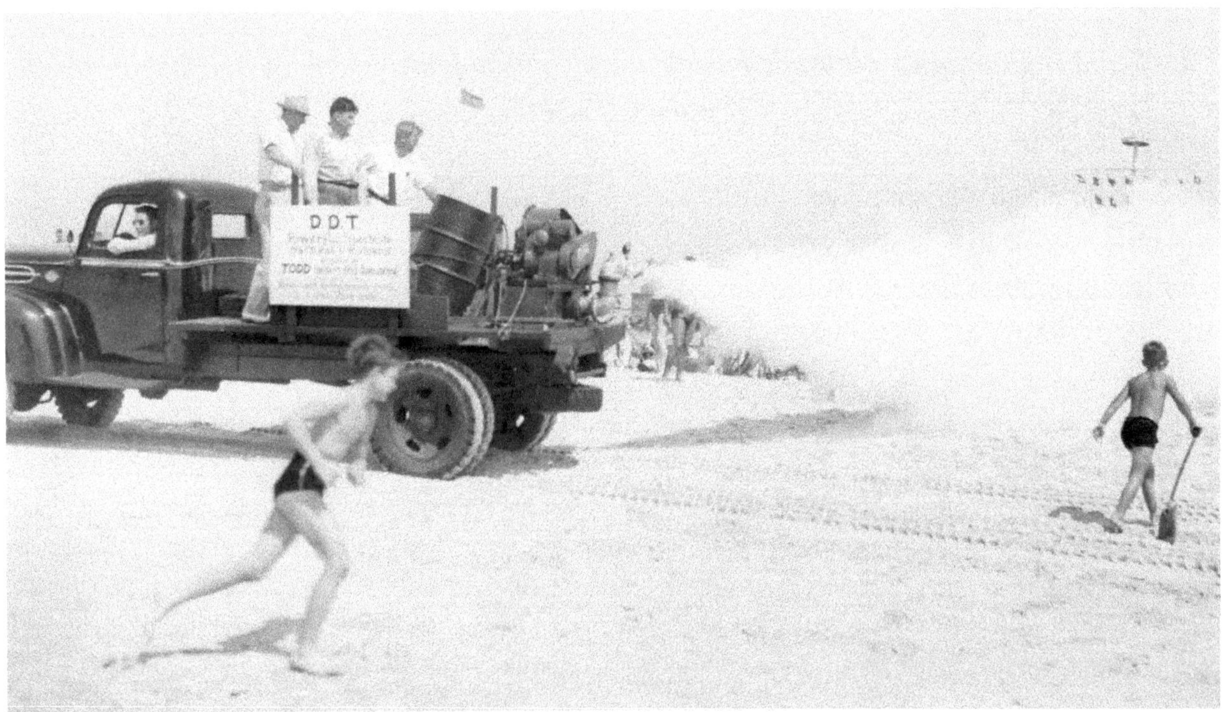

DDT spraying became somewhat controversial global movement

Current Implications

Müller's work with DDT revolutionized pest control, offering a potent tool against diseases spread by insects. While DDT was initially hailed for its effectiveness and played a crucial role in eradicating malaria from several regions, its later association with environmental and health concerns highlighted the complexities of chemical pest control. Müller's discovery laid the groundwork for the development of safer, more sustainable pest management strategies.

Impact and Products

The introduction of DDT fundamentally changed agricultural practices and public health initiatives, contributing significantly to the reduction of disease vectors and the protection of crops. Although the use of DDT has been restricted due to environmental concerns, Müller's pioneering work in the field of synthetic insecticides continues to influence the development of new compounds that balance efficacy with environmental safety.

This discovery was pivotal in the fight against vector-borne diseases such as malaria and typhus, significantly impacting public health.

WALTER RUDOLF HESS, ANTÓNIO EGAS MONIZ (1949)

Defined the complex connections among various lobes of brain and autonomic power centers

1949 the Nobel Prize in Medicine was jointly awarded to Walter Rudolf Hess and António Egas Moniz. Hess was honored for his discovery of the functional organization of the interbrain as a coordinator of the activities of internal organs. At the same time, Moniz was recognized for his development of the prefrontal lobotomy.

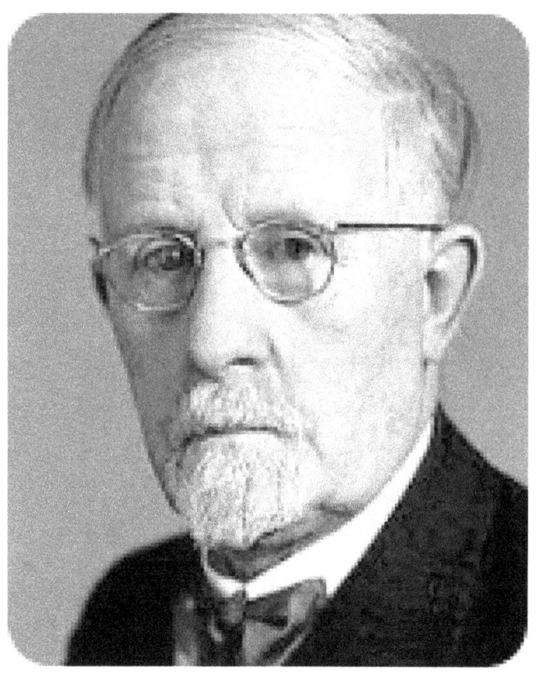 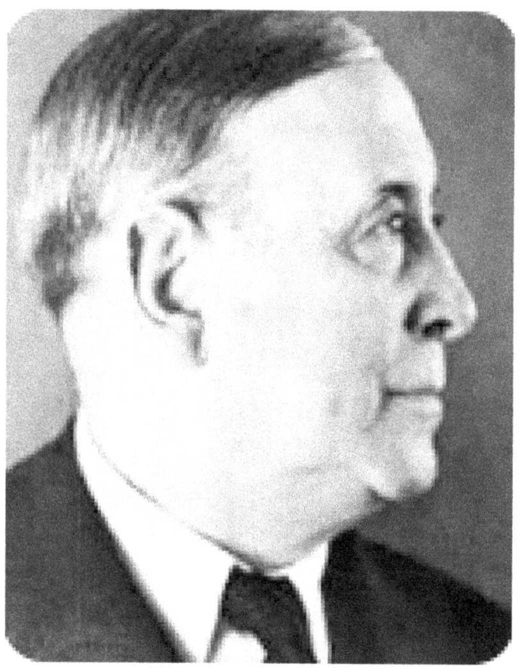

History

Walter Rudolf Hess

Walter Rudolf Hess was born in 1881 in Frauenfeld, Switzerland. His early exposure to physics through his father, a physics teacher, and his natural curiosity about the world around him laid a solid foundation for his future in the sciences. Despite initially practicing as an ophthalmologist due to external circumstances, Hess's passion for research led him back to physiology. His journey took a significant turn in 1912 when he decided to return to physiology research, becoming the Director of the Physiological Institute in Zurich in 1917.

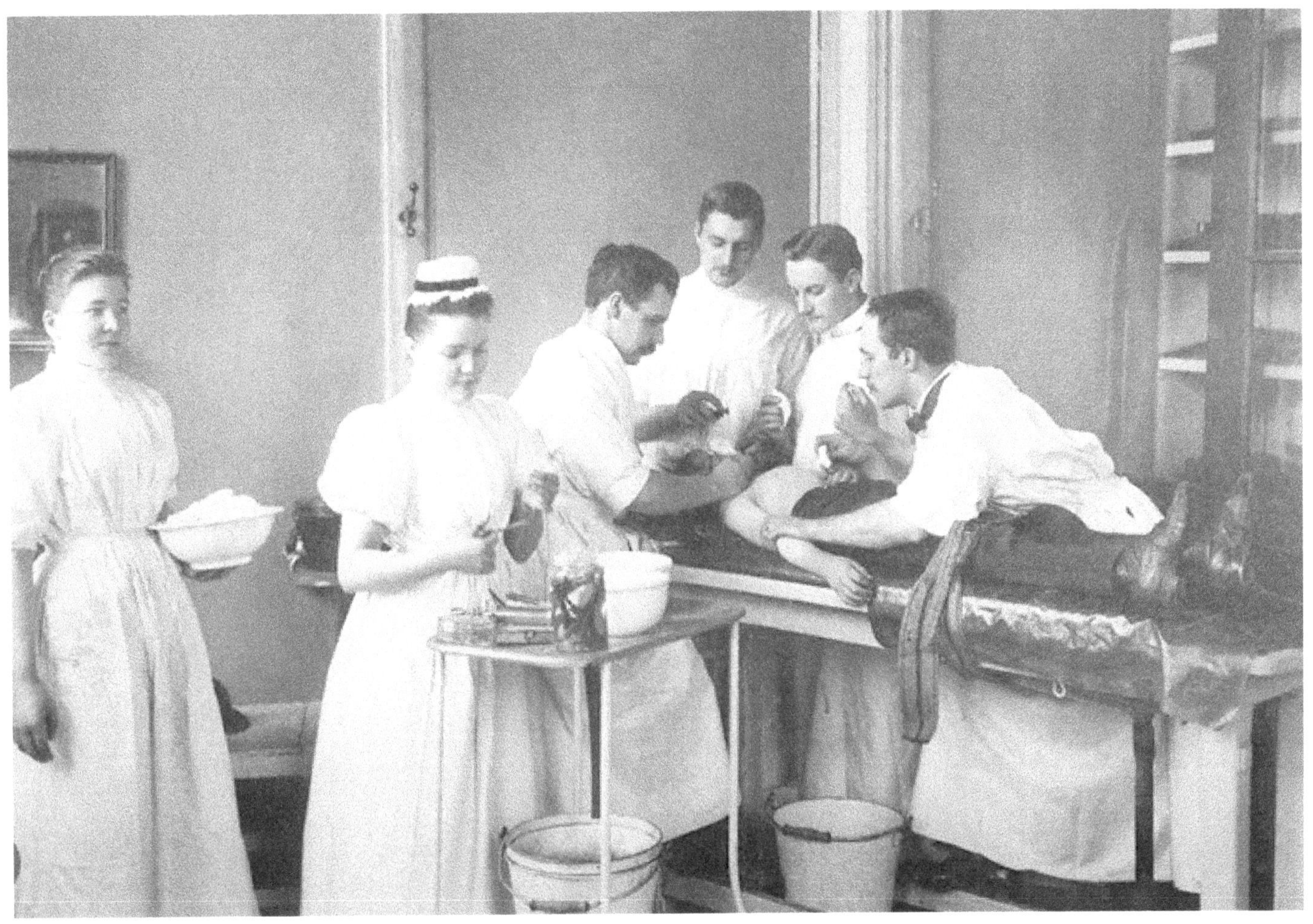

During a lobectomy surgery

Hess's Nobel Prize-winning work involved pioneering studies on the diencephalon of the brain, focusing on understanding how this area governs the physiological functions of internal organs. Through meticulous experiments involving the stimulation of the hypothalamus in animal models, Hess demonstrated the brain's role in controlling various autonomic functions.

António Egas Moniz

António Egas Moniz, born in 1874 in Avanca, Portugal, was initially known for his work in neurology and the development of cerebral angiography. This imaging technique, which he introduced in 1927, allowed for the visualization of the blood vessels in and around the brain, offering new insights into neurological disorders.

Moniz's most controversial contribution, which led to his Nobel Prize, was the development of the prefrontal lobotomy. Introduced in the 1930s as a treatment for severe mental disorders, this surgical procedure was groundbreaking at the time. It sparked a great deal of debate regarding its ethical implications and the nature of psychiatric treatment. Despite the controversy, Moniz's work on lobotomy opened new avenues for the treatment of mental illness and laid the groundwork for the evolution of psychiatric neurosurgery.

Snippets

Walter Rudolf Hess's Pioneering Brain Research: Hess's innovative experiments demonstrated how the diencephalon controls vital physiological processes. By electrically stimulating the hypothalamus in cats, he showed its role in regulating behaviors from sleep to aggression, illustrating the brain's central role in coordinating internal organ functions.

Introduction of Cerebral Angiography by António Egas Moniz: Moniz developed this groundbreaking technique allowing for the visualization of the vascular system in the brain. This significantly advanced the diagnosis and understanding of neurological disorders, marking a key development in medical imaging.

Development of Prefrontal Lobotomy: Moniz's controversial yet pioneering lobotomy procedure aimed to treat severe psychiatric conditions by severing connections in the brain's prefrontal cortex. This approach sparked debates on mental health treatment and the ethics of surgical interventions in psychiatry.

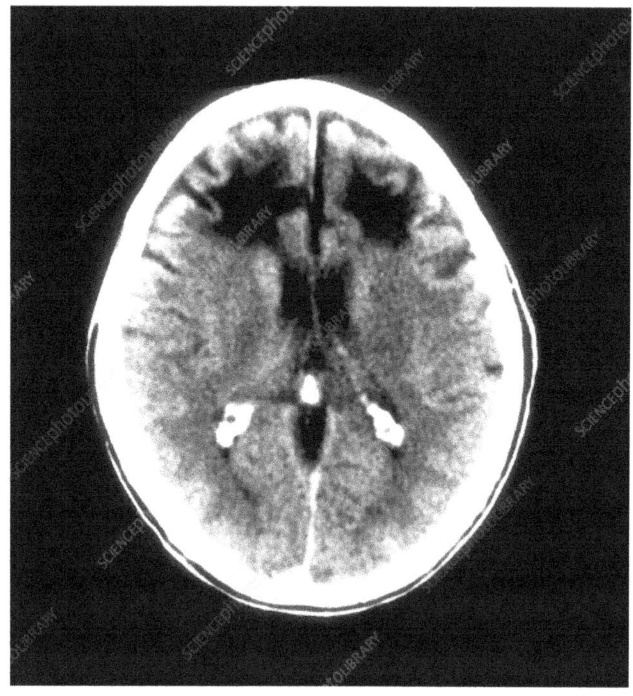

An MRI showing post frontal Lobectomy

Hess's Contributions to Neurophysiology: His work laid foundational knowledge for the understanding of the autonomic nervous system, influencing future research in neurology and psychology, and paving the way for new therapeutic approaches to neurological and psychiatric disorders.

Moniz's Legacy in Psychiatry: Despite the eventual ethical concerns and decline in use, Moniz's work on lobotomy contributed to the evolution of psychiatric treatments and stimulated further research into the biological basis of mental illness.

Early Researchers

Wilder Penfield, a neurosurgeon whose innovative techniques for mapping the functions of various regions of the brain during surgery have had a profound impact on our understanding of brain function and its relation to behavior and sensory perception. Though Penfield's work came slightly after Hess and Moniz, his contributions underscore the collaborative continuum of discovery in neurology.

Another notable pioneer is Paul Broca, a French physician, who in the 1860s identified the part of the brain responsible for producing spoken language, known today as Broca's area. Broca's work was foundational in establishing the relationship between specific brain areas and their functions, a concept that underpins much of modern neuroscience.

Ivan Pavlov, a Russian physiologist known for his research on conditioned reflexes, contributed significantly to the understanding of how behavioral patterns are formed and controlled by the brain. Pavlov's experiments, though focused on the digestive system's physiology, inadvertently revealed key insights into the neural substrates of learning and memory.

Carl Wernicke, a German neurologist, made crucial contributions to our understanding of the brain's language functions. Like Broca, Wernicke identified a brain area—later named Wernicke's area—critical for language comprehension. The discoveries of Broca and Wernicke were pivotal, illustrating that cognitive functions could be localized to specific brain regions.

Current Implications

Neurophysiology and Brain Research: Hess's research on the brain's role in controlling internal organs has paved the way for advanced studies in neurophysiology. Today, understanding the hypothalamus's functions is crucial in research into sleep disorders, obesity, and other conditions related to autonomic nervous system dysfunction.

Psychiatric Treatments and Ethical Considerations: Moniz's development of the prefrontal lobotomy, while largely discontinued, was a precursor to the modern field of psychosurgery. Today, more refined surgical interventions, like deep brain stimulation, are used to treat severe psychiatric disorders, including obsessive-compulsive disorder and major depression, with an emphasis on ethical considerations and patient safety.

Advancements in Medical Imaging: Moniz is also credited with inventing cerebral angiography, a technique that remains fundamental in diagnosing and treating vascular diseases of the brain. This has evolved with technology, leading to more sophisticated imaging methods that provide safer, non-invasive options for exploring cerebral vasculature and diagnosing conditions like aneurysms and arteriovenous malformations.

Integrated Approaches to Mental Health: The historical context of Moniz's lobotomy has underscored the importance of holistic and patient-centered approaches in treating mental health conditions.

Impact and Products

Development of Neuromodulation Techniques: The understanding of brain regions involved in the control of bodily functions and behavior, rooted in Hess's work, has led to neuromodulation techniques like Transcranial Magnetic Stimulation (TMS) and Deep Brain Stimulation (DBS) for treating neurological and psychiatric disorders.

Advancements in Brain Imaging Technologies: Moniz's invention of cerebral angiography laid the groundwork for the development of advanced imaging technologies such as Magnetic Resonance Imaging (MRI) and Computed Tomography (CT) scans, which are crucial for diagnosing brain and vascular diseases.

Psychosurgery and Ethical Standards: The historical context of lobotomy has influenced the establishment of stringent ethical standards and regulations for psychosurgery and other invasive treatments, ensuring patient safety and consent are prioritized in modern psychiatric care.

Hess's and Moniz's work extends beyond scientific implications, impacting technological innovation, clinical practices, education, and ethical standards in treating and understanding neurological and psychiatric conditions.

EDWARD KENDALL, T. REICHSTEIN, PHILIP HENCH (1950)

Astonishing experiments on Adrenal gland and the birth of corticosteroids

In 1950, Edward Calvin Kendall, Tadeus Reichstein, and Philip Showalter Hench were jointly awarded the Nobel Prize in Medicine for their pioneering work on the hormones of the adrenal cortex, specifically their structure and biological effects.

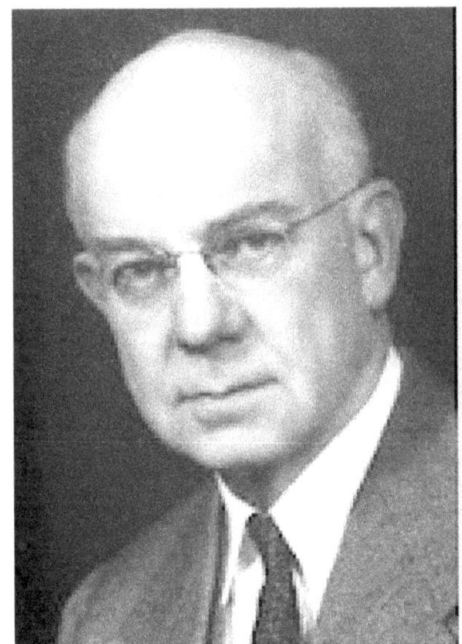

Edward Calvin
Kendall
(1886 - 1972)

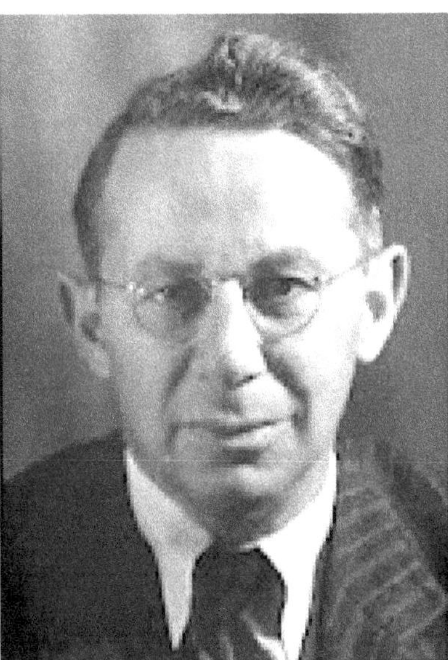

Tadeus Reichstein
(1897 - 1996)

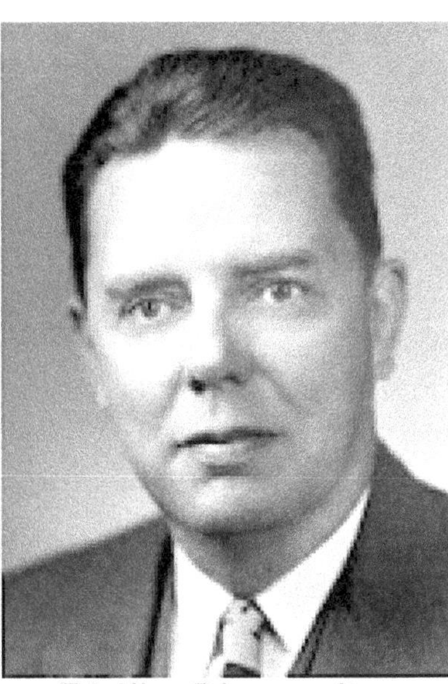

Philip Showalter
Hench
(1896 - 1965)

History

Edward Calvin Kendall was an American chemist born on March 8, 1886. His educational journey took him through Columbia University, where he obtained a Ph.D. in Chemistry. Kendall's work at the Mayo Foundation, affiliated with the University of Minnesota, led to the isolation of thyroxine and several steroids from the adrenal gland cortex, including cortisone, which had profound medical implications.

Tadeus Reichstein, a Polish-Swiss chemist born on July 20, 1897, contributed to the isolation and identification of the hormones of the adrenal cortex. His work, conducted independently but simultaneously with Kendall's, was crucial in the synthetic production of these hormones, which allowed for their physiological effects to be studied in detail.

Philip Showalter Hench, born on February 28, 1896, was an American physician whose clinical observations at the Mayo Clinic were pivotal in suggesting the potential therapeutic effects of adrenal cortex hormones, particularly in treating rheumatoid arthritis. His collaboration with Kendall on the use of cortisone marked a significant leap forward in medical treatment for inflammatory diseases.

Current Implications

The trio's groundbreaking work laid the foundation for the therapeutic use of corticosteroids in medicine. Their discovery of cortisone, a steroid hormone, revolutionized the treatment of rheumatoid arthritis and other inflammatory conditions, providing relief for millions of patients worldwide. This work has had a lasting impact, influencing both the clinical approach to treating chronic diseases and the pharmaceutical development of synthetic steroids.

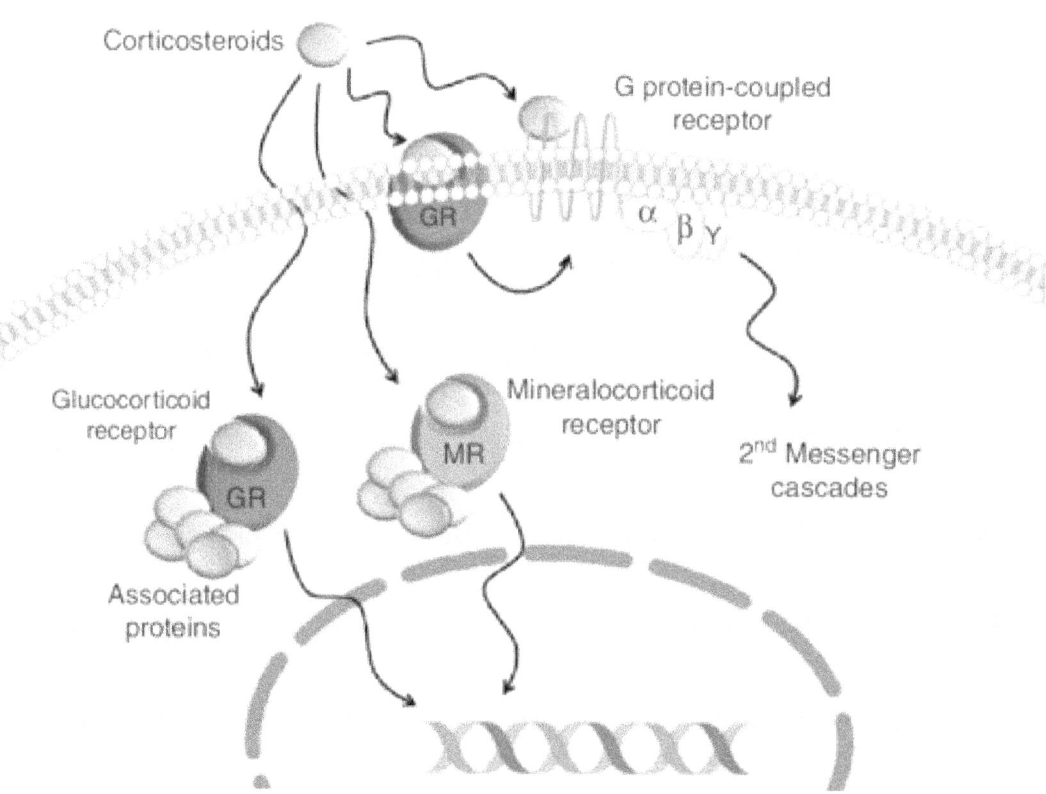

Impact and Products

The development of cortisone and other corticosteroids has become central to treating a wide range of diseases, from autoimmune disorders to asthma and allergic reactions. Their collective contributions not only enhanced the medical community's understanding of adrenal hormones but also opened new avenues for drug development and therapeutic interventions.

Their collective research led to significant advancements in understanding and treating inflammatory diseases, among other conditions.

MAX THEILER (1951)

The famous South African, tamed the global scourge of yellow fever with his vaccine

In 1951, Max Theiler was honored with the Nobel Prize in Medicine for his pioneering work on yellow fever, specifically his development of a vaccine against the disease.

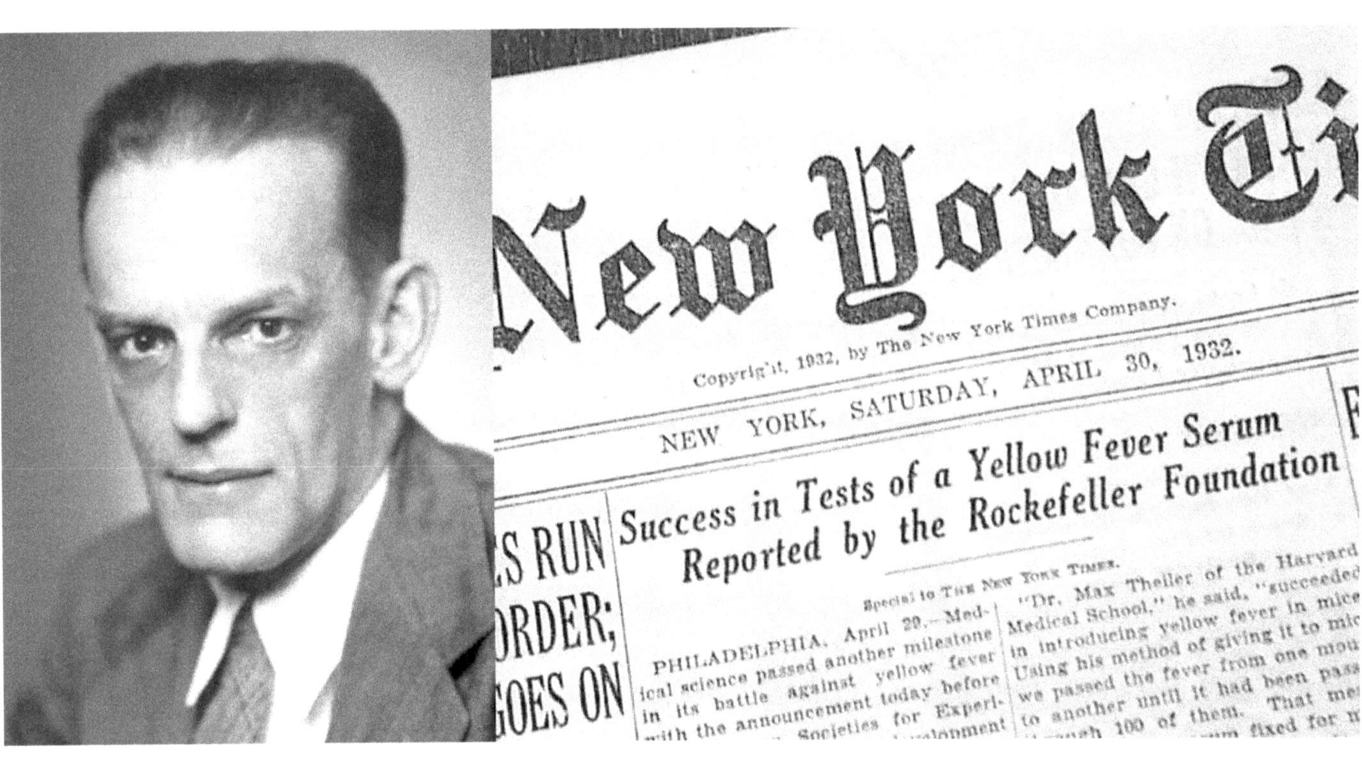

History

Born in Pretoria, South Africa, on January 30, 1899, Theiler's contributions revolutionized the approach to combating yellow fever, a major killer in tropical regions. Theiler's medical journey began with disproving the existing hypothesis that yellow fever was caused by a bacterium, leading to the discovery that it was, in fact, a viral disease. This breakthrough allowed Theiler and his team to focus on developing a vaccine using a weakened form of the virus, which ultimately led to the creation of the 17D vaccine strain.

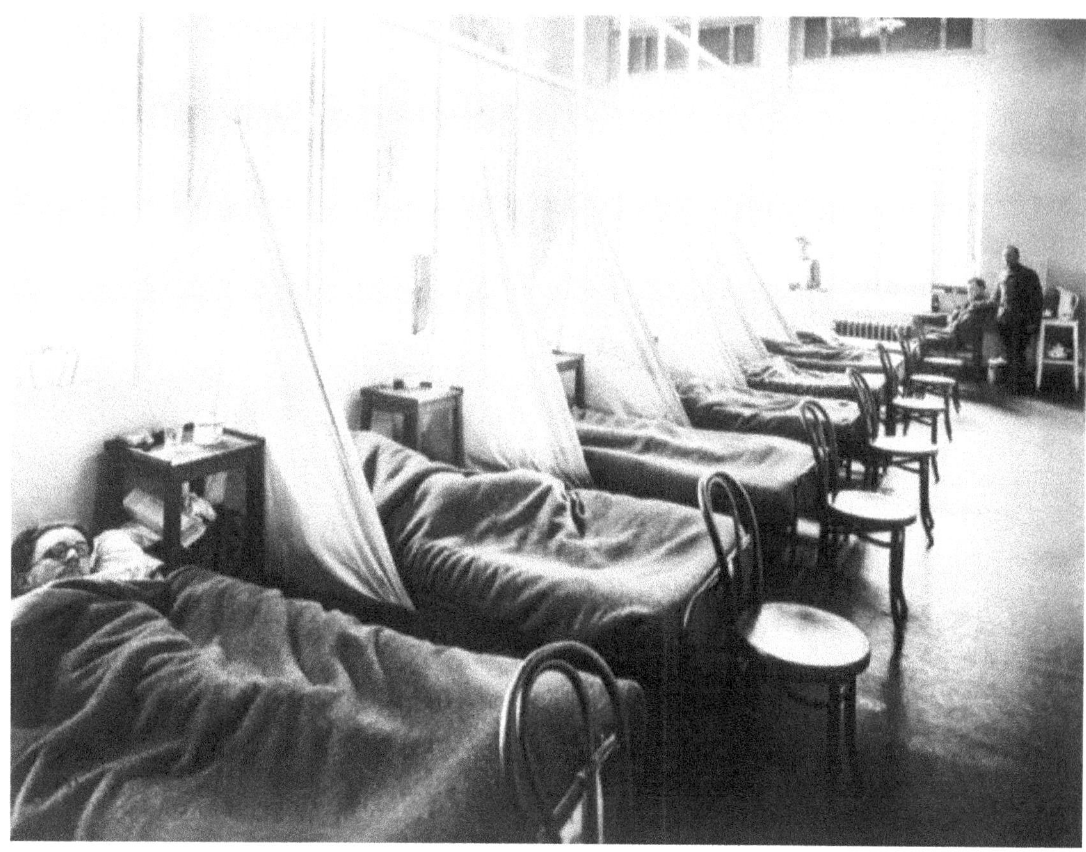

Yellow fever Pandemic scene in US camp hospital

Snippets

The development of the 17D vaccine was a culmination of Theiler's extensive research, including the innovative use of mice to propagate the virus and the subsequent attenuation of the virus in chicken embryos. This vaccine was both safe for humans and highly effective, marking a significant advancement in the fight against yellow fever.

Current Implications

Theiler's yellow fever vaccine had a profound impact on public health, drastically reducing the incidence of the disease and saving countless lives. His work laid the groundwork for future vaccine development and highlighted the importance of virology in medicine. The 17D vaccine remains a critical tool in yellow fever prevention to this day.

Impact and Products

Beyond the yellow fever vaccine, Theiler's research contributed to a broader understanding of viral diseases and vaccine development. His discovery of Theiler's murine encephalomyelitis virus furthered scientific knowledge on viral pathology and immunity. Theiler's legacy is characterized by his innovative approach to research and his dedication to improving global health through vaccination.

SELMAN WAKSMAN (1952)

When the world was at war in 1940s, he conquered tuberculosis with his Streptomycin

In 1952, Selman Waksman, an influential microbiologist, received the Nobel Prize in Medicine for his discovery of streptomycin, marking a monumental advancement in the battle against tuberculosis.

History

Selman Waksman, born on July 22, 1888, in the Russian Empire, emigrated to the United States, setting a course for a distinguished academic and research career at Rutgers University. His education culminated in a Ph.D. in Biochemistry from the University of California in 1918. Waksman's tenure at Rutgers was marked by his leadership in soil microbiology and his focus on the actinomycetes, leading to the landmark discovery of streptomycin.

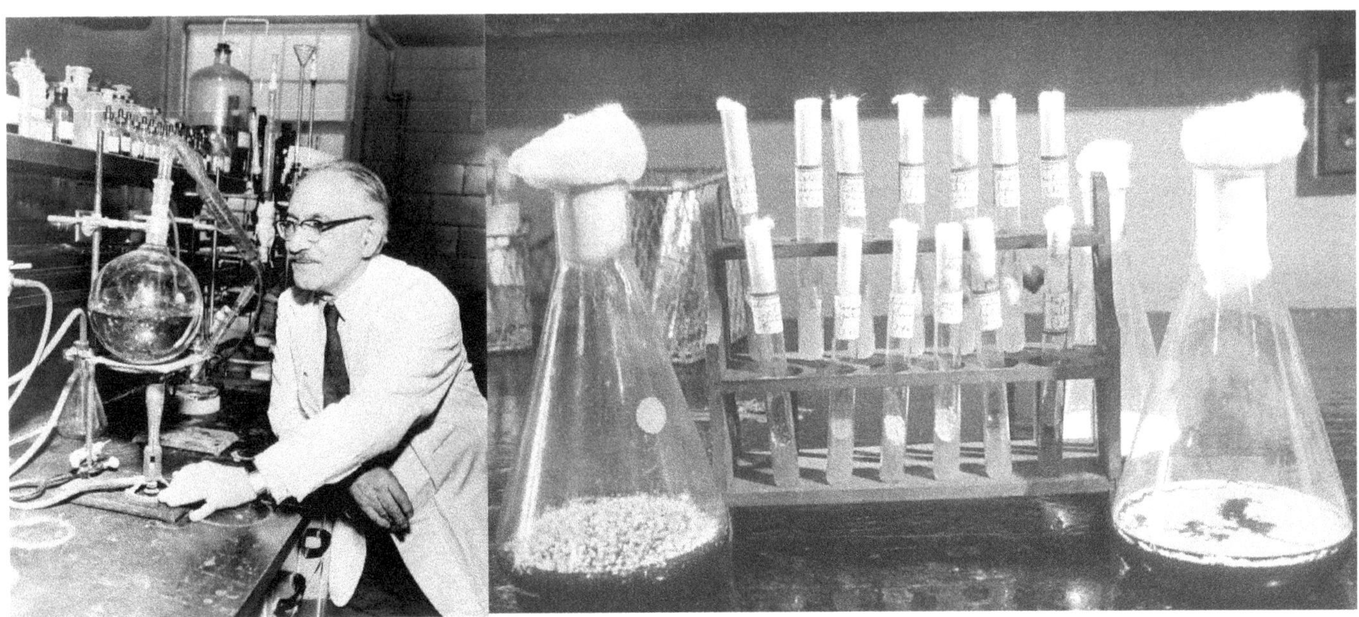

Snippets

The path to discovering streptomycin involved meticulous research into soil microorganisms, where Waksman's expertise in actinomycetes played a crucial role. The breakthrough came when Albert Schatz, a student of Waksman, isolated streptomycin from Streptomyces griseus in 1943. This antibiotic became the first effective treatment against tuberculosis, a disease that had claimed countless lives worldwide.

Current Implications

Waksman's discovery of streptomycin transformed the landscape of medical treatment for bacterial infections, offering a lifeline to tuberculosis patients for the first time. His work not only paved the way for the development of further antibiotics but also emphasized the significance of soil microbiology in pharmaceutical discovery.

Impact and Products

Beyond streptomycin, Waksman's research yielded over 15 antibiotics, significantly broadening the arsenal against infectious diseases. His dedication to microbiology education and research culminated in the establishment of the Waksman Institute of Microbiology at Rutgers University, fostering future generations of scientists. The impact of Waksman's work extends into modern medicine, agriculture, and environmental science, reflecting his legacy in promoting human health and understanding the natural world.

HANS KREBS AND FRITZ LIPMANN (1953)

A crown among Nobel prizes. The confluent cycle of carbohydrate, protein and fat metabolism

In 1953, Hans Krebs and Fritz Lipmann were awarded the Nobel Prize in Medicine for their outstanding contributions to the understanding of cellular metabolism. Their research laid the foundation for biochemistry, influencing countless discoveries and innovations in medicine and biology.

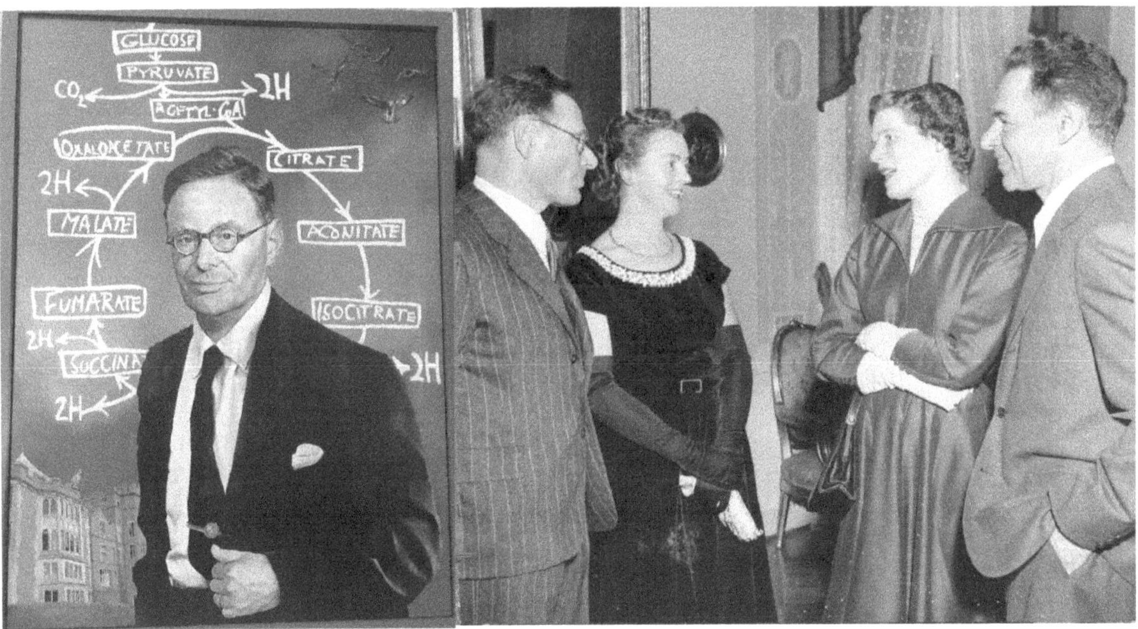

History

Hans Adolf Krebs, born on August 25, 1900, in Hildesheim, Germany, was a pioneer in studying cellular respiration, a critical biochemical process that extracts energy from food and oxygen to fuel organisms. Krebs's journey in science took him through several prestigious institutions in Germany, where he developed his research skills under notable scientists such as Otto Warburg. However, due to the rise of the Nazi regime and his Jewish heritage, Krebs fled to England, where he continued his groundbreaking work at the University of Sheffield and later at the University of Oxford. His most notable discovery, the citric acid cycle (also known as the Krebs cycle), illuminates how organisms generate energy from nutrients.

Fritz Albert Lipmann, sharing the prize with Krebs, was recognized for his discovery of co-enzyme A and its importance in intermediary metabolism. His work complemented Krebs's findings by elucidating how the body utilizes and transforms energy at the molecular level, which is fundamental to understanding cellular metabolism and energy transfer.

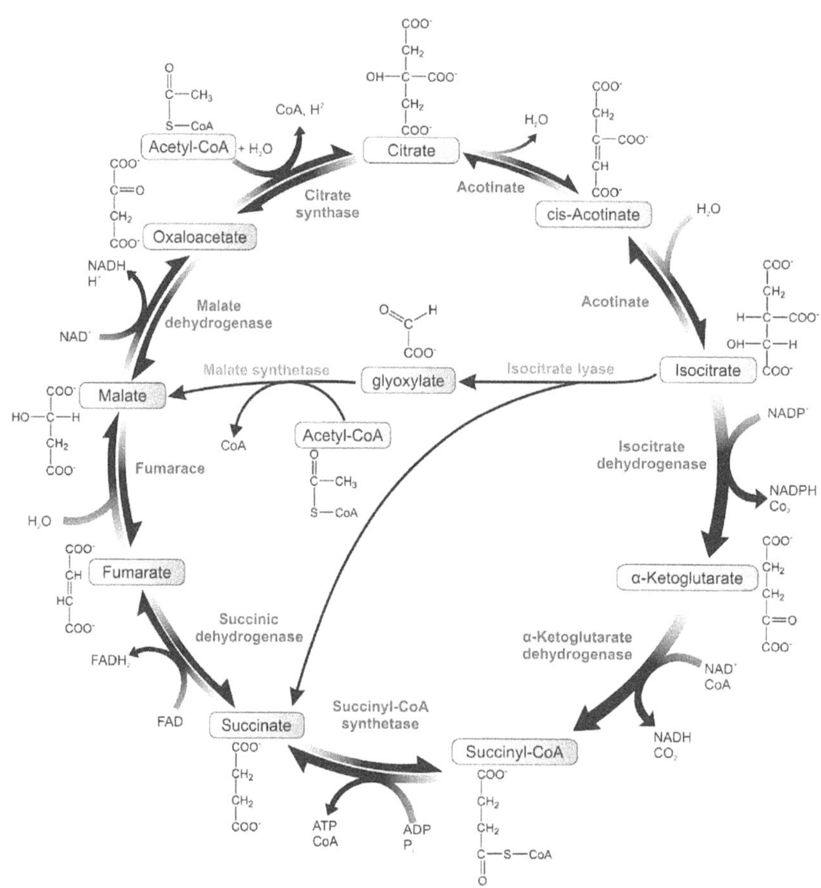

The most famous and complex biochemical cycle of confluence between carbohydrate, fat and protein metabolism.

Current Implications

The discoveries of Krebs and Lipmann have profound implications in modern science and medicine. The Krebs cycle is central to cellular metabolism, explaining how energy is produced and utilized in living organisms. This understanding is crucial for research in various fields, including genetics, physiology, and medical sciences, showing the way for advancements in treating metabolic disorders, cancer research, and developing therapeutic strategies targeting metabolic pathways.

Impact and Products

The work of Krebs and Lipmann has facilitated significant progress in biotechnology and pharmaceutical industries, contributing to the development of drugs targeting metabolic pathways involved in diseases. Their research has also been instrumental in the fields of bioengineering and synthetic biology, where metabolic pathways are engineered for industrial purposes, such as biofuel production and the synthesis of valuable pharmaceutical compounds.

JOHN ENDERS, THOMAS WELLER, FREDERICK ROBBINS
(1954)

The three great masters of virology, who laid the road map for polio vaccine

In 1954, John Franklin Enders, Thomas Huckle Weller, and Frederick Chapman Robbins were awarded the Nobel Prize in Medicine for their landmark discovery that enabled the poliomyelitis viruses to grow in cultures of various types of tissue. This breakthrough was pivotal in the fight against polio, a disease that had caused widespread fear and devastation prior to their work.

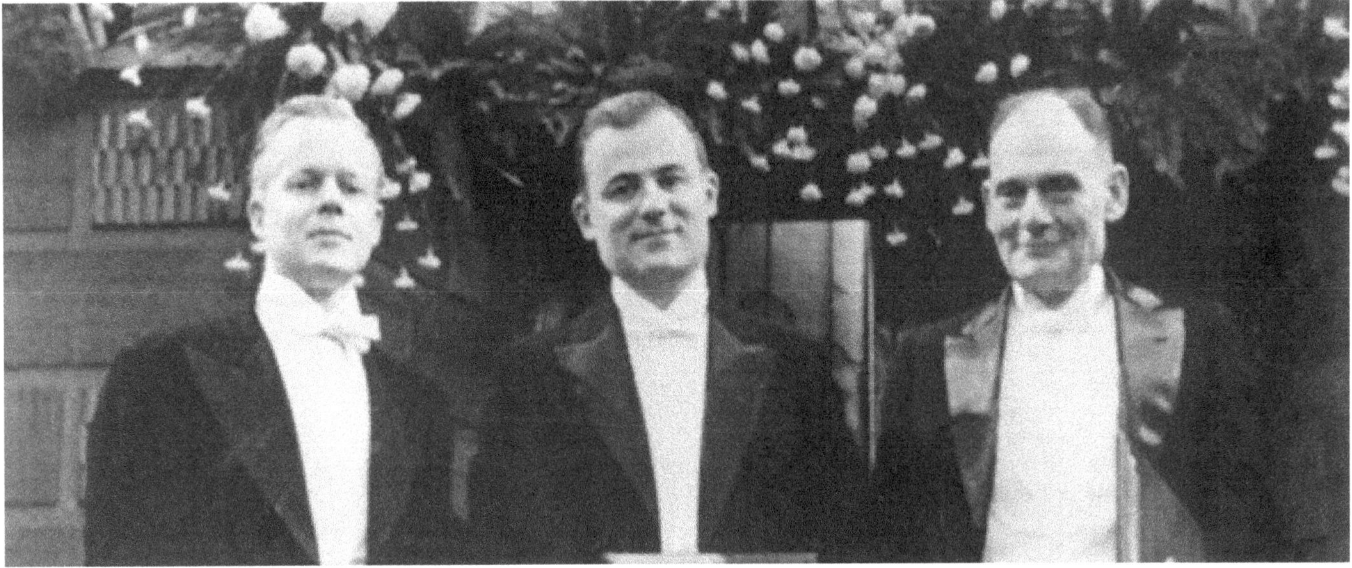

History

- John F. Enders, born on February 10, 1897, in West Hartford, Connecticut, USA, initiated his groundbreaking research at the Children's Medical Center in Boston, MA.
- Thomas H. Weller, born on June 15, 1915, in Ann Arbor, Michigan, joined Enders as a crucial part of the team, contributing his expertise in virology and infectious diseases.
- Frederick C. Robbins, born on August 25, 1916, in Auburn, Alabama, completed the trio, bringing his medical knowledge to the forefront of their collaborative efforts.

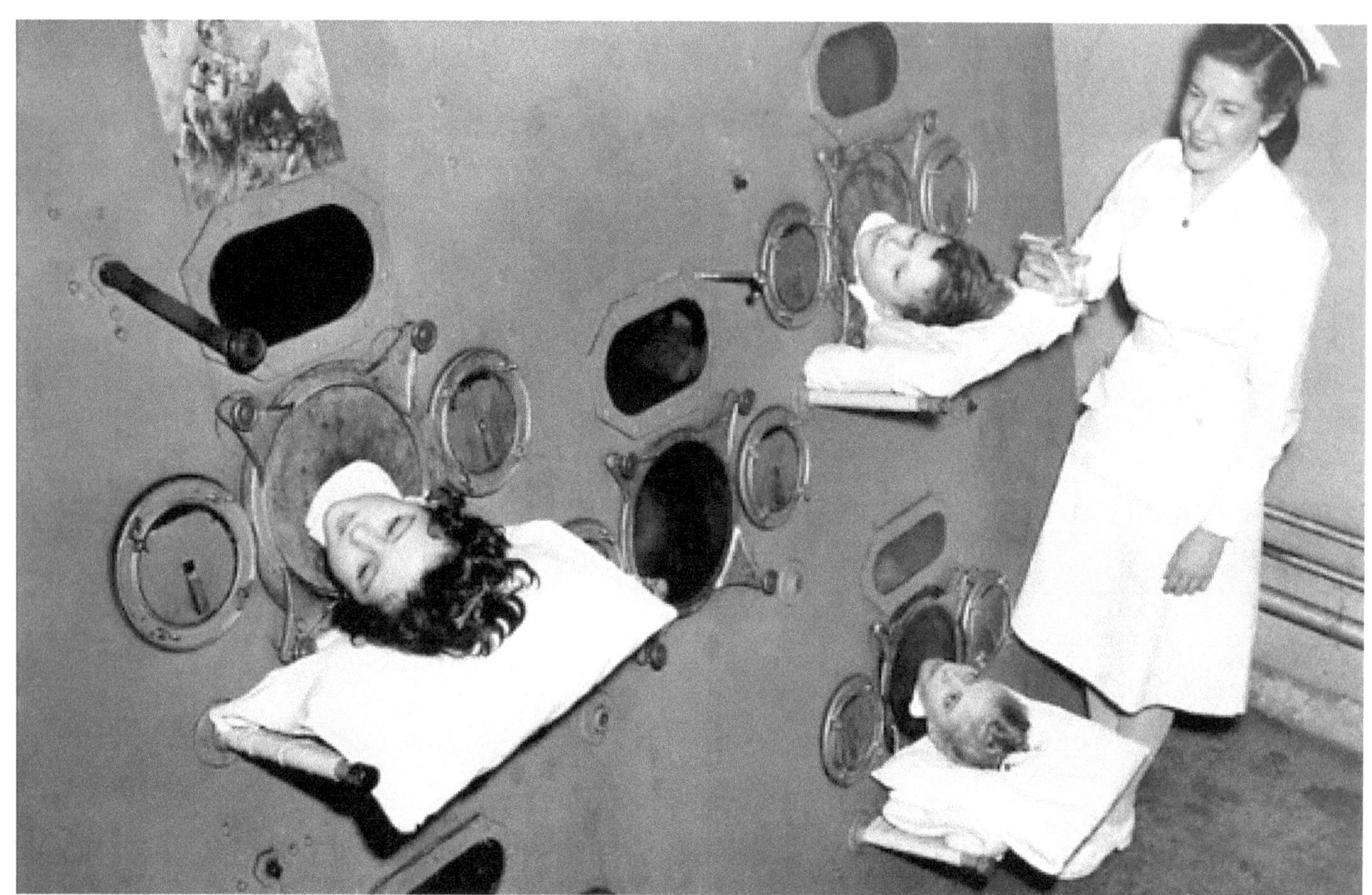

*During the peak of the polio epidemic in the U.S., some hospital wards
had iron lungs where multiple children lived.
(Courtesy of Boston Children's Hospital Archive)*

Snippets

The trio's work marked a significant advancement in virology and medical science, proving for the first time that viruses could be cultured outside a living organism. This achievement opened the door to the development of vaccines, most notably the polio vaccine, which has since led to the near eradication of the disease worldwide. Their method involved the use of human muscle and tissue to culture the poliovirus, an approach that was revolutionary at the time and laid the groundwork for future research in virology.

Current Implications

The work of Enders, Weller, and Robbins has had a lasting impact on public health and the scientific approach to infectious diseases. By enabling the culture of viruses in a laboratory setting, they provided a vital tool for the study of viruses and the development of vaccines, significantly influencing the course of modern medicine and virology.

Impact and Products

The discovery by Enders, Weller, and Robbins has been central to the fight against not only polio but also other viral diseases. Their pioneering techniques for culturing viruses in tissue have been adapted and expanded upon in countless studies since, facilitating the development of numerous vaccines and advancing our understanding of viral infections. Their work represents a monumental achievement in the ongoing effort to combat infectious diseases and protect global health.

AXEL HUGO THEODOR THEORELL (1955)

The Swede, who found the rhythm of life, by defining the intracellular oxidation process

In 1955, Axel Hugo Theodor Theorell was awarded the Nobel Prize in Medicine for his pioneering research on the nature and mode of action of oxidation enzymes.

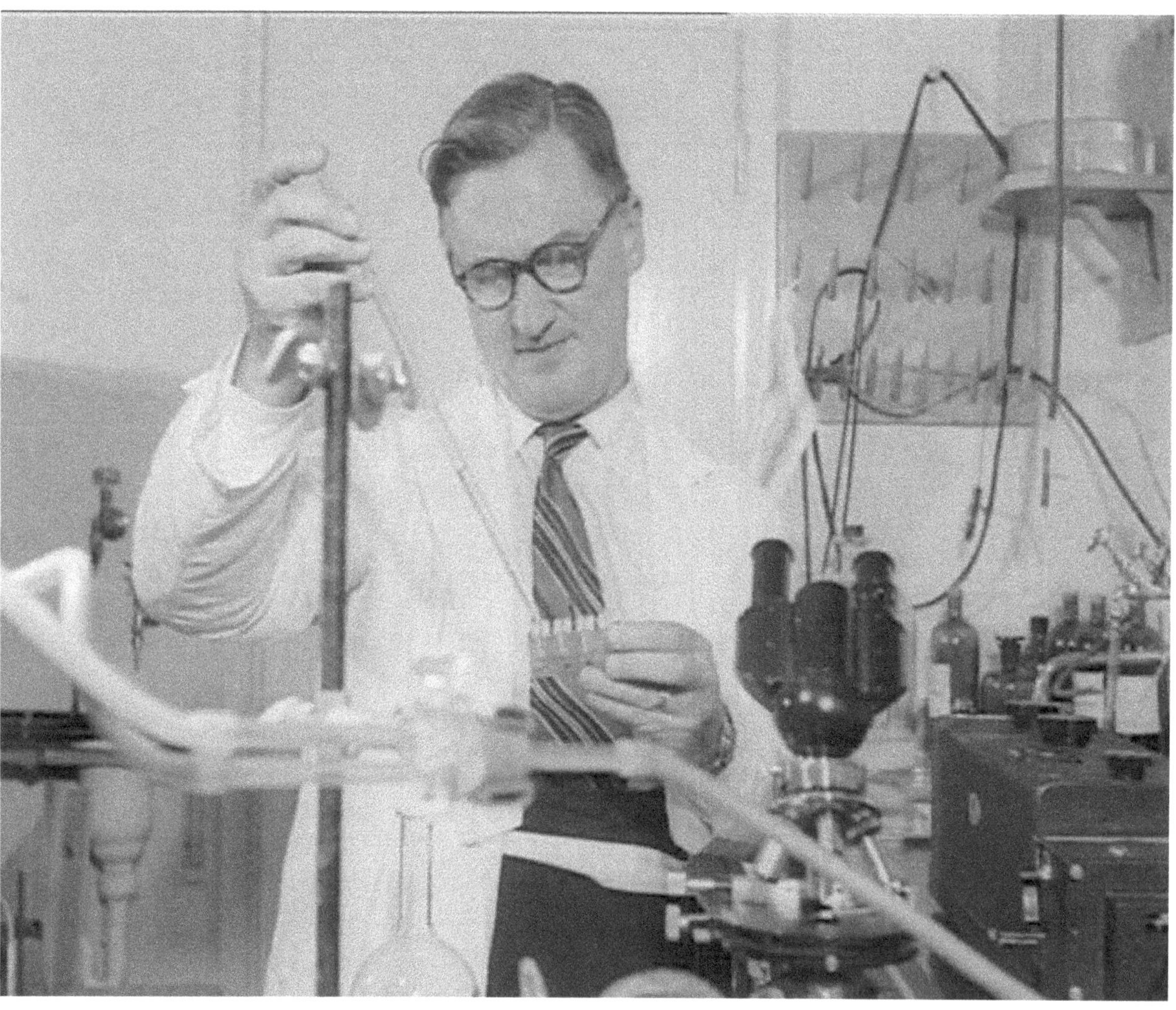

History

Born on July 6, 1903, in Linköping, Sweden, Theorell's work significantly advanced our understanding of enzymatic processes that are crucial for cellular respiration and metabolism.

Theorell's academic journey led him to the Karolinska Institute in Stockholm, where he earned his medical degree in 1930. His career was distinguished by a productive period spent with Otto Warburg in Berlin, where he focused on enzymes related to oxidation processes. Upon his return to Sweden, Theorell continued his research at the Karolinska Institute and later headed the Biochemical Department of the Nobel Medical Institute, founded in 1937.

Snippets

Theorell's groundbreaking discovery involved the identification of the two-part structure of a yellow-colored enzyme, demonstrating the essential roles of flavin mononucleotide and a protein component in the enzyme's function. His work elucidated how iron atoms in enzymes are critical for electron transport, a fundamental aspect of cellular energy production.

Current Implications

Theorell's discoveries laid the groundwork for the biochemical understanding of how enzymes facilitate oxidation-reduction reactions within cells, a process vital for energy conversion and various metabolic pathways. His contributions have had lasting implications for both basic science and applied medical research, influencing the development of treatments for diseases related to metabolic dysfunction.

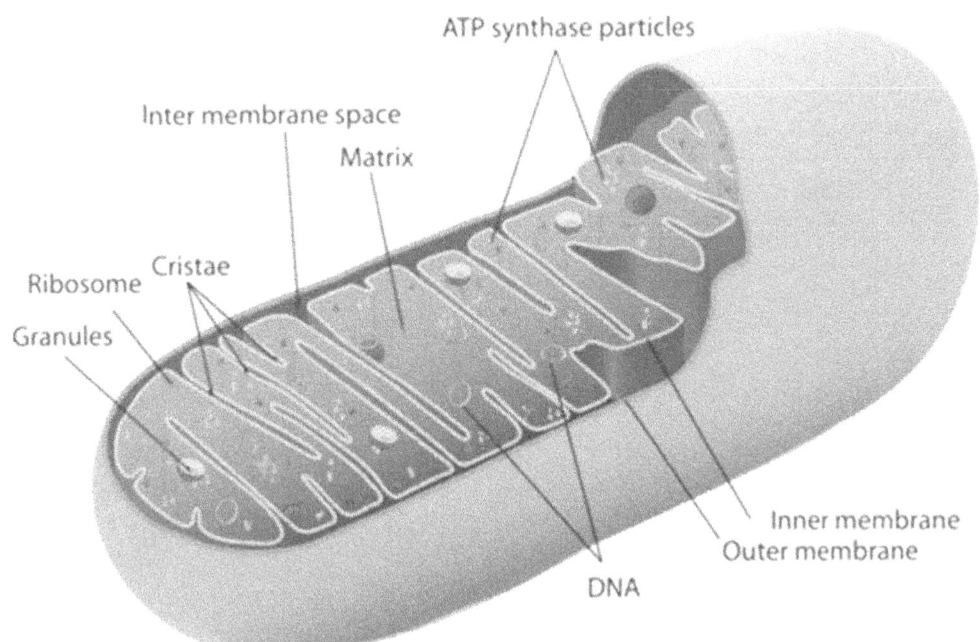

Impact and Products

Theorell's extensive study of enzymes has enriched the field of biochemistry, helping to unravel the complex mechanisms of life at the molecular level. His work continues to inspire current research in enzymology and metabolic diseases, underscoring the importance of understanding enzymatic actions for medical advancement.

ANDRÉ COURNAND, WERNER FORSSMANN, DICKINSON RICHARDS (1956)

The trio who opened the gateway to heart, that brought a tectonic shift in the field of cardiology

André Cournand, Werner Forssmann, and Dickinson Richards were awarded the Nobel Prize in Medicine in 1956 for their groundbreaking work in developing heart catheterization and elucidating pathological changes in the circulatory system.

History

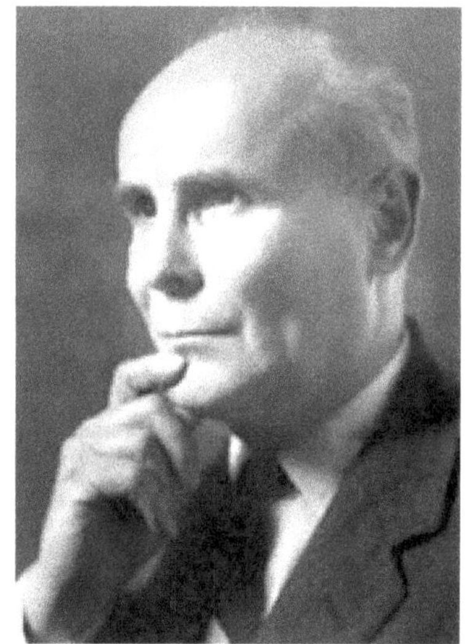

André Cournand

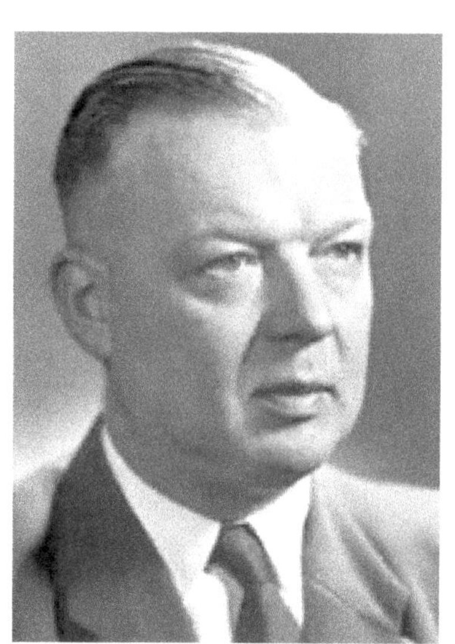

Werner Forssmann

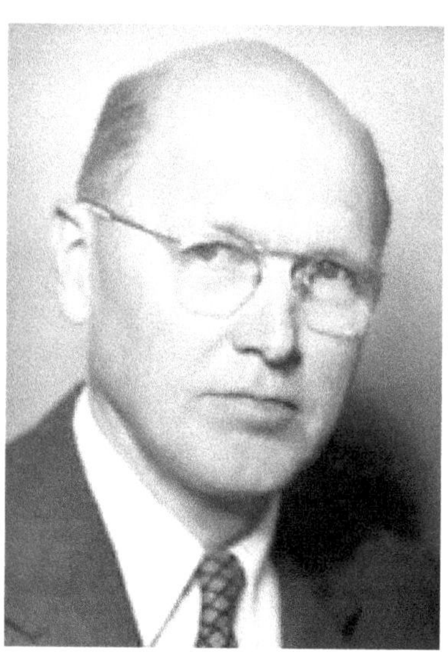

Dickinson W. Richards

André Frédéric Cournand, born in Paris in 1895, began his medical studies before serving in the French Army during World War I. After the war, he resumed his studies, becoming deeply involved in internal medicine and later moving to the United States to further his research at Columbia University and Bellevue Hospital in New York. Cournand's work in the U.S. led him to collaborate with Dickinson Richards on studying the physiology of respiration and the circulatory system.

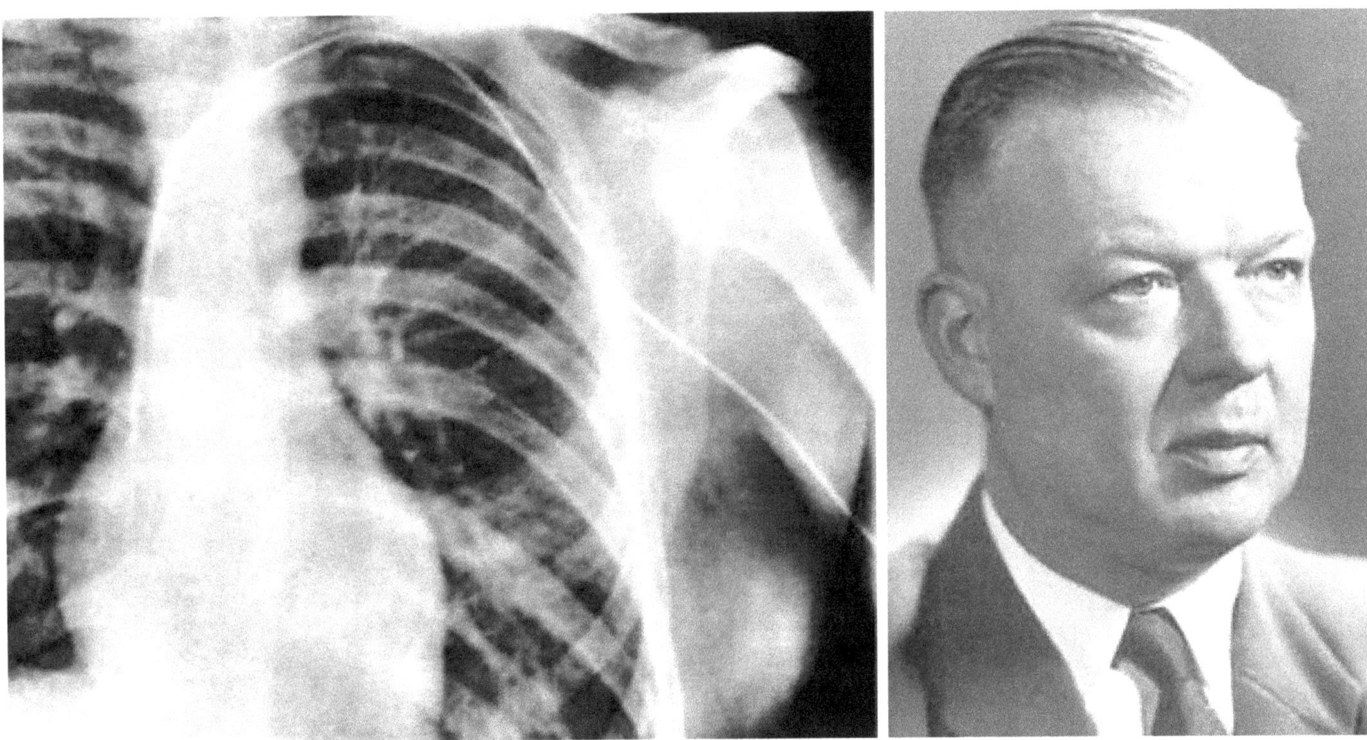

The original X ray of Forssmann experiments on his own heart

Werner Forssmann, born in Berlin in 1904, took a more daring route to medical innovation. As a young medical officer, he performed the first human cardiac catheterization on himself in 1929, inserting a catheter into his own arm and then walking to the X-ray department to photograph the catheter in his heart. Despite the initial skepticism from the medical community, Forssmann's work laid the foundational groundwork for future research in heart catheterization.

Dickinson Woodruff Richards Jr., born in Orange, New Jersey, in 1895, focused his studies on English and Greek at Yale University before turning to medicine at Columbia University's College of Physicians and Surgeons. After serving as an artillery officer in France during World War I, Richards returned to the U.S. to pursue his medical career.

Snippets

Innovation Born from Courage: Werner Forssmann's audacious self-experimentation marked the beginning of cardiac catheterization. By inserting a catheter into his own vein and navigating it into his heart, Forssmann demonstrated the procedure's feasibility, setting the stage for a new era in cardiac diagnostics and treatments.

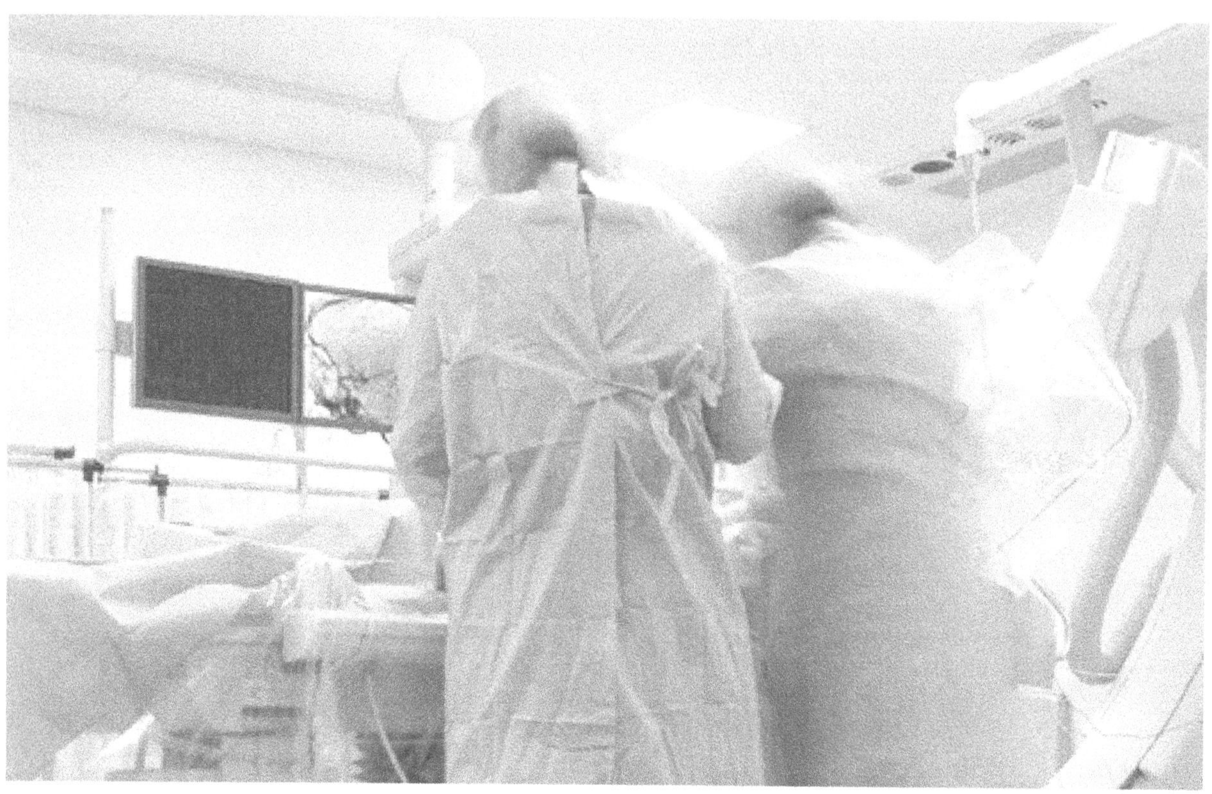

The Nobel trio's genius has taken the field of cardiology to unprecedented summits of success

Collaborative Expansion and Refinement: Building on Forssmann's initial work, Cournand and Richards further developed and refined cardiac catheterization techniques. Their collaboration extended the application of this method, enabling precise measurements of blood pressure within the heart and the oxygen content in blood, thus offering insights into the heart's functioning that were previously unattainable.

Diagnostic Breakthroughs: The trio's work allowed for the introduction of contrast fluid for X-ray images, significantly enhancing the visualization of the heart's structures and any pathological changes. This advancement was instrumental in diagnosing a variety of heart conditions, from congenital heart diseases to more complex circulatory system disorders.

A Foundation for Future Cardiology: The methodology and techniques developed by Cournand, Forssmann, and Richards provided a robust foundation for the future of cardiology, influencing countless diagnostic and treatment strategies. Their pioneering work opened up new pathways for understanding and treating heart diseases, leading to significant improvements in patient care and outcomes.

Early Researchers

Among these early innovators, one must recognize the contributions of pioneers such as Claude Bernard, who in the 19th century performed the first known cardiac catheterization on a horse, demonstrating the possibilities of accessing the heart through the venous system. His work, though not directly related to human cardiac catheterization, opened the minds of future scientists to the potential of direct heart measurement and intervention.

Another significant figure is Alexis Carrel, a Nobel laureate himself, who developed surgical techniques that would later be crucial for cardiac surgery. His work on vascular suturing and organ transplantation laid the groundwork for the surgical approaches needed to address the complications of heart diseases.

Also notable is James B. Herrick, who first described sickle cell anemia but more importantly for cardiology, provided early descriptions of myocardial infarction, highlighting the importance of understanding the circulatory system's pathology. Herrick's work underscored the need for diagnostic tools that could offer direct insights into the heart's functioning, setting the stage for the acceptance of invasive techniques like cardiac catheterization.

Current Implications

Expansion of Catheter-Based Procedures: Beyond diagnostic applications, cardiac catheterization has evolved to enable a wide range of therapeutic procedures, including angioplasty, stenting, and valve repairs, significantly reducing the need for open-heart surgeries.

Personalized Medicine in Cardiology: The detailed data obtained from cardiac catheterization allows for personalized treatment plans, adjusting therapies to the specific needs and conditions of individual patients, enhancing the effectiveness of cardiac care.

Advancements in Imaging Techniques: The integration of cardiac catheterization with advanced imaging techniques, such as intravascular ultrasound (IVUS) and optical coherence tomography (OCT), provides unprecedented views of the interior of blood vessels, aiding in the precise treatment of blockages and other heart diseases.

Development of Wearable Monitoring Devices: Insights from cardiac catheterization have influenced the development of wearable technology that monitors heart health, enabling early detection and intervention for cardiac conditions outside of clinical settings.

Global Health Impact: The technique's adaptability and scalability have facilitated its adoption in varying healthcare settings worldwide, improving access to advanced cardiac care even in resource-limited environments, thus addressing global health disparities in cardiovascular disease treatment.

Regenerative Medicine and Research: Cardiac catheterization plays a crucial role in delivering stem cells and other regenerative therapies directly to damaged heart tissues, opening new avenues for treating heart disease and potentially restoring heart function.

Impact and Products

Catheterization Equipment: The fundamental technology of cardiac catheterization has led to the development of specialized catheters, including pressure-monitoring catheters, balloon catheters used in angioplasty, and electrophysiology catheters for mapping heart electrical activity. Each of these products is tailored for specific diagnostic or therapeutic purposes, showcasing the versatility and innovation spurred by the trio's research.

Interventional Cardiology Devices: Building on the principles of cardiac catheterization, a range of devices for interventional cardiology has been developed. This includes coronary stents to keep arteries open, closure devices for sealing holes in the heart, and transcatheter heart valves for treating valve diseases without open-heart surgery. These devices have revolutionized the treatment of heart disease, offering less invasive options with quicker recovery times.

Diagnostic Imaging Software and Equipment: The integration of cardiac catheterization with imaging technologies has led to the advancement of software and equipment for enhanced visualization of the heart and its blood vessels. Digital subtraction angiography (DSA), computed tomography (CT) angiography, and magnetic resonance imaging (MRI) are examples of how imaging technology has evolved, providing clearer, more detailed cardiac images for accurate diagnosis and treatment planning.

Heart Monitoring Systems: Insights gained from the use of cardiac catheterization have informed the development of advanced heart monitoring systems. These systems, including Holter monitors and implantable loop recorders, allow for continuous monitoring of heart activity, detecting arrhythmias and other conditions that may not be captured during a standard ECG.

Educational Models and Simulation Platforms: The need to train medical professionals in the safe and effective use of cardiac catheterization has led to the creation of sophisticated educational models and simulation platforms. These tools simulate real-life scenarios, allowing practitioners to practice and refine their skills in a controlled environment, thus improving patient safety and procedural outcomes.

Telemedicine and Remote Monitoring Tools: Cardiac catheterization's role in diagnosing heart conditions has also paved the way for the development of telemedicine and remote monitoring tools. Patients with heart conditions can now be monitored remotely, enabling timely interventions and adjustments to treatment plans without the need for frequent hospital visits.

DANIEL BOVET (1957)

The famed Swiss scientist, who countered Histamine and put a full stop to systemic allergy

In 1957, Daniel Bovet was honored with the Nobel Prize in Medicine for his significant contributions to medical science, particularly his discoveries of synthetic compounds that inhibit the action of certain body substances.

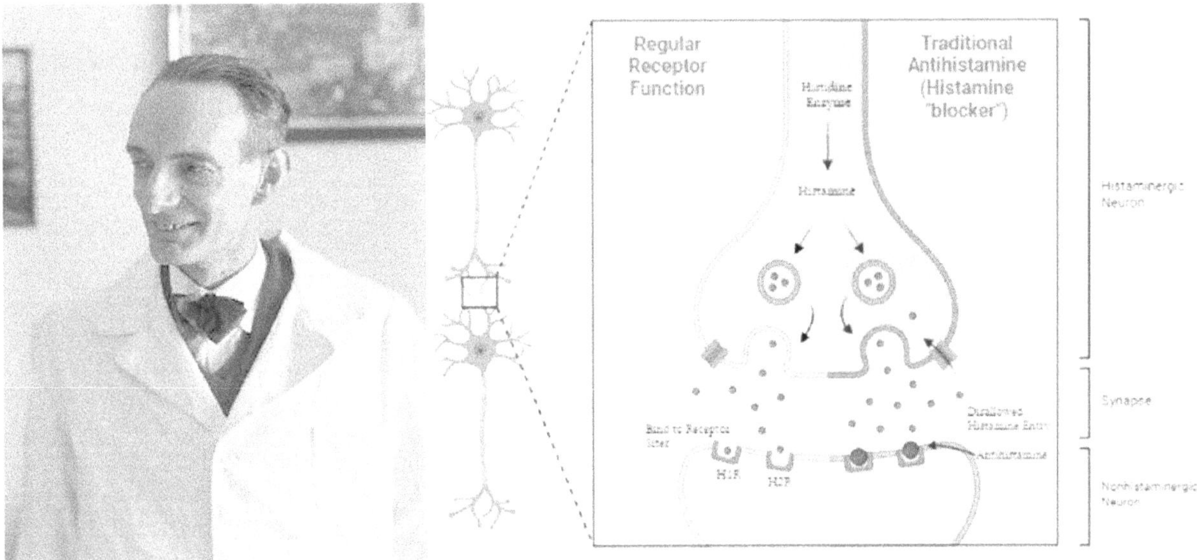

History

Daniel Bovet, born on March 23, 1907, in Neuchâtel, Switzerland, embarked on an illustrious career in pharmacology after completing his doctorate in science at the University of Geneva in 1929. Bovet's pioneering research took place against the backdrop of a career that spanned institutions and countries. It took him from the Pasteur Institute in Paris to his significant tenure in Rome, Italy, where he eventually took citizenship.

Snippets

Bovet's groundbreaking discovery of the first antihistamine in 1937 marked a revolution in the treatment of allergic reactions. His work on antihistamines, which counteract the effects of histamine, paved the way for the development of the first antihistamine drug for humans in 1942. This achievement, alongside his research into sulfa drugs and muscle relaxants, showcases Bovet's role in the development of chemotherapeutic agents that have transformed the approach to allergy treatment and surgery.

Current Implications

The implications of Bovet's discoveries are profound, offering new avenues for the treatment of allergic reactions and enhancing the efficacy of surgical procedures through muscle relaxants. His work in synthesizing curare, a drug used to relax muscles during surgery, exemplifies his contribution to making surgical procedures safer and more predictable.

Impact and Products

Daniel Bovet's legacy is evident in the widespread use of antihistamines and muscle relaxants in modern medicine. His research has not only improved the quality of life for individuals with allergies but also enhanced the safety and effectiveness of anesthesia in surgical settings. Bovet's dedication to advancing pharmacological science has left an indelible mark on the field, influencing generations of researchers and clinicians.

His work notably impacted the vascular system and skeletal muscles, leading to advancements in pharmacology that have had lasting effects on health care and treatment methodologies.

GEORGE BEADLE, EDWARD T. JOSHUA LEDERBERG (1958)

The pioneers who decoded the genetic basis of microbial biochemistry

In 1958, George Wells Beadle, Edward Lawrie Tatum, and Joshua Lederberg were awarded the Nobel Prize in Medicine for their discoveries elucidating the genetic control of biochemical reactions in microorganisms.

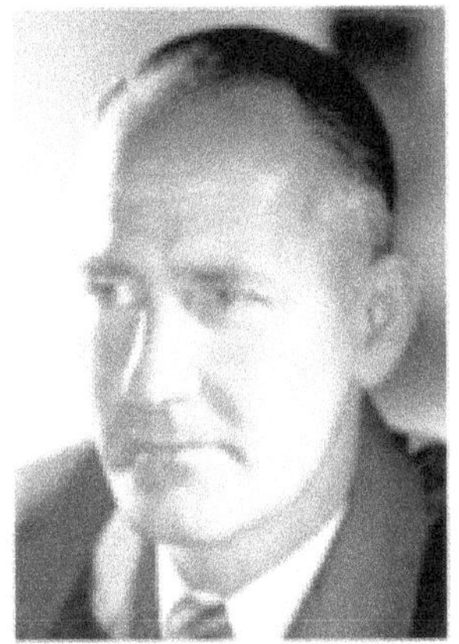

George Wells
Beadle

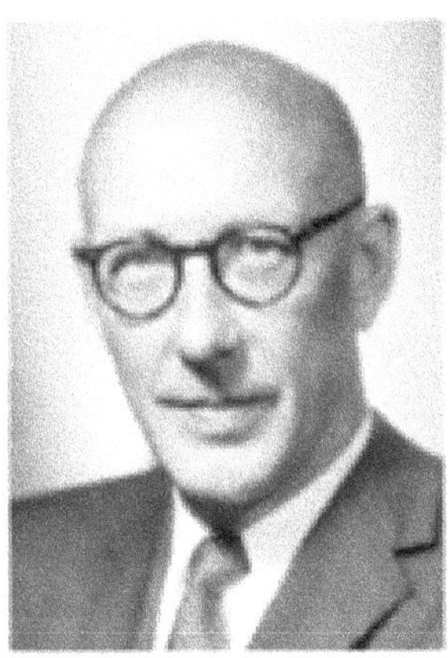

Edward Lawrie
Tatum

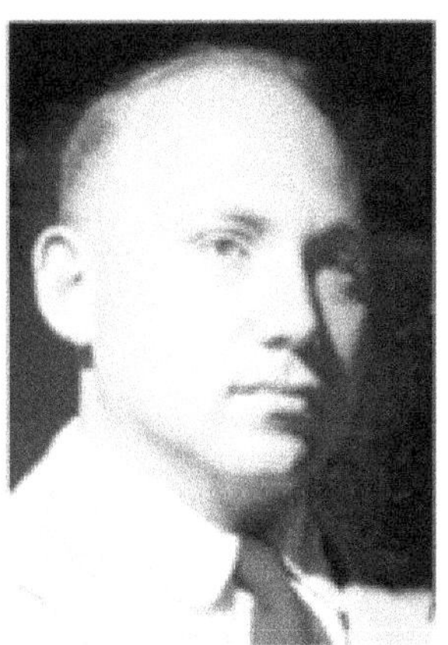

Joshua Lederberg

History

George Wells Beadle, born on October 22, 1903, in Wahoo, Nebraska, USA, and Edward Lawrie Tatum, born on December 14, 1909, in Boulder, Colorado, USA, collaborated on research that demonstrated the role of genes in regulating biochemical events within cells. Their work with the bread mold Neurospora crassa in the early 1940s established the one gene-one enzyme hypothesis, laying the groundwork for the field of molecular biology.

Joshua Lederberg, born on May 23, 1925, in Montclair, New Jersey, USA, was recognized for his discoveries concerning genetic recombination and the organization of the genetic material of bacteria, further broadening the understanding of genetic inheritance and variation.

Current Implications

The groundbreaking work of Beadle, Tatum, and Lederberg has had rooted implications in the fields of genetics, medicine, and biochemistry. Their discoveries have facilitated the development of genetic engineering, the understanding of hereditary diseases, and the exploration of new treatments for genetic disorders, impacting both clinical practices and therapeutic strategies.

Impact and Products

The collective achievements of these laureates have been central to the advancement of medical genetics. The one gene-one enzyme hypothesis and the understanding of bacterial genetics have been instrumental in the development of antibiotics, the study of genetic diseases, and the exploration of genetic therapy options.

This trio of scientists significantly advanced our understanding of genetics and its application to medical science.

SEVERO OCHOA AND ARTHUR KORNBERG (1959)

This genius pair took us to the doorsteps of a new world of DNA and RNA

In 1959, Severo Ochoa and Arthur Kornberg were jointly awarded the Nobel Prize in Medicine for their groundbreaking discoveries in the mechanisms of the biological synthesis of RNA and DNA, the molecules essential for genetic information and cellular processes.

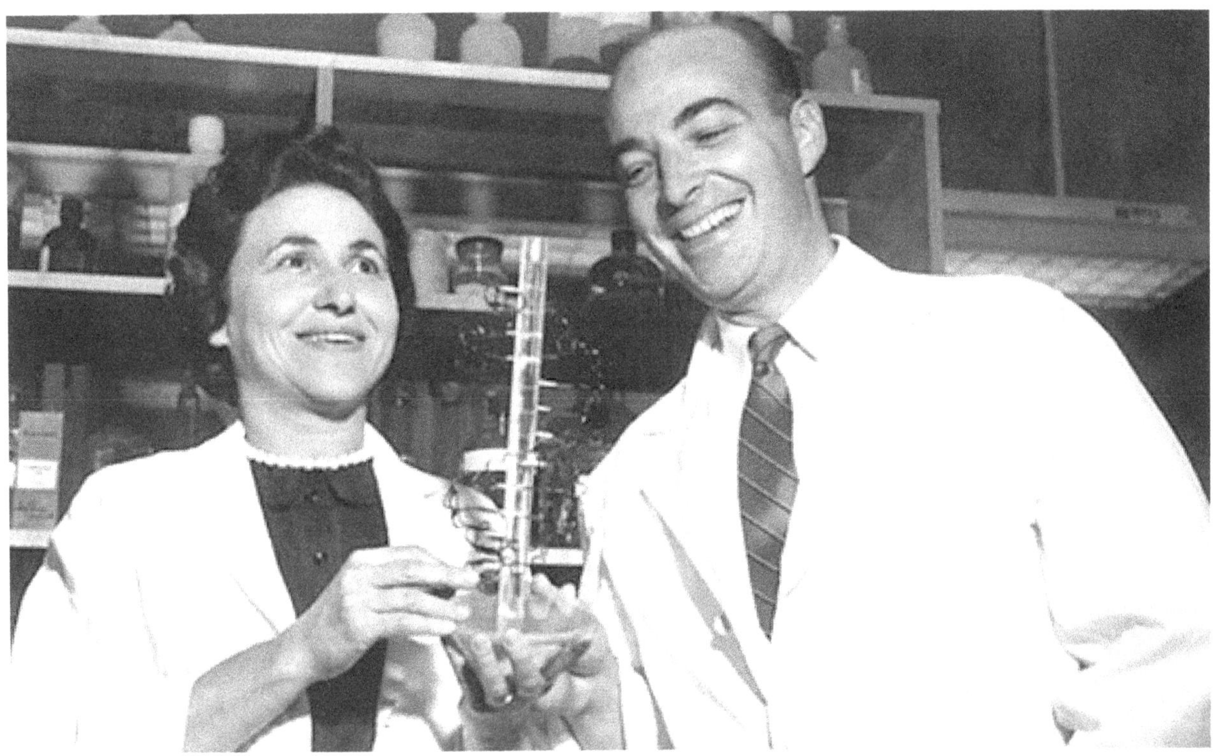

History

Severo Ochoa, born on September 24, 1905, in Luarca, Spain, made significant contributions to understanding how DNA and RNA are synthesized. Working at New York University College of Medicine, Ochoa's work on the enzymatic process of RNA synthesis laid foundational stones for molecular biology.

Arthur Kornberg, born on March 3, 1918, in Brooklyn, New York, and affiliated with Stanford University at the time of the award, discovered DNA polymerase, the enzyme responsible for DNA synthesis. His research provided critical insights into how genetic information is copied and passed from one generation to the next.

Current Implications

The work of Ochoa and Kornberg has profoundly impacted the field of genetics and molecular biology, providing essential knowledge for understanding genetic diseases, genetic engineering, and the development of biotechnological applications. Their discoveries have enabled further research into gene expression, replication, and the manipulation of genetic material, which has numerous medical and scientific applications.

Impact and Products

The discovery of the mechanisms behind the synthesis of RNA and DNA by Ochoa and Kornberg has been pivotal in the advancement of modern biology and medicine. It has facilitated the development of various biotechnological tools and techniques, including genetic editing tools like CRISPR-Cas9, and has contributed to the fight against genetic disorders through gene therapy.

Their work not only enhanced our understanding of life's molecular foundations but also opened new pathways for drug development and therapeutic interventions against a wide array of diseases.

SIR FRANK MACFARLANE BURNET AND PETER MEDAWAR (1960)

A watershed moment in Immunology, the concept of Immune Tolerance & Autoimmunity

In 1960, Sir Frank Macfarlane Burnet and Peter Brian Medawar were jointly awarded the Nobel Prize in Medicine for their discovery of acquired immunological tolerance. This concept has become a foundational principle in the field of immunology and has profound implications for organ transplantation and the treatment of autoimmune diseases.

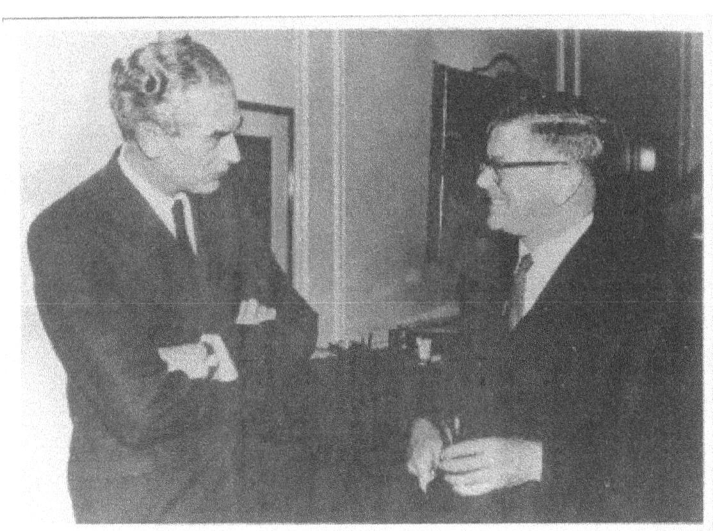

History

Sir Frank Macfarlane Burnet, born on September 3, 1899, in Traralgon, Australia, pursued his medical degree at the University of Melbourne, graduating in 1924. His early research focused on bacteriophages and virus culturing techniques, contributing significantly to virology and immunology. Burnet's career was notably distinguished by his leadership at the Walter and Eliza Hall Institute of Medical Research in Melbourne, where he served as director and professor of experimental medicine at the University of Melbourne.

Peter Brian Medawar, born on February 28, 1915, in Rio de Janeiro, Brazil, was celebrated for his work in graft rejection and the immune response, providing experimental evidence supporting Burnet's theory of acquired immunological tolerance. Medawar's research laid the groundwork for understanding how the immune system distinguishes between self and non-self, a critical factor in the success of organ transplants.

Current Implications

The discovery of acquired immunological tolerance by Burnet and Medawar has had lasting impacts on medicine, particularly in the fields of organ transplantation and autoimmune disease treatment. Their work has enabled the development of therapies that can induce tolerance to transplanted organs, reducing the risk of rejection and improving transplant outcomes.

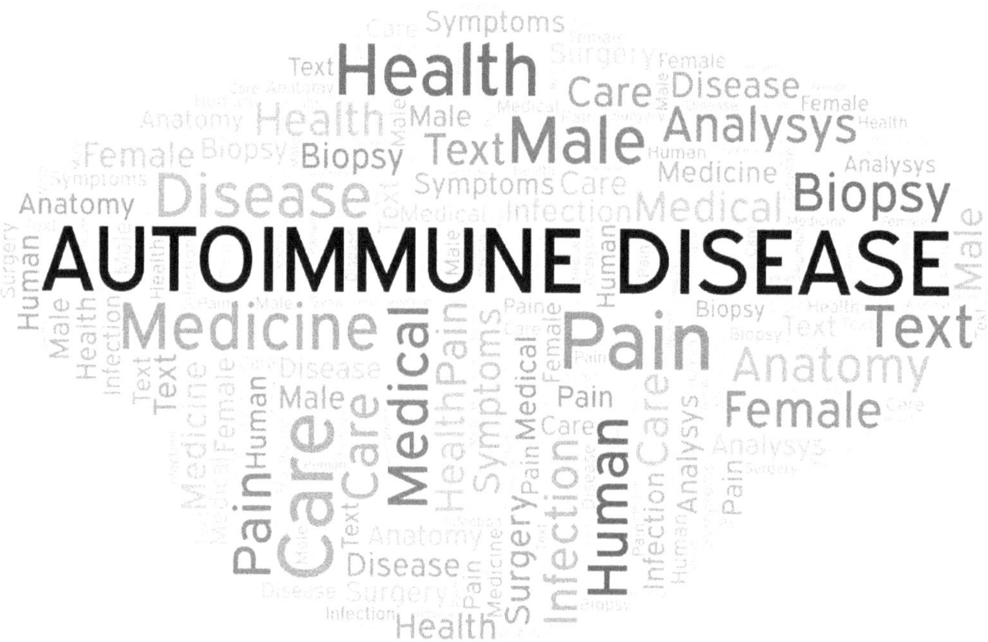

Impact and Products

The principles of immunological tolerance discovered by Burnet and Medawar continue to influence immunological research and clinical practices. Their pioneering work has not only facilitated the advancement of organ transplantation but also opened avenues for novel treatments of autoimmune diseases, where the immune system's tolerance mechanisms can be harnessed or mimicked to prevent the body from attacking its own tissues.

GEORG VON BÉKÉSY (1961)

Father of cochlear biology, who proved how sound waves are converted to nerve impulse

Georg von Békésy was awarded the Nobel Prize in Medicine in 1961 for his discoveries regarding the physical mechanisms of stimulation within the cochlea, a crucial part of the inner ear involved in hearing.

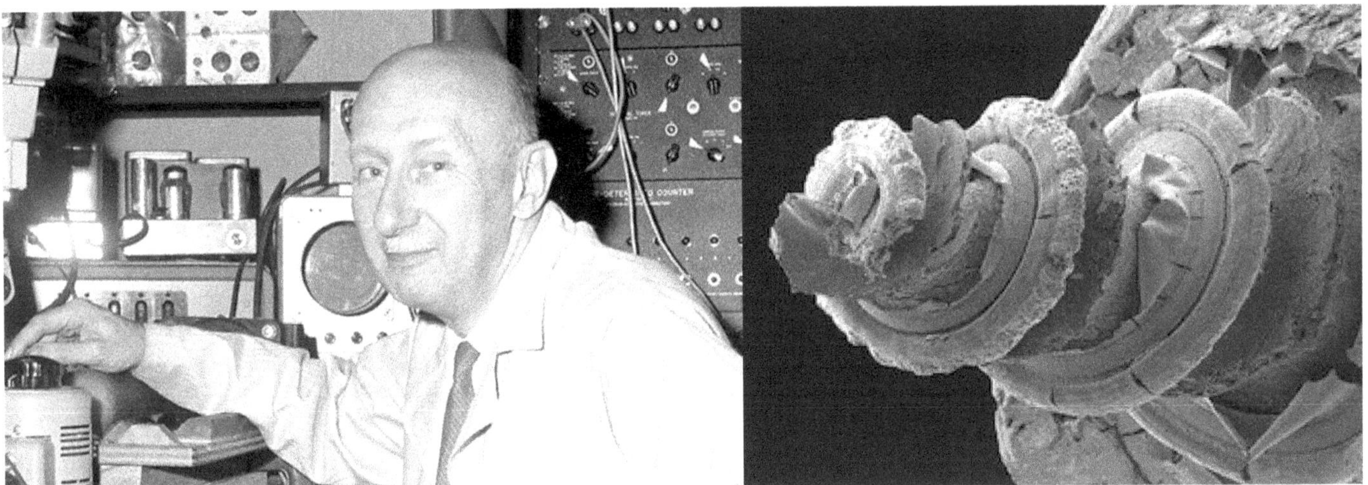

History

Born on June 3, 1899, in Budapest, Hungary, into a diplomatic family, von Békésy was exposed to a variety of cultures and educational systems from a young age. His academic pursuits took him to Munich, Constantinople, and Zurich before he embarked on a study of chemistry at the University of Berne. His transition to physics, culminating in a Ph.D. from the University of Budapest, marked the beginning of his distinguished career.

Von Békésy's professional journey was intertwined with his work at the Hungarian Post Office, where his responsibilities led him to investigate telecommunication systems. This role, seemingly unrelated to physiology, unexpectedly steered him toward the study of the human ear and hearing mechanics. His curiosity about the ear was partly driven by the technical challenges of improving long-distance telephone communication.

In 1946, after the tumult of World War II, von Békésy left Hungary to continue his research in Sweden at the Karolinska Institute. A year later, he moved to the United States, where he joined Harvard University. It was here, in the Psycho-Acoustic Laboratory, that von Békésy embarked on the groundbreaking research that would earn him the Nobel Prize. His innovative experiments on the cochlea of the inner ear laid the foundation for understanding how sound is converted into nerve impulses—a question that had puzzled scientists for decades.

Snippets

Revolutionizing Understanding of the Cochlea: Von Békésy's meticulous research unveiled how the cochlea in the inner ear decodes sound vibrations. By dissecting the cochlea and using innovative techniques like stroboscopic photography, he observed how different frequencies of sound create specific patterns of vibration along the basilar membrane. This finding was crucial in demonstrating the physical mechanism of sound frequency discrimination within the ear.

Tonotopy Concept: His experiments led to the discovery of tonotopy, a principle stating that different parts of the cochlea are activated by different frequencies of sound. High frequencies stimulate areas closer to the base of the cochlea, while lower frequencies affect regions toward the apex. This discovery provided a physical explanation for the perception of pitch and frequency in hearing.

Mechanical Models of the Ear: Von Békésy created mechanical models to simulate the inner ear's function further. These models, which used the human arm to represent nerve supply, replicated how sound waves are processed within the cochlea, offering tangible insights into the complex processes that enable hearing. His innovative approach to modeling the inner ear's mechanics contributed significantly to the field of auditory physiology.

Interdisciplinary Approach: Starting his career in telecommunications, von Békésy's transition to studying the ear's mechanics exemplifies the power of interdisciplinary research. His background in physics and experience in telecommunications provided him with unique perspectives and methodologies, which he successfully applied to unravel the mysteries of hearing.

Early Researchers

Hermann von Helmholtz, a 19th-century physicist and physician known for his theory on the perception of sound. Helmholtz proposed the concept of resonance in the cochlea, suggesting that different parts of the cochlea vibrate in response to different frequencies of sound. Although aspects of his resonance theory were later revised by von Békésy's work, Helmholtz's contributions to the study of acoustics and the physiology of hearing were foundational.

Another significant figure is Lord Rayleigh (John William Strutt), an English physicist who made substantial contributions to acoustics, including the theory of sound propagation and resonance. His work provided a mathematical and physical understanding of sound that was critical for later studies on hearing.

Thomas Young, an English polymath, contributed to the understanding of the mechanics of the human body, including the eye and vision, but his work on wave theory also indirectly influenced auditory science.

Ernst Heinrich Weber and Gustav Theodor Fechner were early experimenters in the psychology of perception, including hearing. Their work on the just-noticeable difference (the smallest change in a stimulus that can be detected) was among the first to quantify sensory experiences, paving the way for psychoacoustics, a field that von Békésy would later contribute to significantly.

Current Implications

Enhanced Diagnostic Techniques: The understanding of cochlear mechanics has led to the development of sophisticated diagnostic tools for hearing impairments. Techniques such as otoacoustic emissions (OAE) testing and auditory brainstem response (ABR) testing rely on principles uncovered by von Békésy, allowing for early detection of hearing loss in infants and adults.

Cochlear Implant Development: Von Békésy's work is directly relevant to the design and function of cochlear implants. These devices, which convert sound into electrical signals that directly stimulate the auditory nerve, are designed with a deep understanding of how different frequencies are processed within the cochlea. This has transformed the lives of many with profound hearing loss, enabling them to perceive sound in a way that closely mimics natural hearing.

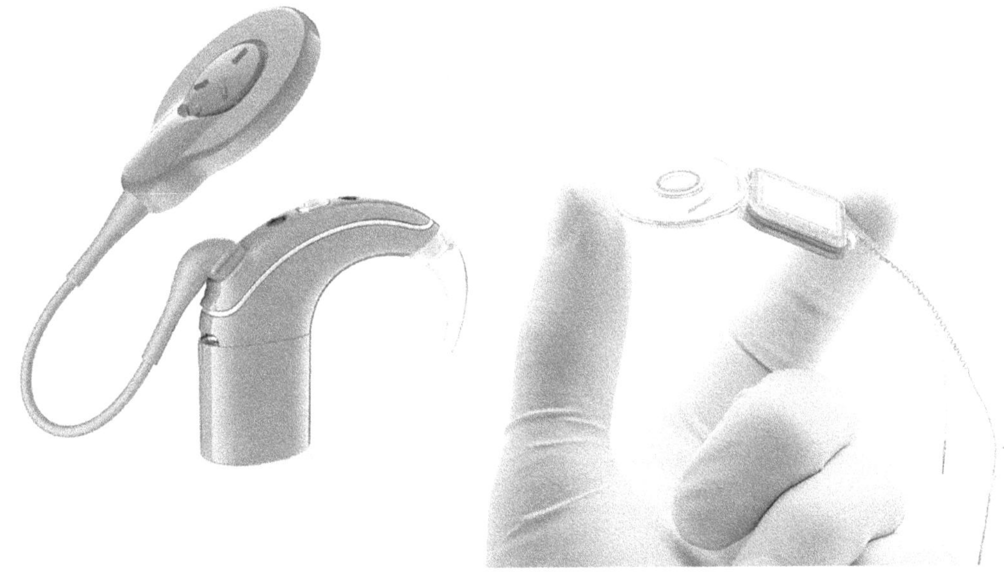

Laid the foundation for modern cochlear transplants

Auditory Neuroscience Research: The exploration of how the inner ear converts sound into neural signals has opened up new avenues in auditory neuroscience, leading to a better understanding of how the brain processes and interprets sound. This research is crucial for developing treatments for auditory processing disorders and improving educational strategies for the hearing impaired.

Hearing Aid Technology: Modern hearing aids are increasingly sophisticated, with many utilizing digital processing to selectively amplify certain frequencies based on the user's specific hearing loss profile. This customization capability stems from an understanding of the cochlea's frequency-specific response to sound, a concept first elucidated by von Békésy.

Psychoacoustics and Sound Design: In the realm of psychoacoustics, von Békésy's findings have implications for how sound is engineered and manipulated in environments ranging from concert halls to headphones. By understanding how sound is perceived, designers can create auditory experiences that are more pleasing, more immersive, and tailored to the human ear's specific sensitivities.

Impact and Products

Advanced Hearing Assessment Tools: Von Békésy's insights into cochlear mechanics have led to the development of advanced auditory assessment tools that offer precise measurements of hearing capabilities and impairments. These tools are fundamental in diagnosing various types of hearing loss and tailoring individual rehabilitation plans.

Next-Generation Cochlear Implants: Building on the foundational understanding of cochlear function, next-generation cochlear implants have been developed to more accurately mimic natural hearing processes. These devices now feature sophisticated algorithms designed to enhance speech recognition in noisy environments, improving the quality of life for users.

Customized Hearing Aids: The evolution of hearing aid technology has been significantly influenced by von Békésy's work. Modern hearing aids not only amplify sound but also process and modify it to match the user's specific hearing loss profile, providing a customized hearing experience. This includes features like directional microphones, noise reduction technologies, and wireless connectivity, all designed to optimize hearing in various environments.

Educational Software and Virtual Models: The principles of cochlear mechanics discovered by von Békésy have been incorporated into educational software and virtual models, providing students and professionals with interactive learning experiences. These tools help demystify the complex processes of hearing and are invaluable for training audiologists and other hearing professionals.

Noise-Canceling Headphones: Inspired by the understanding of how sound is perceived and processed, noise-canceling headphone technology has been refined to more effectively reduce unwanted ambient sounds. This technology uses principles of sound wave interference, a concept that underlies much of auditory physics and has direct links to von Békésy's research.

Tinnitus Management Devices: Insights into the cochlea's function have informed the development of devices and therapies aimed at managing tinnitus, a condition often related to cochlear damage. These include sound therapy devices that use specific sounds to minimize the perception of tinnitus, offering relief to those affected.

Speech Therapy Tools: Understanding the cochlear mechanics has also impacted the field of speech therapy, particularly in the development of tools and methods for helping individuals with hearing loss and speech defects. These tools often utilize visual or tactile feedback mechanisms based on how sound frequencies are processed within the ear.

FRANCIS CRICK, JAMES WATSON, MAURICE WILKINS (1962)

The triplet claimed the Nobel for demonstration of double helix in DNA

Francis Crick, James Watson, and Maurice Wilkins were awarded the Nobel Prize in Medicine in 1962 for their groundbreaking work in discovering the molecular structure of nucleic acids and its significance for information transfer in living material.

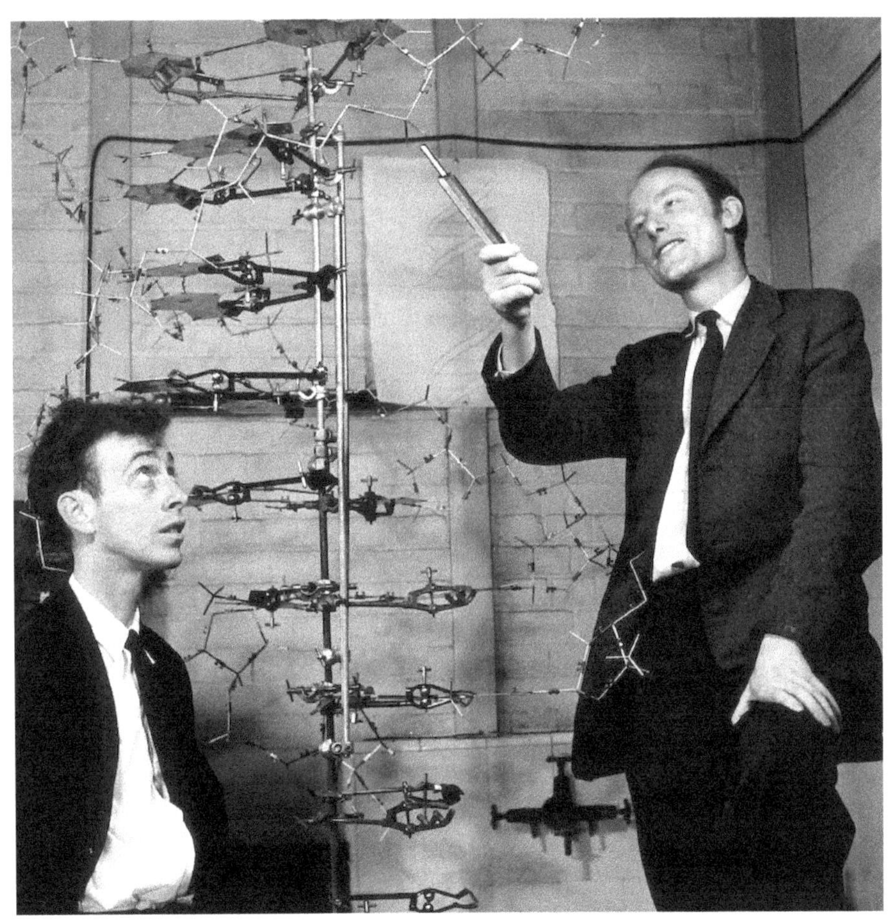

History

Francis Crick, born in 1916 in Northampton, England, had a background in physics and biophysics. He joined the Medical Research Council Unit at the Cavendish Laboratory in Cambridge, where he would eventually meet James Watson. Crick's initial research focused on X-ray diffraction.

James Watson, an American geneticist born in 1928, arrived in Cambridge in 1951 after studying at the University of Chicago and Indiana University. Eager to uncover the secrets of the gene,

Watson's interest in DNA led him to collaborate with Crick, despite their differing scientific backgrounds.

Maurice Wilkins, born in New Zealand in 1916, worked at King's College London. His work involved X-ray diffraction studies of DNA, which would later provide crucial evidence supporting the double helix model. Wilkins's contribution to understanding DNA's structure was foundational, yet his role is often overshadowed by the more publicized partnership of Watson and Crick.

Snippets

The Double Helix Model: In 1953, Watson and Crick proposed the double helix structure of DNA, suggesting that DNA is composed of two strands that wind around each other, with pairs of bases (adenine with thymine, and cytosine with guanine) forming the rungs of a spiraling ladder. This model was crucial for understanding how genetic information is stored and replicated.

X-ray Diffraction Evidence: Maurice Wilkins and Rosalind Franklin's work on X-ray diffraction was pivotal in confirming the double helix structure. Franklin's photograph, known as Photo 51, provided critical evidence of the helical structure of DNA, although her contributions were only fully recognized posthumously.

Impact on Science: Their discovery has had a profound and wide-ranging impact, paving the way for advancements in genetics, molecular biology, and biotechnology. It has been fundamental to the development of DNA sequencing, genetic engineering, and our understanding of genetic diseases and evolution.

Legacy and Controversy: While the discovery has been celebrated for its monumental contribution to science, it has also been scrutinized for the dynamics between the involved parties, especially the acknowledgment of Rosalind Franklin's critical contributions. The story of the double helix is as much about scientific ingenuity as it is about the complexities of collaboration and recognition in scientific research.

Forgotten Heros

Rosalind Franklin stands out as a pivotal yet often overlooked character. Her work with X-ray diffraction provided crucial evidence that underpinned the model proposed by Watson and Crick. Franklin's famous "Photo 51," an X-ray diffraction image of DNA, demonstrated the helical str ucture of DNA with clarity and precision.

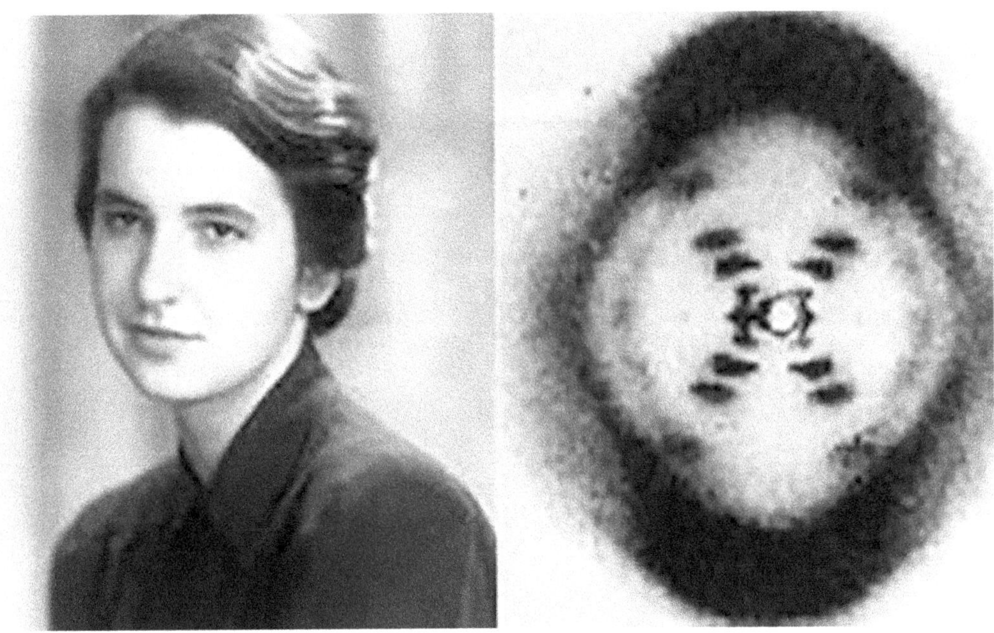

Rosalind Franklin & Photo 51

Another significant figure is Raymond Gosling, a doctoral student who worked closely with Franklin. It was Gosling who actually took Photo 51 under Franklin's guidance, and his role in capturing this critical piece of evidence is often overshadowed by his more famous colleagues.

Aaron Klug, a later collaborator with Franklin, continued her work on the structural analysis of viruses and eventually won a Nobel Prize for Chemistry in 1982. While Klug's work was recognized, his contributions underscore the continuity of research that began with Franklin and others who laid the groundwork for molecular biology.

Jerry Donohue, a lesser-known chemist, also played a crucial role. His advice to Watson on the correct tautomeric forms of the DNA bases was critical for the accurate modeling of the DNA structure. Donohue's contribution was a key piece of the puzzle that allowed Watson and Crick to correct their model and ultimately solve the structure of DNA.

Current Implications

Genetic Research and Medicine: The elucidation of DNA's structure has been foundational for genetic research, enabling the sequencing of the human genome. This knowledge has facilitated advances in personalized medicine, allowing for treatments tailored to individual genetic profiles, significantly impacting cancer treatment, rare diseases, and other genetic disorders.

Biotechnology and Synthetic Biology: Understanding DNA's structure has propelled developments in biotechnology, including the engineering of microorganisms to produce pharmaceuticals, biofuels, and other useful compounds. Synthetic biology, which aims to redesign organisms for specific purposes, also relies heavily on insights derived from DNA's double helix.

Forensic Science: DNA fingerprinting, based on understanding DNA's unique structure and sequence variations among individuals, has transformed forensic science. It provides a powerful tool for identifying individuals in criminal investigations and resolving paternity and ancestry questions.

Evolutionary Biology: The discovery has deepened our understanding of evolutionary processes, allowing scientists to trace the genetic lineage of species and understand their evolutionary relationships. This insight is crucial for studying biodiversity and the mechanisms of evolution.

Agriculture: Advances in genetic engineering, informed by the structure of DNA, have led to the development of genetically modified organisms (GMOs) that are more resistant to pests, diseases, and environmental stresses. This has significant implications for food security and agricultural sustainability.

Ethics and Society: The ability to manipulate DNA has raised ethical, legal, and social issues, including concerns about genetic privacy, the use of genetic information, and the implications of gene editing technologies like CRISPR-Cas9. These discussions are critical as society navigates the benefits and challenges of genetic and genomic research.

Impact and Products

CRISPR-Cas9 Gene Editing: This revolutionary technology, which allows for precise editing of the DNA sequence in living organisms, stems from an understanding of DNA's structure and function. CRISPR-Cas9 has applications in medicine, agriculture, and research, enabling the correction of genetic defects, the creation of disease-resistant crops, and the study of genes' roles in health and disease.

Synthetic Genomics: Advances in synthetic biology have led to the creation of synthetic genomes, with the potential to design organisms that produce pharmaceuticals, biofuels, and other valuable compounds more efficiently. This field relies heavily on the foundational knowledge of DNA's structure and the mechanisms of gene expression and regulation.

Direct-to-Consumer Genetic Testing: The availability of genetic testing kits has democratized access to genetic information, allowing individuals to learn about their ancestry, genetic predispositions to certain health conditions, and traits. This consumer product directly stems from the understanding of DNA as the blueprint of life.

Vaccine Development: The structural understanding of DNA has accelerated vaccine development, most notably in the rapid creation of mRNA vaccines for COVID-19. These vaccines use a synthetic segment of the virus's genetic material to elicit an immune response, showcasing a direct application of molecular biology in public health.

Data Storage: Research into using DNA as a medium for data storage is an innovative application of understanding DNA's structure. DNA offers a compact, durable medium with a vast capacity for storing information, which could revolutionize data storage technologies in the future.

Forensic Developments: Beyond DNA fingerprinting, the field of forensic science has seen advancements in techniques such as phenotyping, where predictions about physical appearance and ancestry are made based on DNA samples. This application has significant implications for law enforcement and historical research.

ALAN HODGKIN, ANDREW HUXLEY AND JOHN ECCLES, (1963)

Crossed new frontiers in the Molecular basis of Neurobiology, Ionic channels & action potentials

The Nobel Prize in Medicine in 1963 was awarded to Sir John Carew Eccles, Alan Lloyd Hodgkin, and Andrew Fielding Huxley for their discoveries concerning the ionic mechanisms involved in excitation and inhibition in the peripheral and central portions of the nerve cell membranc.

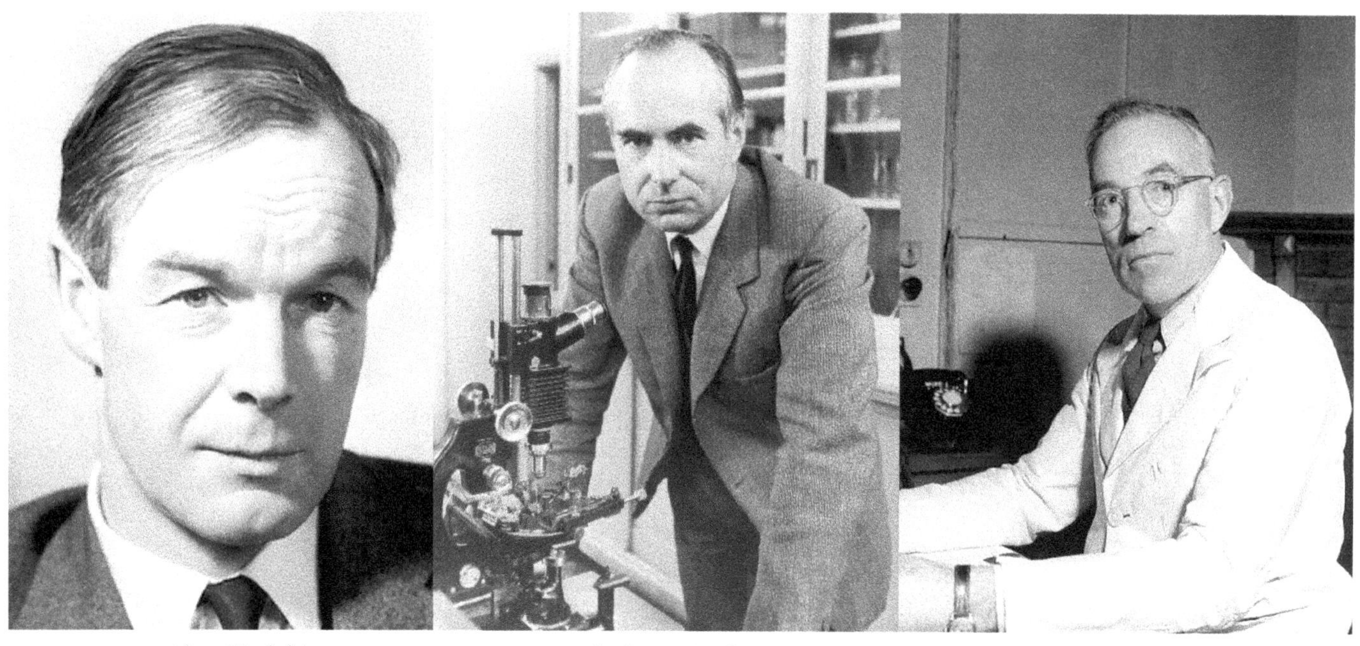

| Alan Hodgkin | Andrew Huxley | John Eccles |

History

Sir John Eccles, born in Melbourne, Australia, in 1903, pursued his fascination with the human brain and nervous system throughout his career. Moving from Australia to Oxford as a Rhodes Scholar, Eccles's research journey was profoundly influenced by his work on synaptic transmission and neuronal communication, leading to significant insights into how neurons communicate and the role of synapses in this process.

Alan Lloyd Hodgkin, born in 1914 in Banbury, England, and Andrew Fielding Huxley, born in 1917 in Hampstead, London, started on their collaborative research journey during their time together at the

University of Cambridge. Their work was primarily focused on understanding the electrical activities of neurons. By experimenting with the giant axon of the squid, they were able to elucidate the dynamic changes in ionic concentrations that underlie nerve impulse propagation, a discovery that laid the foundation for modern neurophysiology.

Eccles's work complemented Hodgkin and Huxley's findings by exploring the mechanisms of synaptic transmission, particularly the distinction between excitatory and inhibitory synapses and their role in neuronal communication. His experiments further elucidated how synaptic inputs are integrated by neurons to produce coordinated responses, enhancing our understanding of the complex signaling that underlies brain function.

Snippets

Ionic Movements and Action Potentials: Demonstrated how specific ionic movements across the neuron's membrane are essential for generating action potentials, the fundamental electrical signals for nerve communication.

Understanding Synaptic Function: Revealed the critical role of synapses in transmitting nerve impulses between neurons, essentially dictating how information is relayed within the nervous system.

Differentiation of Synapses: Their work highlighted the existence of two main types of synapses: excitatory, which stimulate nerve cell activity, and inhibitory, which reduce or prevent nerve cell activity. This distinction is crucial for the modulation and integration of sensory inputs and motor outputs.

Mechanism of Nerve Impulse Propagation: Explored how action potentials are propagated along neurons, providing insight into the rapid transmission of information across different parts of the nervous system.

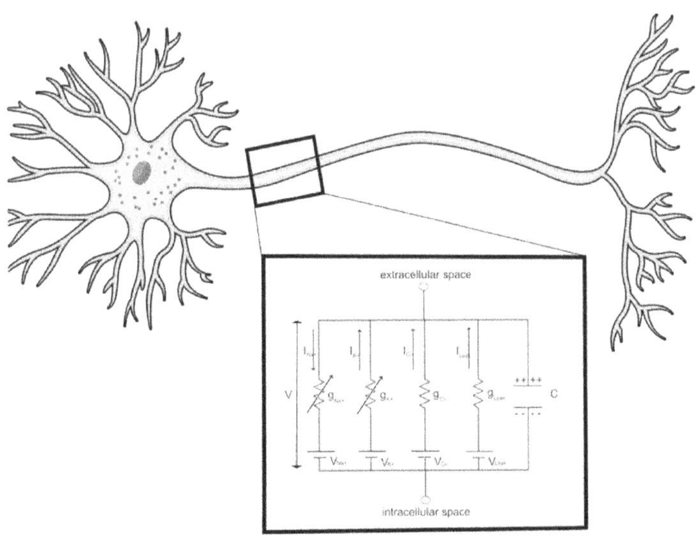

Synaptic Plasticity Insight: Although not directly part of their initial findings, their research laid the groundwork for understanding synaptic plasticity—the ability of synapses to strengthen or weaken over time, which is key to learning and memory.

Basis for Neurological Treatments: The trio's discoveries have informed the development of treatments for neurological conditions by targeting specific ionic channels and neurotransmitter systems affected in diseases like epilepsy and anxiety disorders.

Early Researchers

Julius Bernstein, a German physiologist who, in the late 19th and early 20th centuries, proposed the "membrane theory" of electrical conduction in neurons. His work on the bioelectric potentials in living tissues set the stage for the later detailed studies of nerve impulse conduction by Hodgkin, Huxley, and Eccles.

Another notable pioneer is Luigi Galvani, an Italian physician and physicist from the 18th century, whose experiments with frog legs were among the first to demonstrate the electrical basis of nerve impulses. Although his interpretation of "animal electricity" was not fully accurate, his observations sparked further research into bioelectricity, ultimately leading to the development of electrophysiology.

In more recent times, the contributions of Bernard Katz to the field of synaptic transmission cannot be overstated. His work, alongside Eccles, on the quantal hypothesis and neurotransmitter release mechanisms provided a molecular understanding of how neurons communicate across synapses. Katz's experiments elucidated the role of acetylcholine as a neurotransmitter and laid the foundation for the study of chemical synapses.

Current Implications

Neurological Disorders: Their research has significantly enhanced our understanding of neurological disorders such as epilepsy, Alzheimer's disease, and multiple sclerosis. By understanding the mechanisms of nerve cell function and signal transmission, researchers are better equipped to develop targeted treatments and interventions for these conditions.

Neuropharmacology: The trio's work has also influenced the field of neuropharmacology, enabling the development of drugs that specifically target ion channels and neurotransmitter systems. This has led to more effective medications with fewer side effects for treating psychiatric disorders, chronic pain, and other conditions related to nerve function.

Neural Engineering and Neuroprosthetics: Insights into how neurons transmit signals have propelled advancements in neural engineering, including the development of neuroprosthetic devices that can restore lost functions, such as cochlear implants for hearing loss or retinal implants for vision impairment. These devices rely on the principles of nerve impulse transmission to interface effectively with the nervous system.

Computational Neuroscience: The Hodgkin-Huxley model, a mathematical description of the action potential in neurons, has become a cornerstone of computational neuroscience. It allows researchers to simulate neural behavior and understand complex neural networks, contributing to the development of artificial intelligence and machine learning algorithms inspired by the functioning of the brain.

Education and Training: The legacy of Eccles, Hodgkin, and Huxley extends into neuroscience education, where their discoveries are fundamental to the curriculum. Students and professionals alike learn about their contributions as a basis for further study and research in neurobiology and related fields.

Impact and Products

Advanced Diagnostic Tools: Their discoveries have led to the development of sophisticated diagnostic tools for neurological and neuromuscular disorders. Techniques like electromyography (EMG) and nerve conduction studies, which assess the health of muscles and the nerve cells that control them, rely on understanding the electrical activity of nerve cells. These tools are crucial for diagnosing conditions such as peripheral neuropathy and myopathy.

Neuromodulation Devices: Inspired by the understanding of how nerve signals are transmitted, neuromodulation devices such as deep brain stimulators have been developed. These devices deliver electrical impulses to specific parts of the brain to treat neurological conditions such as Parkinson's disease, essential tremor, and dystonia, offering life-changing improvements for many patients.

Pain Management Therapies: Understanding the ionic mechanisms behind nerve impulse transmission has led to better-targeted pain management therapies. Transcutaneous Electrical Nerve Stimulation (TENS) devices, for example, use low-voltage electrical currents to relieve pain, a method that stems from a deeper understanding of how nerve cells communicate pain signals.

Ion Channel Research and Drug Development: The trio's work has catalyzed research into ion channels, leading to the development of drugs that target these channels to treat a variety of conditions. For instance, certain antiepileptic drugs work by modifying ion channel activity to prevent seizures. This area of drug development continues to expand as researchers discover new therapeutic targets based on ion channel function.

KONRAD BLOCH AND FEODOR LYNEN (1964)

Drew the molecular blue print of cholesterol and lipid metabolism

In 1964, Konrad Bloch and Feodor Lynen were jointly awarded the Nobel Prize in Medicine for their pivotal discoveries concerning the mechanism and regulation of cholesterol and fatty acid metabolism. This work laid the foundation for our understanding of vital biochemical pathways.

History

Konrad Bloch, born on January 21, 1912, in Neisse, Germany, embarked on his academic and research journey that led him to significant findings in lipid metabolism after moving to the United States and obtaining his Ph.D. at Columbia University.

Feodor Lynen, born on April 6, 1911, in Munich, Germany, made his mark in biochemistry through his research on the metabolism of cholesterol and fatty acids.

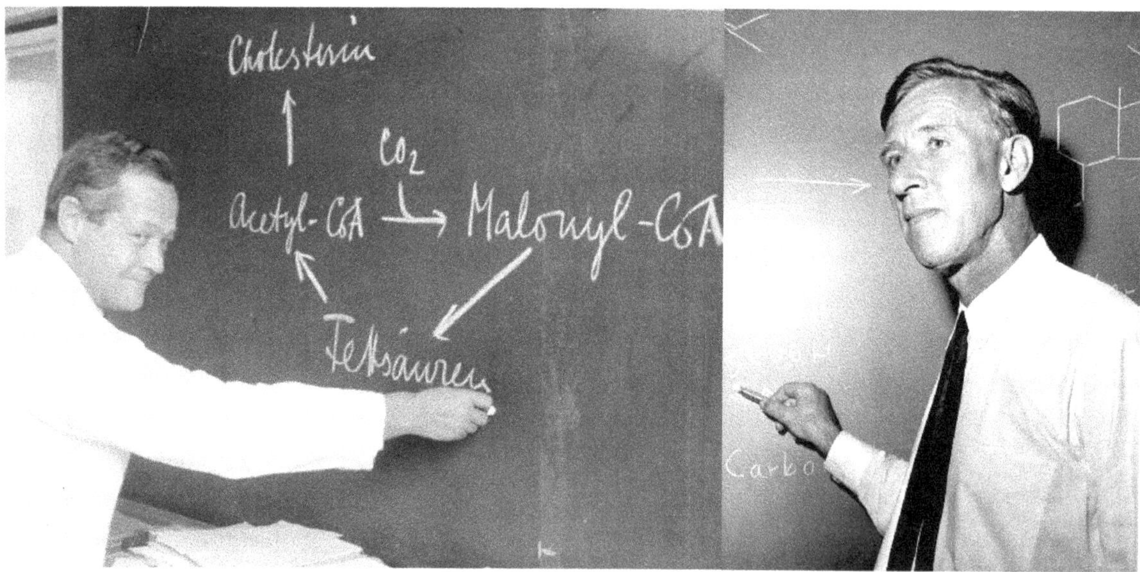

Snippets

Bloch's work, particularly on the biosynthesis of cholesterol and unsaturated fatty acids, highlighted the complex processes governing lipid metabolism.

Lynen's academic pursuits at the University of Munich culminated in groundbreaking work that detailed the biochemical pathways essential for the synthesis of cholesterol and fatty acids, significantly advancing our understanding of cellular metabolism.

Current Implications

The discoveries by Bloch and Lynen have had a profound impact on the field of biochemistry, shedding light on the metabolic processes that are crucial for the maintenance of cellular and physiological functions. Their work has informed research in various medical and scientific areas, including the development of treatments for cholesterol-related conditions and metabolic disorders.

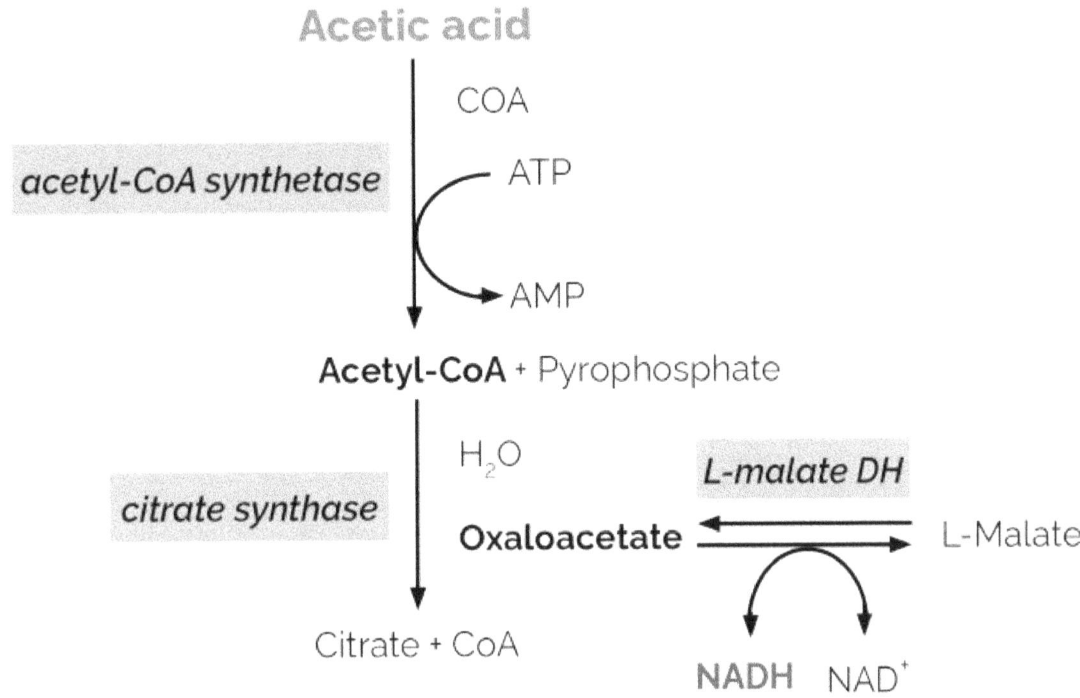

They decoded the Acetyl COA which represents a critical node in metabolism due to its intersection with all the three key metabolic pathways and transformations namely Carbohydrate, Protein and Fat

Impact and Products

Their research has been instrumental in developing strategies for managing and treating diseases related to lipid metabolism, such as cardiovascular diseases. The detailed understanding of cholesterol and fatty acid metabolism provided by their work continues to influence scientific research and healthcare practices, contributing to advancements in drug development and therapeutic interventions.

FRANÇOIS JACOB, ANDRÉ LWOFF, JACQUES MONOD (1965)

Vital new studies on genetic control of enzymes

In 1965, François Jacob, André Lwoff, and Jacques Monod were collectively awarded the Nobel Prize in Medicine for their pioneering contributions to molecular biology, specifically for their discoveries on the genetic control of enzyme and virus synthesis.

History

François Jacob, born on June 17, 1920, in Nancy, France, André Lwoff, born on May 8, 1902, in Ainay-le-Château, France, and Jacques Monod, born on February 9, 1910, in Paris, France, were instrumental figures in the early days of molecular biology.

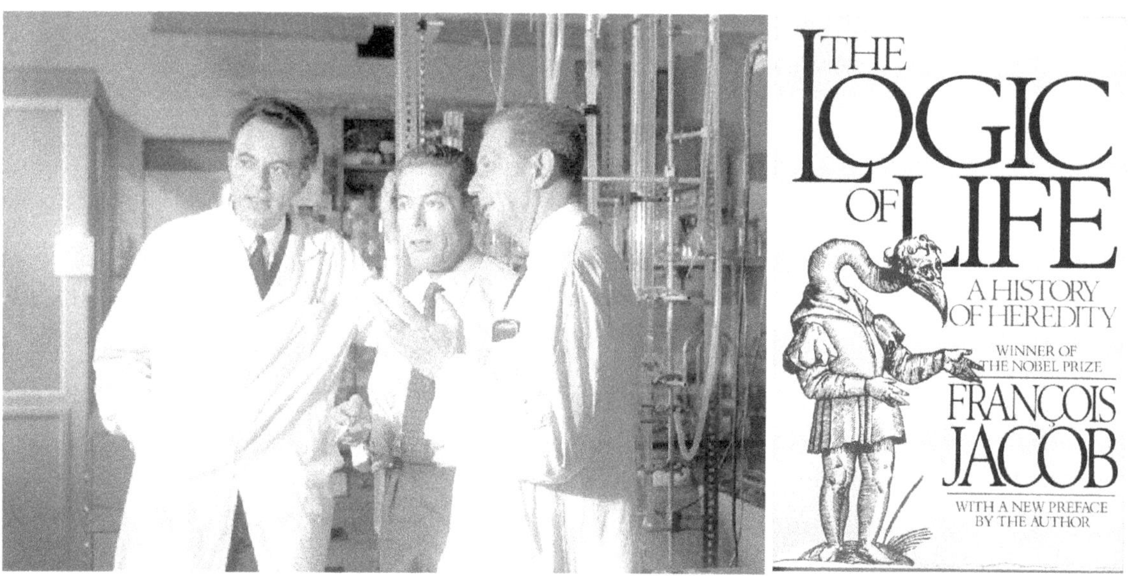

Their work at the Pasteur Institute brought to light the complex mechanisms by which genetic information controls the synthesis of enzymes and viruses, laying the groundwork for modern genetics and molecular biology.

Snippets

Jacob and Monod's elucidation of the operon model was a landmark discovery, demonstrating how genes are turned on or off in bacteria, a process that is fundamental to the genetic regulation of cells. Lwoff's contributions to understanding the lysogeny in bacteria, where viruses can exist in a dormant state within their host, further expanded the horizons of microbiology and virology.

Current Implications

The discoveries made by Jacob, Lwoff, and Monod have had profound implications for our understanding of gene regulation and cellular processes. Their work has been crucial in developing genetic engineering and biotechnology, allowing scientists to manipulate genetic material for research, medical, and industrial purposes.

Impact and Products

The advancements in genetic engineering, biotechnology, and the treatment of genetic disorders are directly linked to the foundational work of Jacob, Lwoff, and Monod. Their research has paved the way for the development of gene therapy, genetically modified organisms, and numerous biotechnological innovations that have revolutionized medicine and industry.

PEYTON ROUS AND CHARLES HUGGINS (1966)

The clandestine connect between the virus and cancers were exposed

In 1966, Peyton Rous and Charles Huggins were awarded the Nobel Prize in Medicine for their groundbreaking work in cancer research. Rous was recognized for his discovery of tumor-inducing viruses, and Huggins for his discoveries concerning the hormonal treatment of prostatic cancer.

History

Peyton Rous, born on October 5, 1879, in Baltimore, Maryland, USA, embarked on a path that led him to discover the Rous sarcoma virus, the first virus known to cause cancer in animals. His work at the Rockefeller University in New York played a pivotal role in establishing virology as a field and linking viruses to cancer.

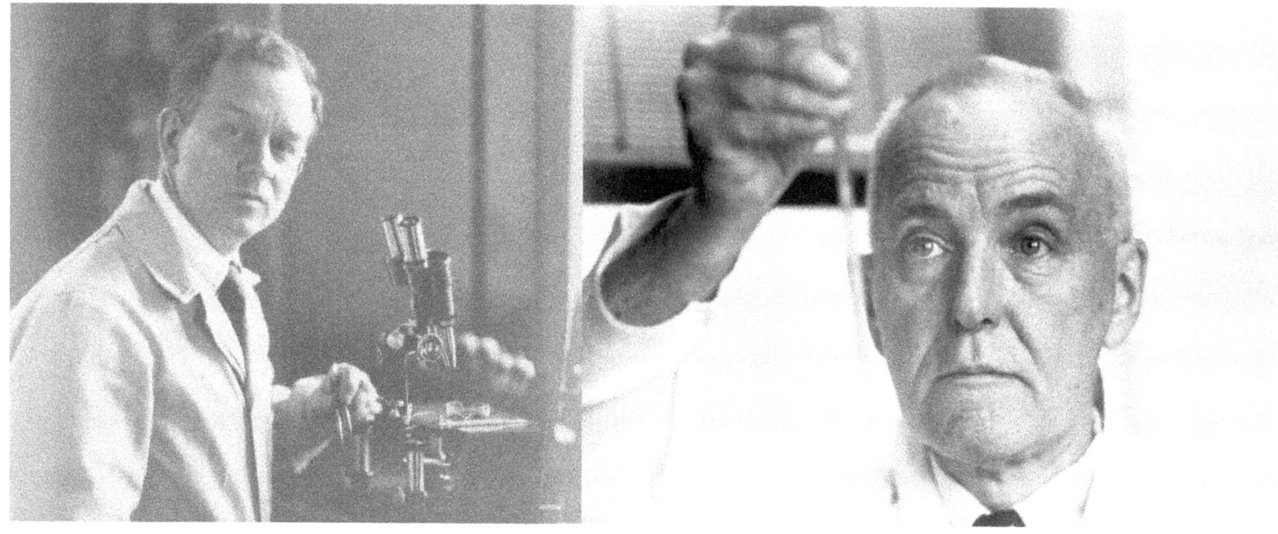

Charles Huggins, born on September 22, 1901, in Halifax, Nova Scotia, Canada, made significant strides in understanding and treating prostate cancer at the University of Chicago. His research demonstrated the effectiveness of hormonal therapy in treating prostate cancer, fundamentally changing the approach to cancer treatment.

Snippets

Rous's research into chicken tumors led to the identification of the Rous sarcoma virus, providing the first evidence that viruses can cause cancer. This discovery opened new avenues for cancer research and the understanding of oncogenic viruses.

Huggins work on the hormonal treatment of prostate cancer introduced the concept of cancer therapy targeting specific hormonal pathways. His approach laid the groundwork for targeted therapy, a cornerstone of modern cancer treatment.

Current Implications

The discoveries by Rous and Huggins have had profound implications for cancer research and treatment. Rous's work on tumor-inducing viruses has contributed to our understanding of viral oncology and the development of vaccines and treatments for virus-related cancers.

Impact and Products

The work of Rous and Huggins has significantly advanced the fields of virology and oncology, influencing cancer diagnosis, treatment, and prevention strategies. Their contributions have paved the way for targeted therapies and the development of cancer vaccines, marking a significant milestone in the fight against cancer.

RAGNAR GRANIT, HALDAN HARTLINE, GEORGE WALD (1967)

Illuminating the neural mechanism of human vision and optics

In 1967, Ragnar Granit, Haldan Hartline, and George Wald were awarded the Nobel Prize in Medicine for their discoveries concerning the primary physiological and chemical visual processes in the eye.

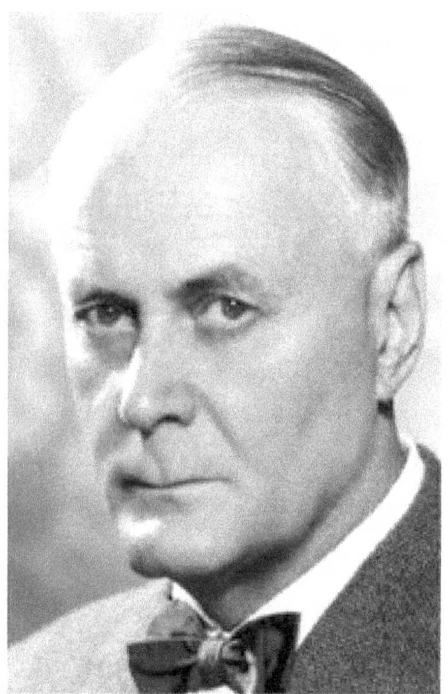

Ragnar Granit

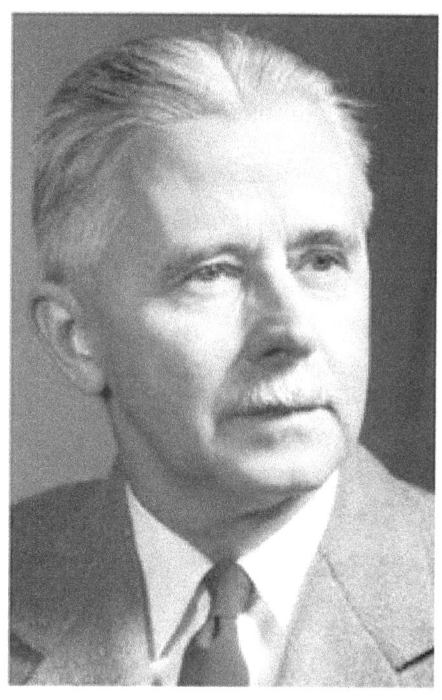

Haldan Hartline

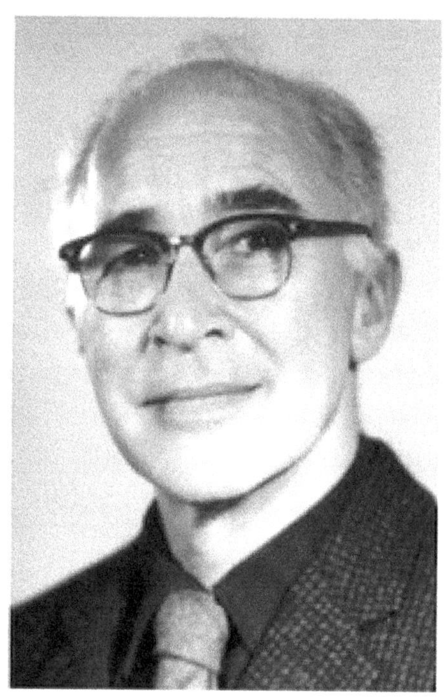

George Wald

History

Ragnar Granit, born on October 30, 1900, in Helsinki, Finland, conducted pioneering research on the neurophysiological mechanisms of vision. Haldan Keffer Hartline, born on December 22, 1903, in Bloomsburg, Pennsylvania, USA. George Wald, born on November 18, 1906, in New York City, USA, joined Granit in laying the groundwork for elucidating how visual information is translated into neural signals in the eye.

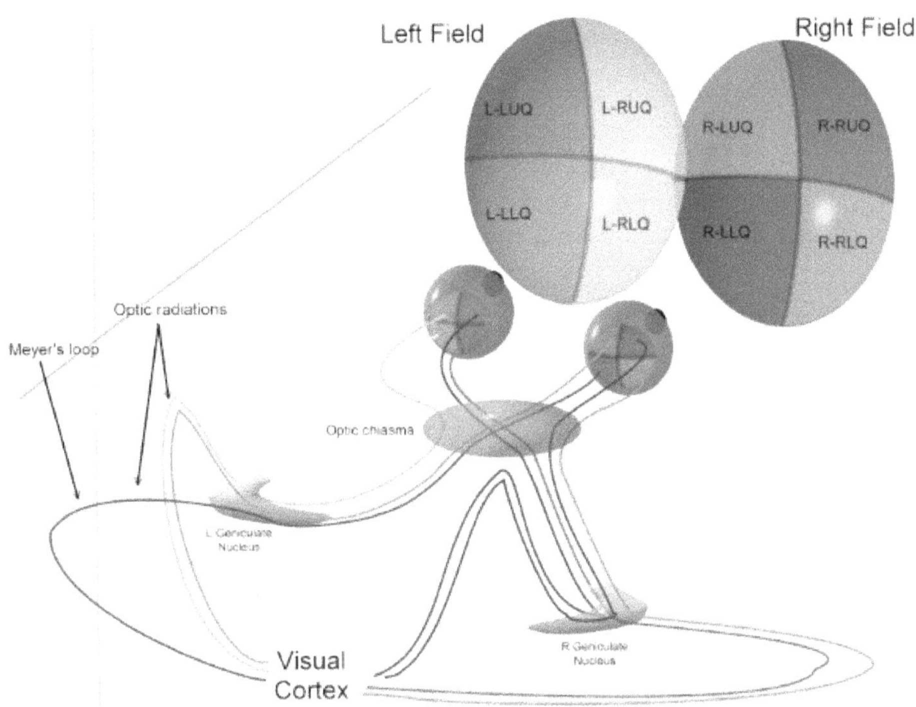

The optical receptors and pathway

Snippets

Granit's work on the different types of photoreceptor cells in the retina and their roles in color vision provided insights into how the eye detects and differentiates colors. Hartline's research focused on the electrical responses of the retina to light stimuli, pioneering the study of how the eye communicates with the brain. Wald discovered the role of vitamin A in the retina and its importance in converting light into visual signals, a process essential for vision in low-light conditions.

Current Implications

The groundbreaking research by Granit, Hartline, and Wald has had profound implications for various fields, including neurology, ophthalmology, and even artificial vision systems. Their discoveries have paved the way for advances in understanding and treating vision disorders, as well as in the development of technologies that mimic human vision.

Impact and Products

The work of Granit, Hartline, and Wald continues to influence the study of vision and the brain. Their contributions have led to better diagnostic and therapeutic tools for eye diseases and have enhanced our understanding of the complex processes underlying visual perception. Their legacy is evident in the ongoing research and innovations in the field of vision science and neurophysiology.

Their collective work significantly advanced our understanding of how the eye perceives and processes light, marking a major milestone in the field of neurophysiology and vision science.

ROBERT HOLLEY, H. KHORANA, MARSHALL NIRENBERG (1968)

This trio worked in tandem to unleash the secrets of transfer RNA and protein synthesis

In 1968, Robert Holley, Har Gobind Khorana, and Marshall Nirenberg won the Nobel Prize in Medicine for cracking the genetic code and explaining how proteins are made in cells.

History

Robert Holley, born in 1922 in Urbana, Illinois, completed his groundbreaking research at Cornell University. Har Gobind Khorana, Indian-American born in Multan in 1922, in what is now Pakistan, worked at the University of Wisconsin. Marshall Nirenberg, born in 1927 in New York City, made his key discoveries at the National Institutes of Health.

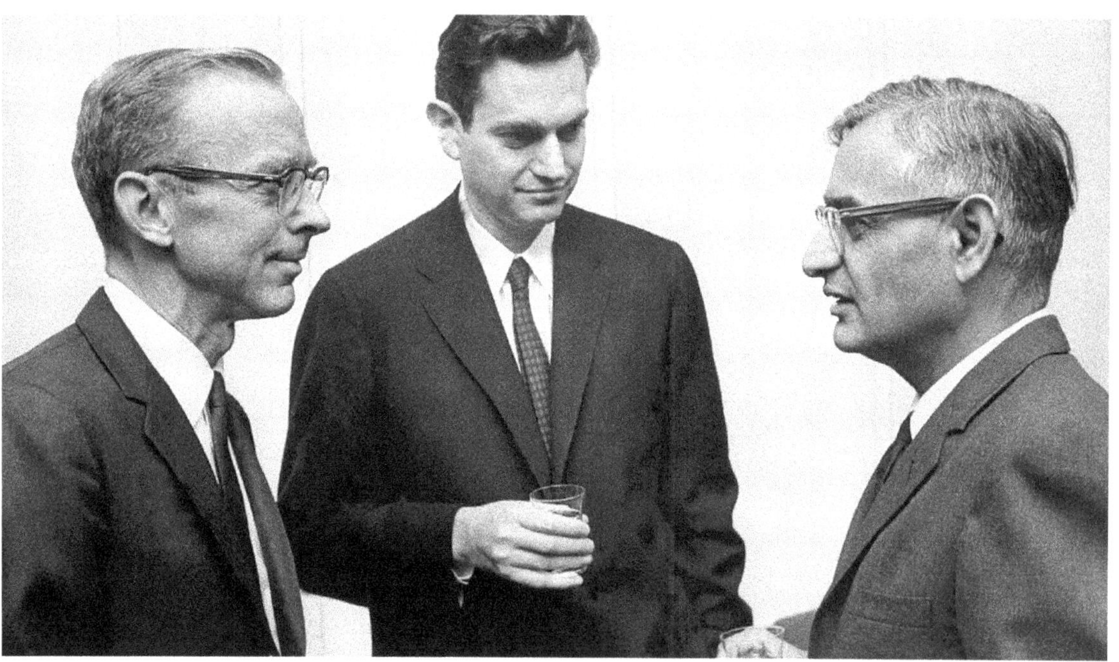

Robert Holley   *Marshall Nirenberg*   *Har Gobind Khorana*

Snippets

Holley identified the structure of transfer RNA, the molecule that helps translate genetic code into proteins. Khorana synthesized artificial genes, demonstrating how DNA's instructions are spelled out. Nirenberg showed how the sequences of DNA lead directly to the production of specific proteins.

Together, they mapped out the process by which genetic information is turned into the proteins essential for life.

Current Implications

Their research has had a huge impact on biology and medicine. Understanding the genetic code has led to advances in genetic engineering, the development of new drugs, and treatments for genetic diseases. It's the foundation of biotechnology and the fight against countless medical conditions.

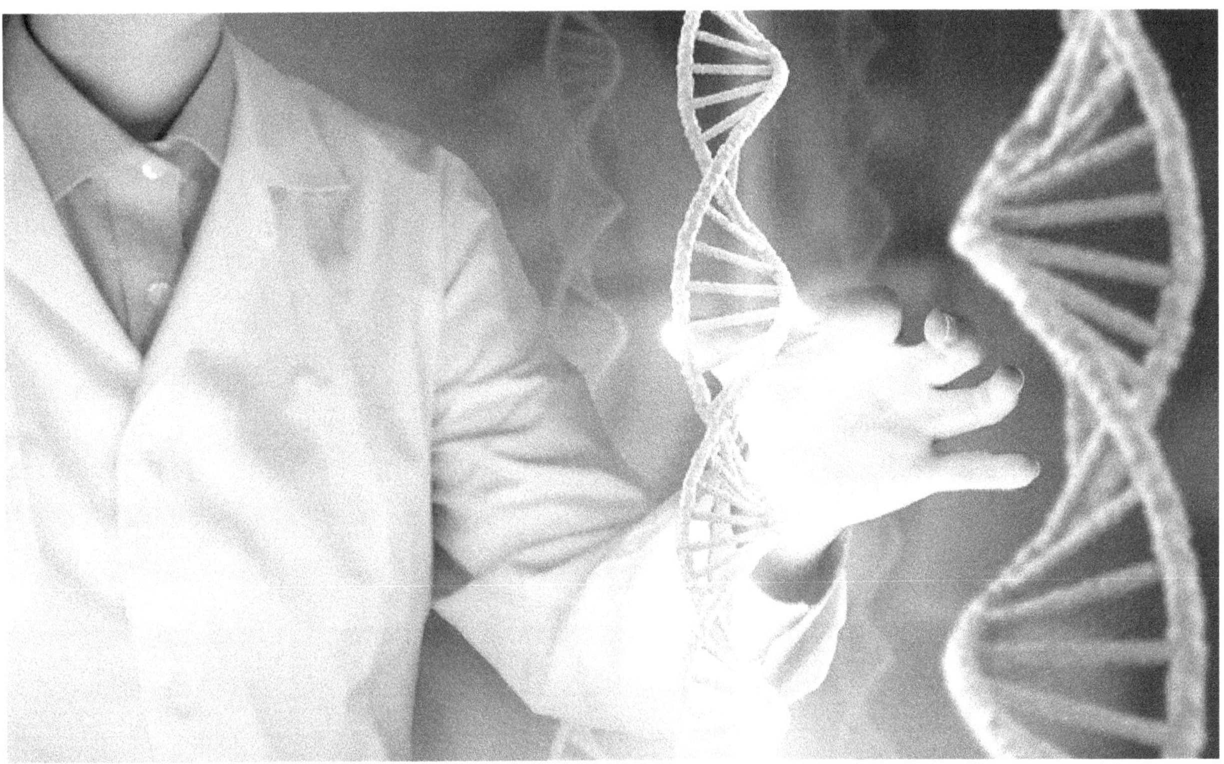

Impact and Products

Thanks to Holley, Khorana, and Nirenberg, we now have the tools to manipulate genes, leading to better crops, new medical therapies, and even the potential to cure genetic disorders. Their work is a cornerstone of modern science, affecting everything from agriculture to gene therapy.

Their discoveries showed how genetic instructions are translated into the proteins that perform various functions in living organisms.

MAX DELBRÜCK, ALFRED HERSHEY, SALVADOR LURIA
(1969)

Molecular mechanisms of viral multiplication, a fore runner for vaccine creation

In 1969, Max Delbrück, Alfred D. Hershey, and Salvador E. Luria were awarded the Nobel Prize in Medicine for their groundbreaking work on the replication mechanisms and genetic structures of viruses. Their collective research has been foundational in the field of molecular biology, particularly in understanding how viruses multiply and how genetic information is transferred in bacterial cells.

History

Max Delbrück, born on September 4, 1906, in Berlin, Germany, was a key figure in the development of molecular genetics. Alfred D. Hershey, born on December 4, 1908, in Owosso, Michigan, USA, and Salvador E. Luria, born on August 13, 1912, in Turin, Italy, were both instrumental in advancing our understanding of virology and genetics. Their collaborative efforts have significantly influenced the scientific community's approach to studying viruses and genetic material.

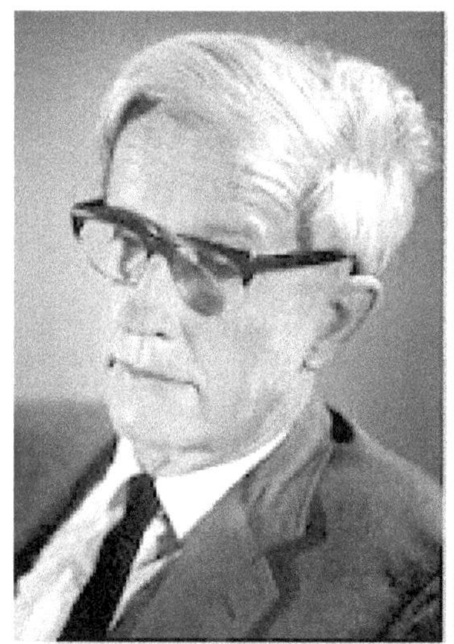

Max Delbrück
(1906 - 1981)

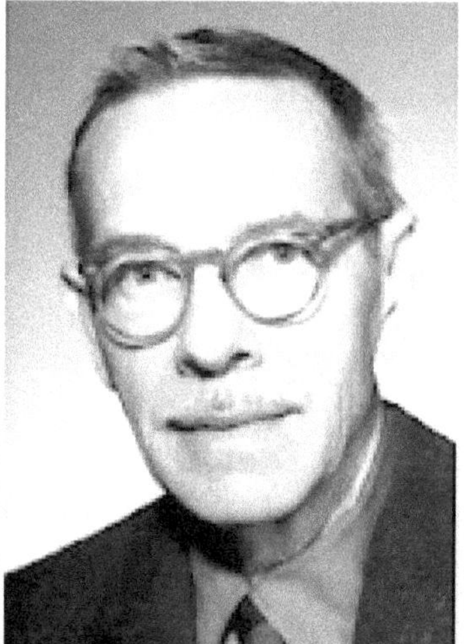

Alfred D. Hershey
(1908 - 1997)

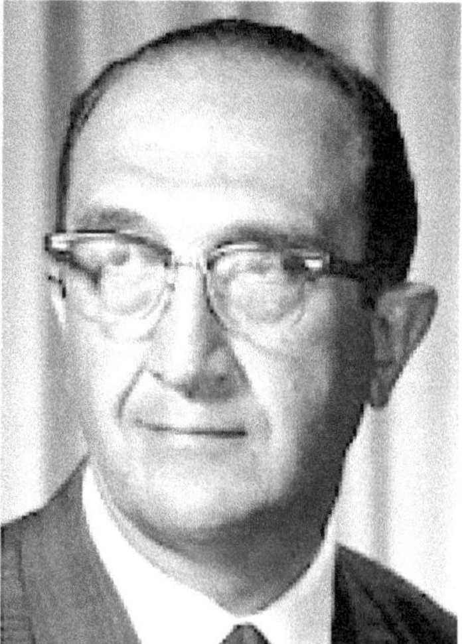

Salvador E. Luria
(1921 - 1991)

Snippets

Delbrück, Hershey, and Luria's research provided profound insights into the nature of viruses, particularly bacteriophages—viruses that infect bacteria. Their work included the famous Hershey-

Chase experiment, which demonstrated that DNA is the material that carries genetic information. Luria's work, alongside Delbrück, established that mutations in bacteria occurred randomly, not as a result of adaptive responses to the environment, which was a significant advance in the study of genetics.

Current Implications

The discoveries made by these three scientists have had lasting impacts on both basic science and practical applications. Their work laid the groundwork for genetic engineering, the development of vaccines, and the treatment of viral infections. Understanding the genetic structure of viruses and their replication mechanisms continues to be crucial in the fight against infectious diseases.

Impact and Products

Today, the contributions of Delbrück, Hershey, and Luria are reflected in the continued exploration of genetic manipulation techniques, the development of gene therapy, and advances in combating bacterial and viral pathogens. Their pioneering work has showed the way for significant medical and biotechnological advancements, contributing to the development of new therapies and the enhancement of public health.

SIR BERNARD KATZ, ULF VON EULER, JULIUS AXELROD (1970)

Strengthening the foundations of Neuropharmacology

In 1970, Sir Bernard Katz, Ulf von Euler, and Julius Axelrod were jointly awarded the Nobel Prize in Medicine for their crucial discoveries regarding the transmission of nerve impulses. Their work unveiled the processes behind the storage, release, and inactivation of neurotransmitters, elements vital for nerve communication.

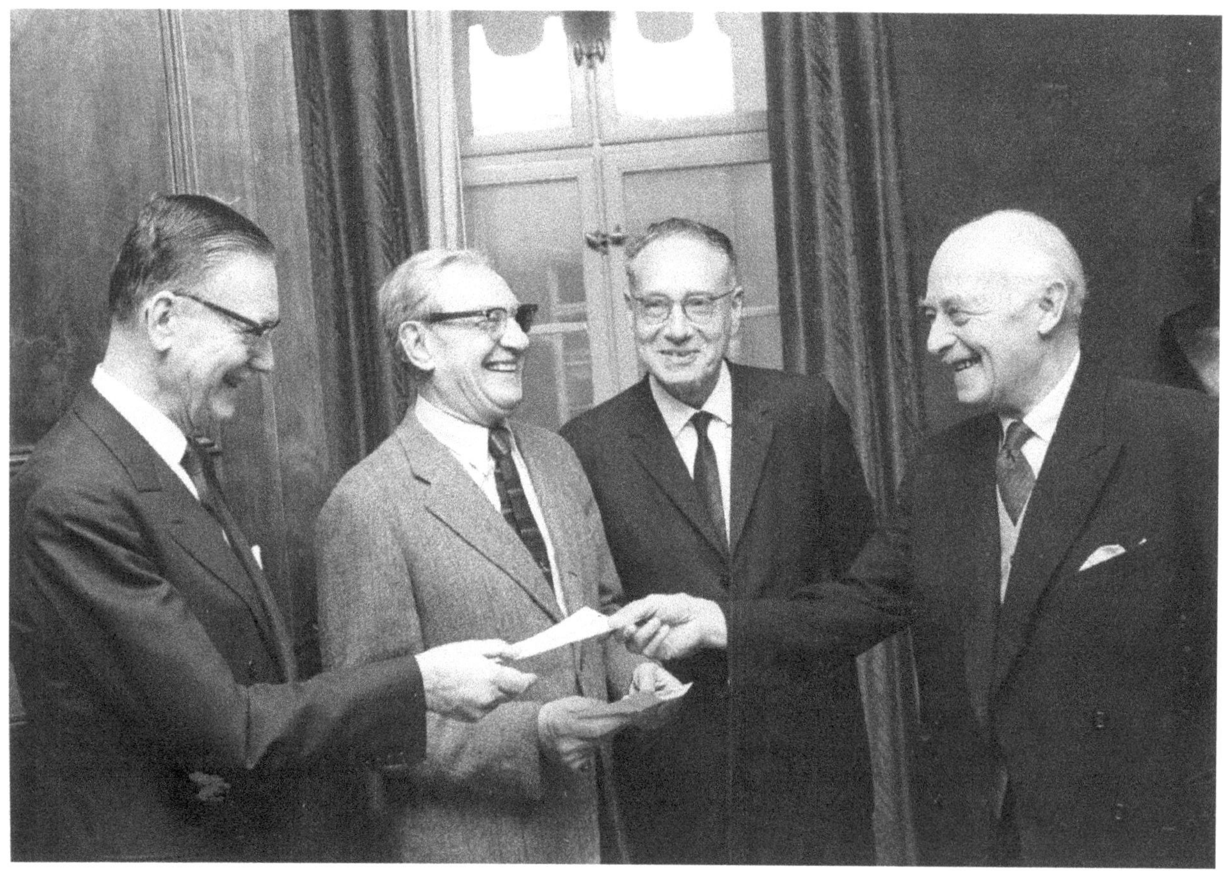

History

Sir Bernard Katz, born on March 26, 1911, in Leipzig, Germany, made significant strides in understanding how neurotransmitters are released from nerve endings. Ulf von Euler, born on February 7, 1905, in Stockholm, Sweden, discovered noradrenaline as a neurotransmitter in the sympathetic nervous system and elucidated how it is stored within nerves. Julius Axelrod, born on May 30, 1912, in New York City, USA, contributed by exploring how neurotransmitters like noradrenaline are metabolized and deactivated in the nervous system.

Snippets

Their collective research efforts provided a deep dive into the chemical basis of nerve transmission, highlighting the role of specific neurotransmitters in signaling between nerve cells and between nerves and muscles. Katz's work, for instance, demonstrated the process by which acetylcholine, a neurotransmitter, is released at synaptic junctions, influencing muscle activation and inter-neuronal communication.

Current Implications

The pioneering work of Katz, von Euler, and Axelrod laid the groundwork for modern neuropharmacology, influencing the development of drugs targeting neurological and psychiatric disorders. Understanding the mechanics of neurotransmitter release and inactivation has been crucial for therapies addressing issues ranging from depression to hypertension.

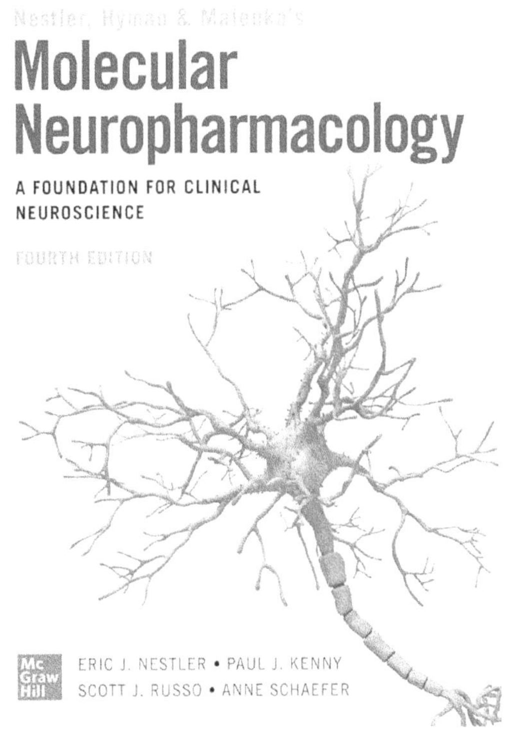

The legacy of these three laureates in revealing the complexities of neurotransmission underscores much of the contemporary approaches to treating mental health disorders, pain management, and neurodegenerative diseases.

EARL SUTHERLAND JR. (1971)

Cyclic AMP: The original second messenger

Earl W. Sutherland Jr. was awarded the Nobel Prize in Medicine in 1971 for his groundbreaking discoveries concerning the mechanisms of hormone action, particularly through secondary messengers like cyclic adenosine monophosphate (cAMP).

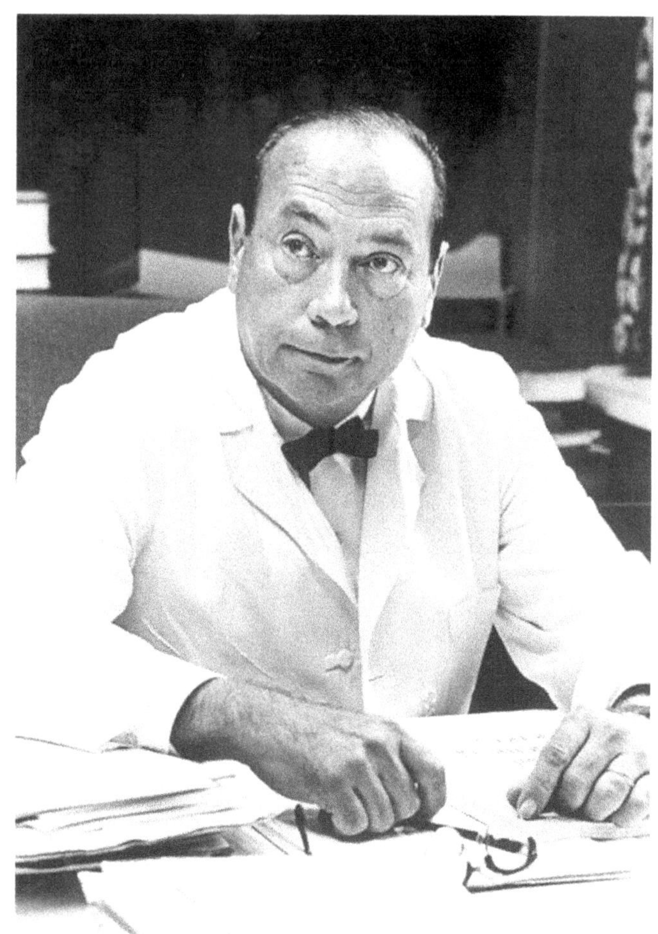

History

Earl W. Sutherland Jr.'s journey in biochemistry and pharmacology began in Burlingame, Kansas, where he was born in 1915. He pursued his undergraduate degree at Washburn College before attending medical school at Washington University in St. Louis, where he obtained his M.D. in 1942. It was at Washington University that Sutherland delved into research, laying the foundation for his future discoveries.

Post-World War II, Sutherland's career took him to several prestigious institutions, where he held various teaching and research positions. His early work at Washington University School of Medicine involved research in biochemistry, laying the groundwork for his later contributions to understanding hormonal mechanisms.

In 1953, Sutherland's career path took him to Cleveland, where he accepted a position as professor of pharmacology and chairman of the department of pharmacology at Case Western Reserve University. It was here, in collaboration with Theodore W. Rall and others, that Sutherland embarked on the research that would lead to the discovery of cyclic AMP (cAMP) as a secondary messenger in cells, a pivotal moment in the field of biochemistry and pharmacology

Sutherland's move to Vanderbilt University in 1963 as professor of physiology provided him with the opportunity to delve deeper into his research on cAMP, supported by financial backing from the American Heart Association. His work at Vanderbilt until 1973 further solidified his contributions to our understanding of cellular processes and hormone action.

Snippets

Discovery of cAMP: Sutherland discovered cyclic AMP (cAMP) and its role as a secondary messenger in cells, revolutionizing our understanding of how hormones signal cellular processes.

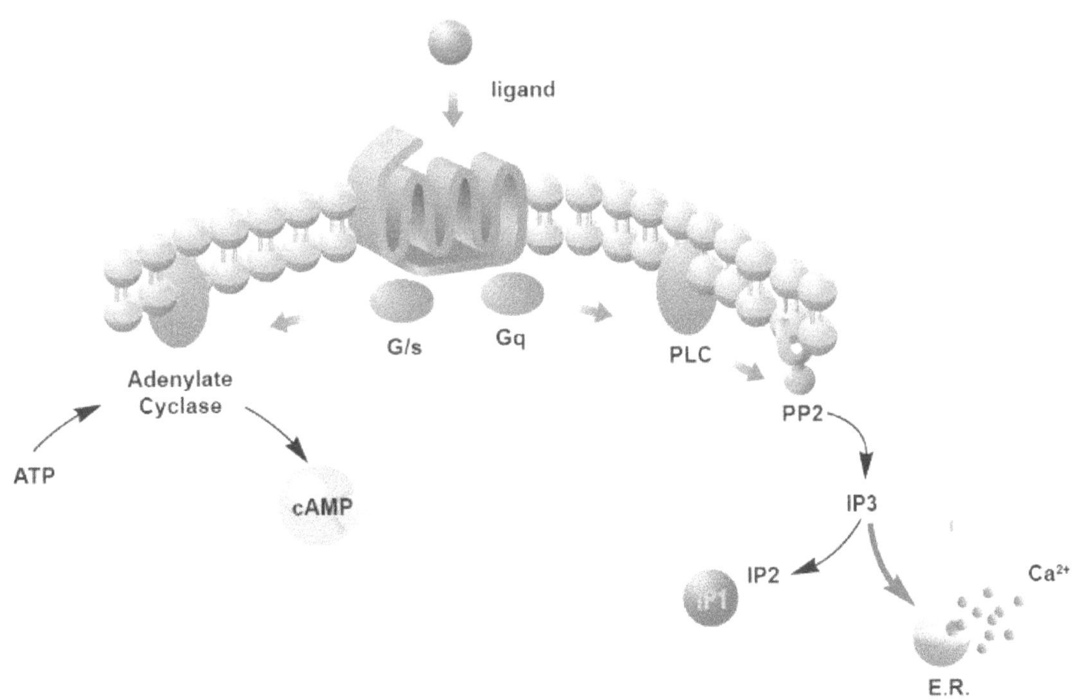

Research Background: Before his landmark discovery, Sutherland was involved in glycogen metabolism research, contributing to foundational knowledge in biochemistry.

Collaboration: While at Case Western Reserve University, he worked with Theodore W. Rall, leading to pivotal insights into hormone action mechanisms.

Methodological Innovation: Sutherland's innovative approach to studying hormone pathways using liver cell homogenates marked a departure from the focus on intact cells, allowing for more detailed analyses.

Implications for Glycogenolysis: His research clarified the role of liver phosphorylase in glycogenolysis, demonstrating the enzyme's regulation by phosphorylation and the influence of hormones like epinephrine and glucagon.

Early Researchers

Carl and Gerty Cori, whose research into the enzymatic conversion of glycogen paved the way for deeper investigations into metabolic regulation and hormone action. Their elucidation of the glycogenolysis pathway established a foundational understanding of how hormones could regulate metabolic processes, an area that Sutherland's work would greatly expand upon.

Bernard Katz made substantial contributions to the understanding of neurotransmission, exploring the synaptic mechanisms that underlie nerve signal transmission. His work on neurotransmitter release mechanisms offered insights into how cells communicate, influencing Sutherland's investigations into secondary messengers.

Another significant contributor was Rosalind Franklin, whose work, though primarily known for DNA structure discovery, also included pioneering insights into the molecular structures of viruses. Her techniques and approaches to molecular biology laid the groundwork for understanding complex biological processes at the molecular level, contributing to the broader field of cell signaling research.

Current Implications

Advancements in Drug Development: Understanding cAMP's role in cellular signaling has led to the development of drugs targeting specific pathways influenced by cAMP, offering new treatments for diseases like heart failure and certain types of cancer.

Improved Understanding of Disease Mechanisms: Research into cAMP has enhanced our understanding of the molecular mechanisms underlying various diseases, including diabetes, by elucidating how hormonal signals regulate glucose metabolism.

Innovations in Neuropharmacology: Insights into cAMP's function have informed the development of neuropharmacological agents that modulate neurotransmitter systems for treating psychiatric disorders such as depression and anxiety.

Enhancements in Cell Therapy: Knowledge of cAMP signaling pathways contributes to cell therapy strategies for regenerative medicine, including stem cell differentiation and tissue repair.

Development of Diagnostic Tools: The discovery of cAMP's role in cell signaling has facilitated the creation of diagnostic assays that measure cAMP levels as biomarkers for certain hormonal imbalances and diseases.

Contribution to Vaccine Research: Understanding how cAMP influences immune cell function has implications for vaccine development, particularly in enhancing immune responses to pathogens.

Impact and Products

Targeted Therapies for Cardiovascular Diseases: The understanding of cAMP's role in heart function has led to the development of targeted therapies for treating heart diseases. By manipulating cAMP levels, researchers have been able to create drugs that improve heart muscle contraction and treat heart failure more effectively.

cAMP Modulators for Metabolic Disorders: Insight into cAMP's involvement in metabolic processes has facilitated the development of modulators that target metabolic disorders. For instance, drugs that influence cAMP pathways are being explored to treat type 2 diabetes by enhancing insulin release and improving metabolic balance.

Diagnostic Kits for Hormonal Disorders: The elucidation of cAMP's role in hormone signaling has spurred the creation of diagnostic kits that measure hormone levels for diagnosing and monitoring treatment of hormonal disorders. These kits offer a non-invasive and rapid assessment of patient hormone levels, aiding in personalized medicine.

Research Tools for Cell Signaling Studies: The fundamental understanding of cAMP as a secondary messenger has led to the development of various research tools and assays. These tools allow scientists to study cAMP levels and its effects in different cellular contexts, advancing our knowledge of cell signaling pathways.

Innovations in Immunotherapy: The role of cAMP in regulating immune responses has opened new avenues in immunotherapy research. By targeting cAMP pathways, novel immunotherapeutic strategies are being developed to boost the immune system's ability to fight cancer and other diseases.

Cosmetics and Skin Care Products: Research into cAMP's effects on skin cells has led to its application in cosmetics and skin care products. By influencing cell growth and differentiation, products aiming to improve skin health and appearance are being formulated based on cAMP-related mechanisms.

These developments underscore the lasting impact of Sutherland's work, demonstrating the wide-ranging applications of his discovery in improving human health through enhanced therapeutic options and diagnostic tools.

GERALD EDELMAN AND RODNEY PORTER (1972)

Unveiling the complex "Y" architecture of antibody structure

Gerald Edelman, an American scientist, and Rodney Porter, a British biochemist, were jointly awarded the Nobel Prize in Medicine in 1972. Their award recognized their independent but complementary discoveries concerning the chemical structure of antibodies, key components of the immune system that protect the body against pathogens.

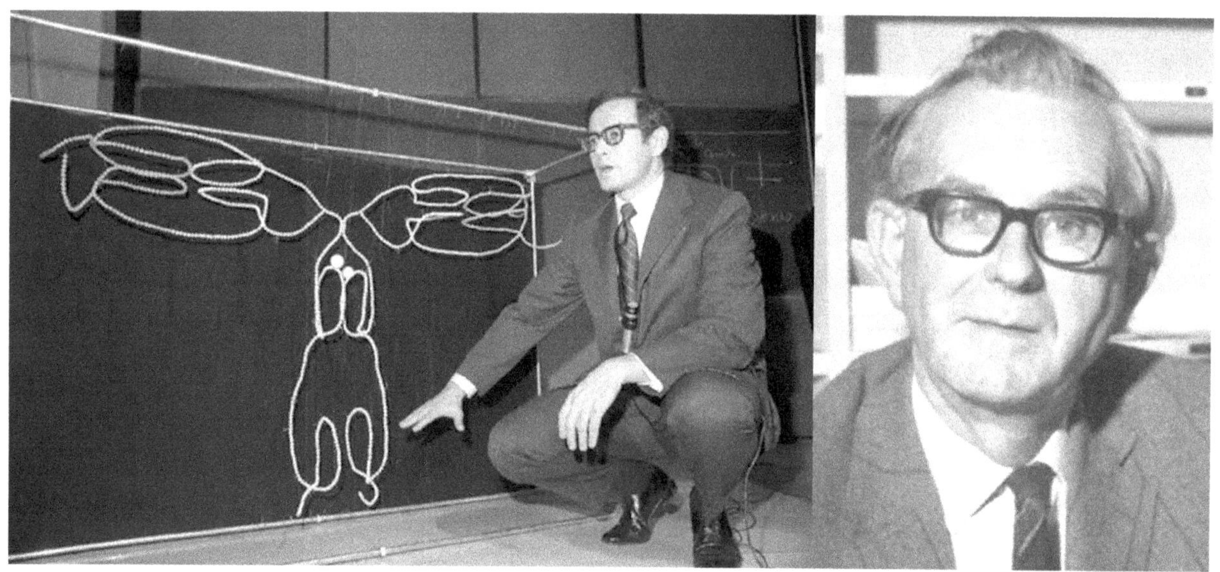

Gerald Edelman

Rodney Porter

History

Gerald Edelman, born in New York City in 1929, started on a medical career that led him from an M.D. degree at the University of Pennsylvania to a transformative period in the Army Medical Corps in Paris. It was during this time that Edelman's interest in the immune system deepened, prompting him to pursue a Ph.D. in physical chemistry at Rockefeller University upon his return to the United States. At Rockefeller, Edelman focused his research on antibodies, laying the groundwork for his Nobel Prize-winning discovery. His work not only elucidated the structure of antibodies but also expanded into neurobiology and consciousness later in his career.

Rodney Porter, born in Newton-le-Willows, Lancashire, England, in 1917, brought a complementary perspective to the study of antibodies through his biochemistry background. After earning his Ph.D.

at the University of Cambridge, Porter's career included significant periods at the National Institute for Medical Research in London and, subsequently, at St. Mary's Hospital Medical School. Porter's innovative approach involved enzymatically fragmenting immunoglobulin molecules to understand their structure better, an endeavor that, alongside Edelman's work, provided a comprehensive understanding of antibody architecture.

Edelman and Porter's work, though conducted independently, converged on a critical aspect of immunology that has since underpinned significant advances in medicine and biology. Their legacy is a testament to the enduring value of deep, focused research into the mechanisms of life and the human body's defense systems.

Snippets

Discovery of Antibody Structure: Gerald Edelman and Rodney Porter independently unveiled the complex structure of antibodies. Their work shed light on how antibodies, the body's defenders against pathogens, are organized at the molecular level, providing a foundation for modern immunological research and therapeutic applications.

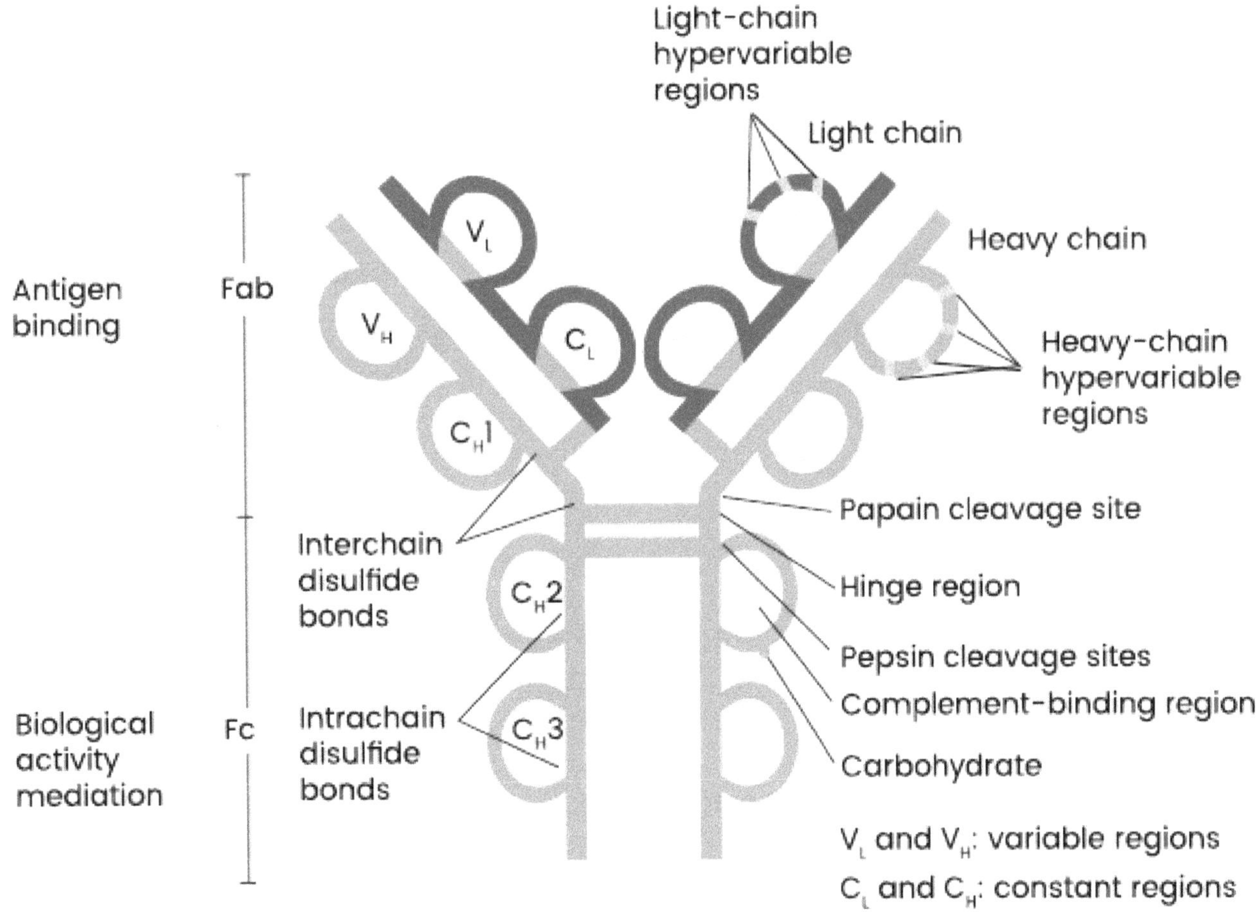

Image source & courtesey www.sinobiological.com

Edelman's Path: Starting his career with a focus on the physical chemistry of antibodies, Edelman's innovative research techniques led to a detailed understanding of antibody molecules, contributing to the model of antibody structure that is widely accepted today.

Porter's Approach: Porter's methodology involved the enzymatic cleavage of antibodies into smaller fragments, allowing for a clearer analysis of their structure. This approach was instrumental in elucidating the quaternary structure of antibodies, which consists of two light and two heavy chains linked by disulfide bonds.

Legacy and Impact: The work of Edelman and Porter has had a lasting impact on the field of immunology, influencing the development of diagnostic tools, therapeutic antibodies, and vaccines. Their discoveries continue to inform research on immune response mechanisms and the design of immunotherapies for a wide range of diseases.

Early Researchers

One such figure is Paul Ehrlich, a German scientist known for his "side-chain theory," which posited that cells have specific receptors that bind to toxins or nutrients, a precursor to the concept of antibodies and their specificity.

Niels Kaj Jerne is another influential figure who laid the groundwork for understanding the immune system's complexity. Jerne's "network theory" of the immune system introduced the idea that the immune system regulates itself through a network of antibodies that recognize not only foreign antigens but also other antibodies. This theory added a new layer of understanding to the immune system's regulatory mechanisms, influencing subsequent research in immunology.

Elvin A. Kabat, through his meticulous work on the immunochemistry of antibodies in the mid-20th century, significantly advanced the understanding of antibody diversity and structure before the detailed elucidations by Edelman and Porter. Kabat's research on the variability and specificity of antibodies contributed to the emerging picture of how the immune system recognizes and responds to an almost infinite variety of antigens.

Current Implications

Advancement in Immunotherapies: Their discoveries have paved the way for the development of targeted immunotherapies, which harness the body's immune system to fight diseases, particularly cancer. Monoclonal antibodies, engineered to target specific antigens on cancer cells, have become a cornerstone of modern cancer treatment.

Vaccine Development: Understanding the structure and function of antibodies has been crucial in designing more effective vaccines. This knowledge helps scientists create vaccines that elicit strong, protective immune responses against pathogens.

Autoimmune Disease Treatment: Insights into antibody structure and function have led to new treatments for autoimmune diseases, where the immune system mistakenly attacks the body's own cells. Therapies that modulate the immune response can help manage conditions like rheumatoid arthritis and lupus.

Diagnostics: The detailed understanding of antibodies has revolutionized diagnostic techniques, allowing for the precise detection of pathogens and biomarkers of disease. This has improved the diagnosis and monitoring of infectious diseases, cancers, and autoimmune disorders.

Research Tools: Antibodies are indispensable tools in biomedical research, used in a wide array of applications from detecting proteins in cells and tissues to purifying specific molecules for study. The ability to produce antibodies that recognize specific targets has enabled countless discoveries in biology and medicine.

Impact and Products

Monoclonal Antibody Therapies: Beyond their use in oncology, monoclonal antibodies have been developed to treat a myriad of diseases, including chronic inflammatory conditions, asthma, and infectious diseases. These therapies specifically target disease mechanisms, offering treatments with fewer side effects compared to traditional drugs.

Precision Diagnostic Platforms: The understanding of antibodies' structure and function has led to the creation of highly specific diagnostic platforms. These include tests for early detection of diseases like Alzheimer's and Parkinson's by identifying biomarkers specific to these conditions.

Biosensors: Antibodies serve as critical components in biosensor devices used for environmental monitoring, food safety, and biosecurity. These sensors rely on the specific binding properties of antibodies to detect contaminants and pathogens with high accuracy.

Therapeutic Vaccines: The insights gained from antibody research have fueled the development of therapeutic vaccines, particularly for treating chronic infections and cancers. These vaccines aim to elicit an immune response specifically targeted at eliminating infected or cancerous cells.

Allergy Treatments: Understanding how antibodies mediate allergic reactions has led to the development of targeted treatments for allergies. These treatments work by blocking the action of specific antibodies responsible for allergic responses, providing relief for conditions like severe asthma and food allergies.

Research and Development: In the research sector, customized antibodies are essential tools for probing the function of genes and proteins in various biological processes. This has implications for drug discovery and basic science research, enabling the identification of potential therapeutic targets.

These developments continue to improve diagnostic capabilities, treatment options, and our overall understanding of complex diseases, showcasing the lasting impact of their Nobel Prize-winning discovery.

KARL VON FRISCH, K. LORENZ, NIKOLAAS TINBERGEN
(1973)

The crucial concepts of animal thinking and the hidden link with human behavior

In 1973, Karl von Frisch, Konrad Lorenz, and Nikolaas Tinbergen were awarded the Nobel Prize in Medicine for their pioneering work in ethology, the study of animal behavior.

History

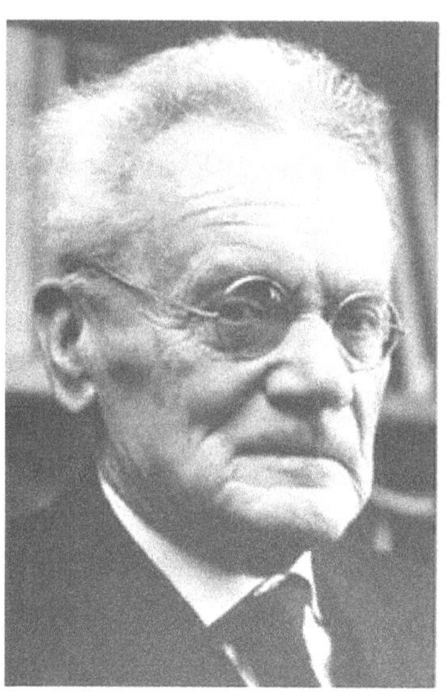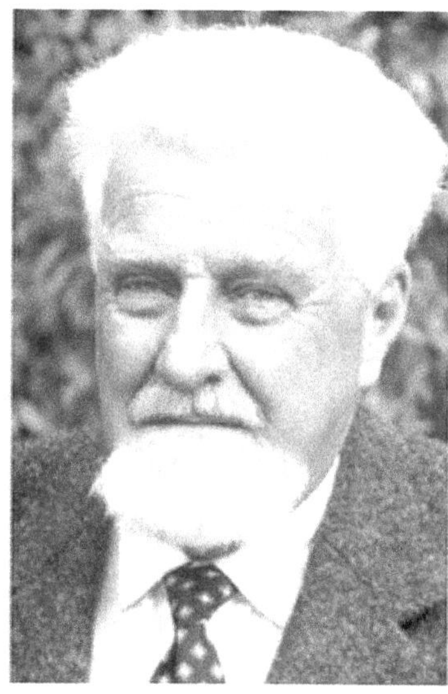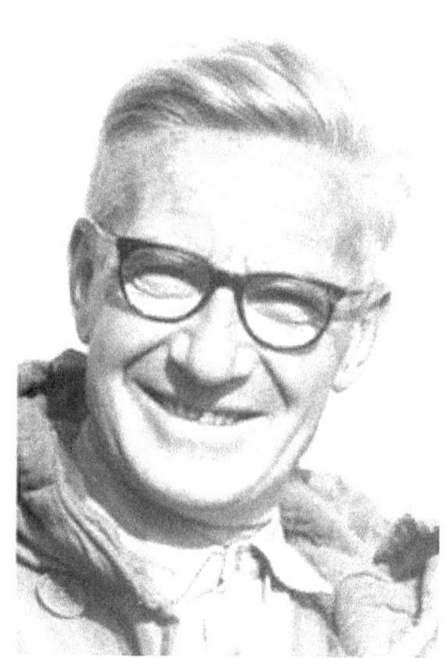

Karl von Frisch, born on November 20, 1886, in Vienna, Austria, was renowned for his study of honeybee communications and sensory perceptions. Konrad Lorenz, born on November 7, 1903, in Vienna, Austria, explored animal behavior patterns, particularly imprinting in birds. Nikolaas Tinbergen, born on April 15, 1907, in The Hague, Netherlands, contributed foundational knowledge on animal instincts and their environmental triggers.

Snippets

Von Frisch deciphered the "dance" of honeybees as a means of communication, revealing how bees convey information about the direction and distance of food sources. Lorenz's observations of greylag geese led to the concept of imprinting, demonstrating how young animals form attachments during a critical period after birth. Tinbergen's experiments on stickleback fish highlighted the role of external stimuli in triggering specific behavior patterns, such as aggression during mating seasons.

Current Implications

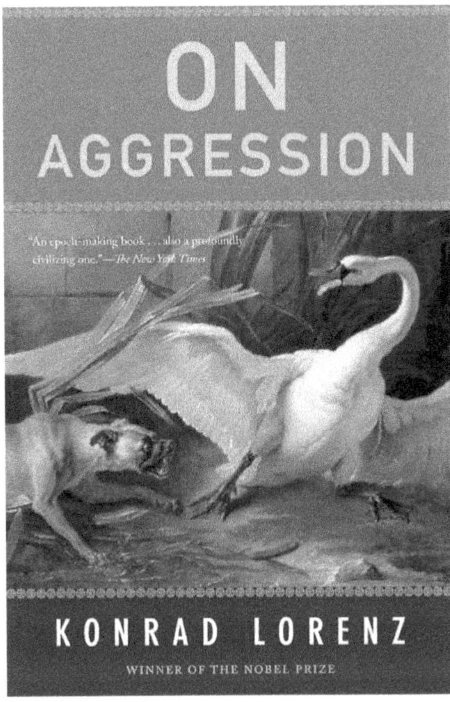

The trio's work has had profound implications beyond ethology, influencing psychology, neuroscience, and even environmental conservation. Their discoveries about animal behavior patterns have provided insights into human behavior, learning processes, and the importance of early developmental stages.

Impact and Products

The research by Frisch, Lorenz, and Tinbergen laid the groundwork for future studies in behavioral science, contributing to the development of behavioral ecology, cognitive ethology, and the interdisciplinary field of biosemiotics.

Their research shed light on how animals perceive and interact with their environments, leading to significant insights into animal and human psychology.

ALBERT CLAUDE, CHRISTIAN DE DUVE, G. EMIL PALADE (1974)

Great Intracellular visionaries who discovered all cytoplasmic organelles

The 1974 Nobel Prize in Medicine was awarded to Albert Claude, Christian de Duve, and George Emil Palade for their discoveries concerning the structural and functional organization of the cell. Their pioneering work illuminated the intricate world of cellular organelles, fundamentally advancing the field of cell biology.

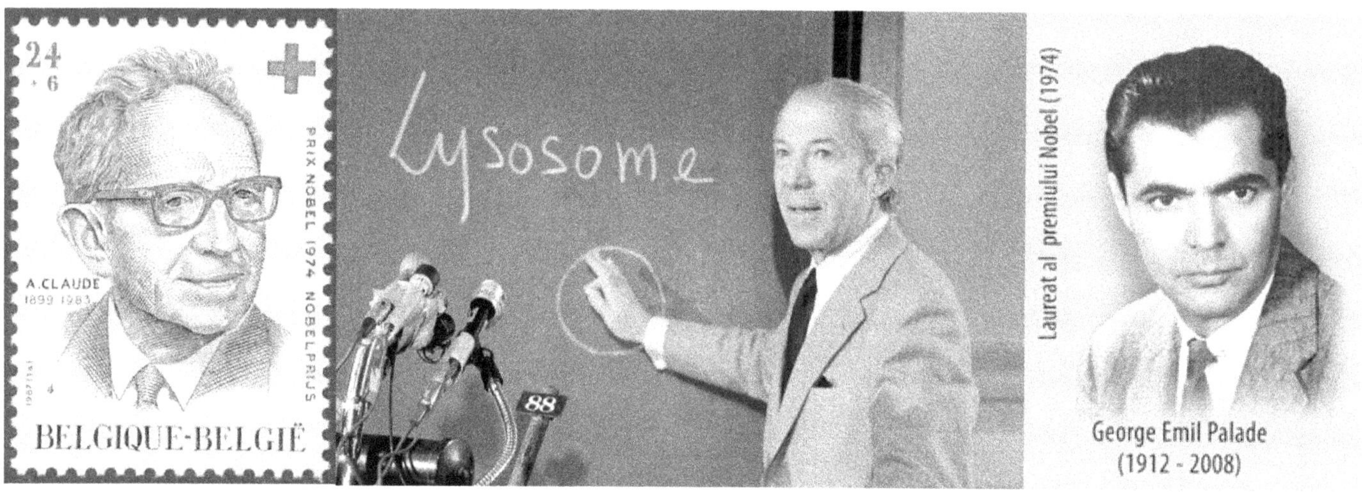

History

Albert Claude was born in Longlier, Belgium, in 1898. After receiving his M.D. from the University of Liège, he moved to the United States in 1929 to work at the Rockefeller Institute for Medical Research in New York. There, he began his pioneering work in cell biology, employing centrifugation and electron microscopy to study cellular components, leading to the discovery of the endoplasmic reticulum and mitochondria.

Christian de Duve, born in 1917 in the United Kingdom but raised in Belgium, also made significant contributions to cell biology. After receiving his M.D. from the Catholic University of Louvain, he delved into biochemistry and cellular biology, where he discovered lysosomes and peroxisomes, contributing to our understanding of cellular metabolism and the enzymatic machinery within cells.

George Emil Palade, born in Iași, Romania, in 1912, emigrated to the United States after World War II. He completed his Ph.D. in 1946 and joined the Rockefeller Institute, where he met Albert Claude.

Palade's use of electron microscopy helped identify the ribosome and provided detailed views of the cell's internal structure, including the mitochondria and the endoplasmic reticulum.

Snippets

Cellular Organelle Discovery: Albert Claude utilized electron microscopy and cell fractionation to identify the endoplasmic reticulum and mitochondria, revealing the complex internal organization of cells.

Lysosomes and Peroxisomes: Christian de Duve discovered lysosomes and peroxisomes, highlighting their roles in cellular metabolism and the detoxification process, respectively.

Ribosomes and Cell Structure: George Emil Palade's work detailed the structure and function of ribosomes and further elucidated the endoplasmic reticulum's role in protein synthesis, enhancing our understanding of cell physiology.

Foundation of Cell Biology: Their collective contributions provided a detailed view of the cell's functional compartments, laying the groundwork for the field of modern cell biology.

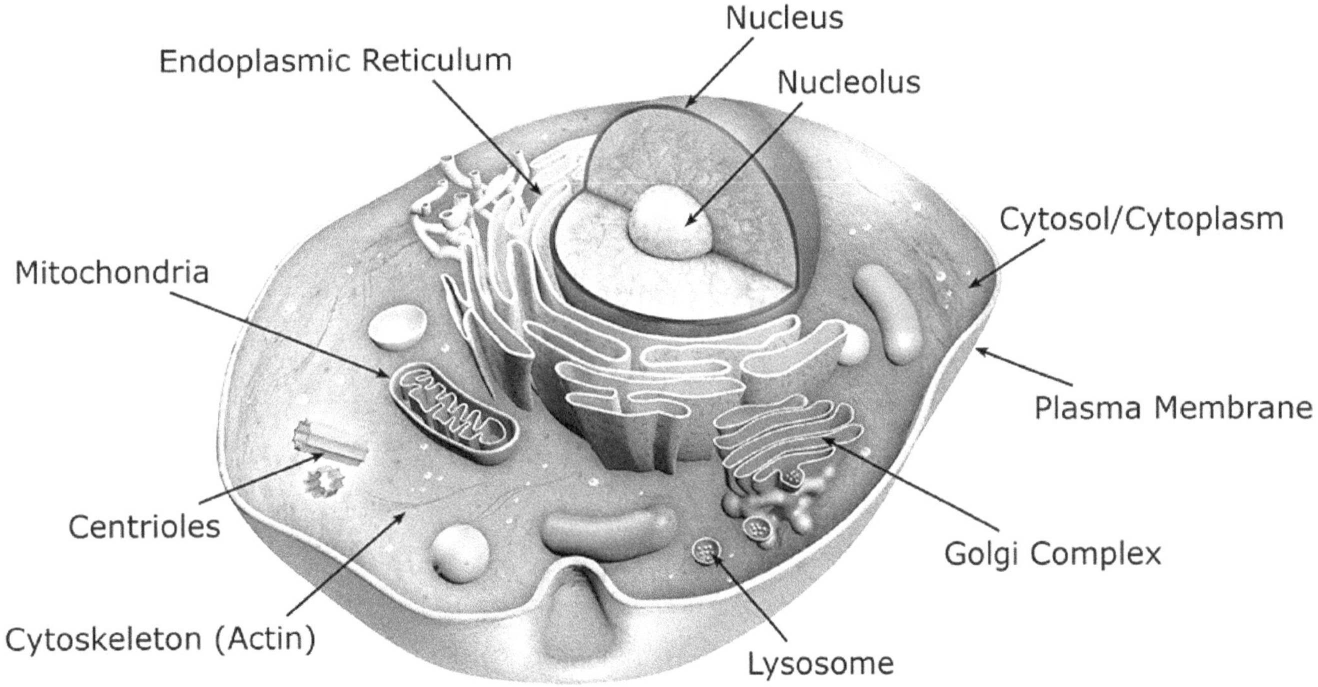

Early Researchers

Antonie van Leeuwenhoek, a 17th-century Dutch tradesman and scientist, who is often credited with the invention of the microscope. His pioneering use of handcrafted microscopes allowed him to be the first to observe and describe single-celled organisms, sperm cells, blood cells, and microbial life, effectively laying the groundwork for microbiology.

Another significant contributor was Robert Hooke, an English natural philosopher who, in 1665, coined the term "cell" after observing the structure of cork through a microscope. His observations, published in "Micrographia," were among the first to describe the cellular nature of living tissue, marking a pivotal moment in biological science.

Matthias Schleiden and Theodor Schwann further built upon these early observations to formulate the cell theory in the 1830s, stating that all living things are composed of cells and that the cell is the basic unit of life. Their work unified the study of plants and animals under one theoretical umbrella, emphasizing the importance of the cell in the larger context of biology.

Jan Evangelista Purkyně, a Czech anatomist and physiologist, made significant contributions to cell theory with his early observations of animal cells and the discovery of Purkinje cells in the cerebellum. His work in the early 19th century contributed to the growing understanding of cellular structure and function in various tissues.

Current Implications

Biomedical Research: Their pioneering work on cellular organelles underpins much of today's biomedical research, particularly in understanding how cells process signals, produce proteins, and regulate their internal environments. This knowledge is crucial for investigating the cellular basis of diseases.

Cancer Research: Understanding the function and structure of organelles like the endoplasmic reticulum and lysosomes is critical in cancer research. It aids in identifying how cancer cells proliferate, evade death, and interact with their environment, opening avenues for targeted cancer therapies.

Drug Development: Insights into cellular organelles have facilitated the development of drugs that target specific cellular processes, such as protein synthesis in the endoplasmic reticulum or waste processing in lysosomes. This specificity can lead to more effective treatments with fewer side effects.

Gene Therapy: Knowledge of cell biology is fundamental to the development of gene therapy techniques, where therapeutic DNA is introduced into patient cells. Understanding how cells process and express genes allows for more effective and safer gene therapy strategies.

Biotechnology and Synthetic Biology: The detailed understanding of cellular machinery has propelled advances in biotechnology and synthetic biology, including the engineering of microbes to produce pharmaceuticals, biofuels, and other valuable products.

Diagnostics: The discovery and characterization of organelles have led to improved diagnostic methods for various diseases. For instance, changes in organelle function or structure can serve as biomarkers for specific conditions, aiding in early detection and treatment.

Impact and Products

Cellular Imaging Technologies: Their work has spurred advancements in imaging technologies, such as high-resolution electron microscopy and live-cell imaging systems. These technologies allow scientists and medical professionals to visualize cellular processes in unprecedented detail, facilitating new discoveries in cell biology and disease mechanisms.

Organelle-Specific Therapies: Insights into the function of specific organelles have led to the development of therapies targeting these cellular components. For example, drugs designed to modulate lysosomal function are being used to treat lysosomal storage diseases, a group of rare genetic disorders.

Cell Culture Systems: Understanding cellular structures and their functions has been instrumental in developing advanced cell culture systems, including 3D cultures and organoids. These systems more accurately mimic the in vivo environment, improving the study of diseases, drug testing, and tissue engineering.

Diagnostic Biomarkers: The identification and characterization of organelles have enabled the use of organelle-specific biomarkers in diagnostic tests. For instance, biomarkers related to mitochondrial dysfunction are used in diagnosing certain metabolic and neurodegenerative diseases.

Biotechnological Tools: The research by Claude, de Duve, and Palade has contributed to the creation of biotechnological tools, such as engineered enzymes derived from lysosomes for industrial applications, including waste processing and the synthesis of bioproducts.

Educational Materials and Models: Their discoveries have enriched educational content and models for teaching cell biology. Detailed models of cells and organelles based on their work are now fundamental tools in biology education, helping students visualize and understand cellular components and their functions.

The impact of their work extends far beyond these examples, continuously influencing the development of new technologies and therapeutic approaches that enhance our ability to diagnose, treat, and understand human diseases at the cellular level.

DAVID BALTIMORE, R. DULBECCO, HOWARD TEMIN (1975)

Molecular basis of virus- tumor interaction that led to the discovery of Reverse transcriptase

In 1975, David Baltimore, Renato Dulbecco, and Howard Temin received the Nobel Prize in Medicine for their work on how tumor viruses interact with the genetic material of cells. Their research has been crucial for understanding the genetic changes that can lead to cancer.

History

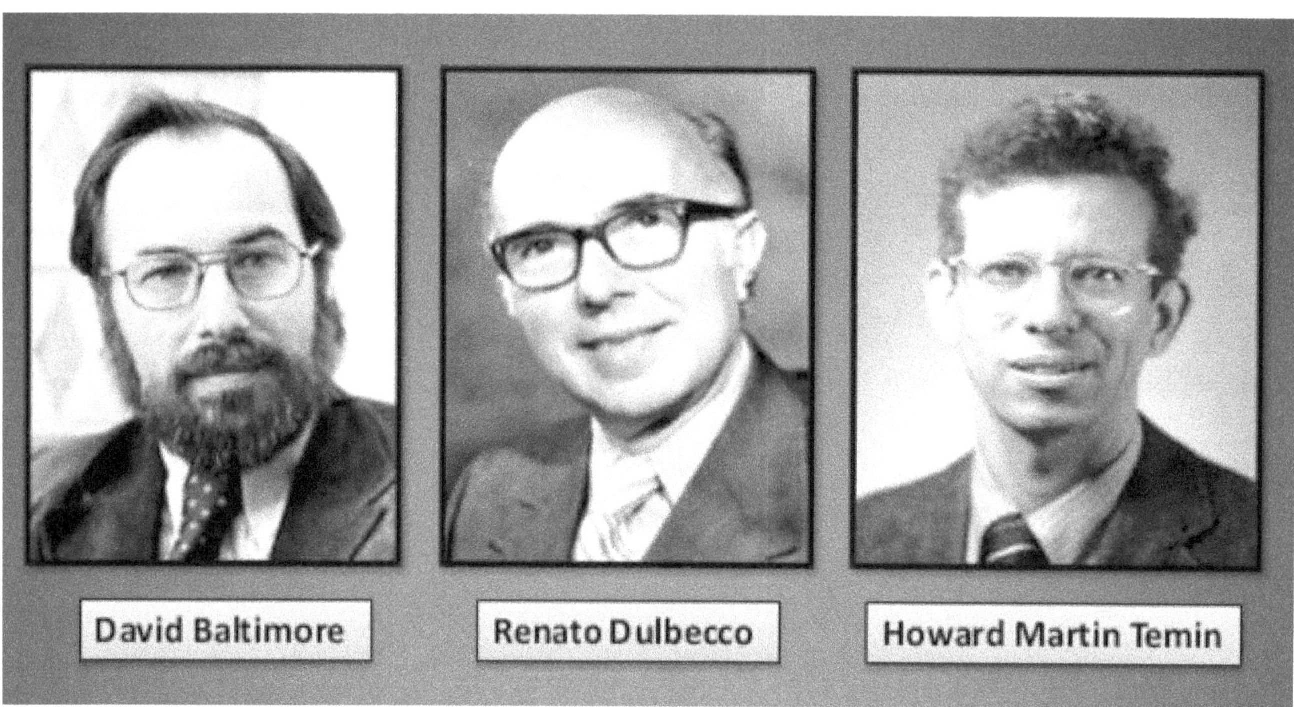

David Baltimore, born March 7, 1938, in New York City, discovered reverse transcriptase, showing how DNA can be made from RNA. Renato Dulbecco, born February 22, 1914, in Italy, and Howard Temin, born December 10, 1934, in Philadelphia, were honored for showing how viruses can insert their DNA into the DNA of host cells, altering cell behavior and sometimes causing cancer.

Snippets

Their discoveries included the process by which RNA viruses replicate by converting their RNA into DNA in the host cell, challenging previously held beliefs about genetic information flow. Dulbecco's experiments showed that the DNA of tumor viruses becomes part of the DNA of infected cells, a fundamental step in understanding cancer's genetic basis.

Current Implications

This work has been vital in cancer research and virology, leading to new methods for studying genetic diseases and developing antiviral drugs. It has improved our understanding of how viral infections can lead to cancer and other diseases.

Impact and Products

The findings by Baltimore, Dulbecco, and Temin have influenced biotechnology, genetics, and the development of cancer treatments. Their discovery of reverse transcriptase, in particular, has been instrumental in genetic engineering and research into viral diseases, contributing significantly to medical science and treatment strategies.

BARUCH BLUMBERG AND DANIEL CARLETON GAJDUSEK (1976)

Phenomenal discovery of hepatitis B virus and cure for Infectious prion disease Kuru,

History

In 1976, Baruch Blumberg and Daniel Carleton Gajdusek received the Nobel Prize in Medicine for their groundbreaking work on infectious diseases. Their research significantly advanced the medical field's understanding of how certain diseases are transmitted and managed.

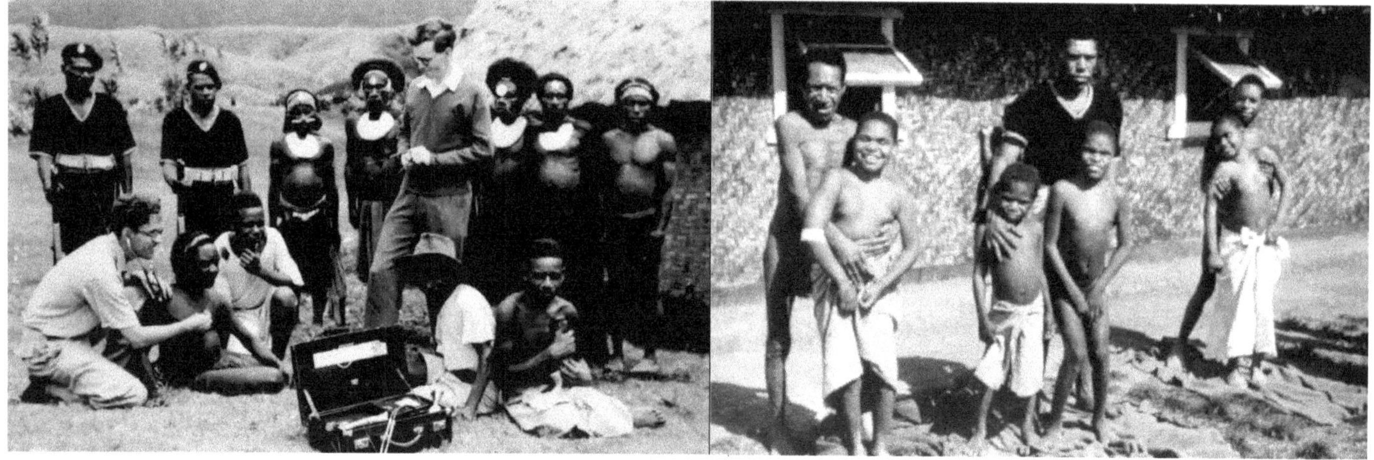

D. Carleton Gajdusek collecting blood from school children at the Okapa Patrol Post. Kuru Research field in Papua New guinea.

Baruch Blumberg, born July 28, 1925, in New York City, was instrumental in discovering the hepatitis B virus, leading to the development of both a diagnostic test and a vaccine. Daniel Carleton Gajdusek, born September 9, 1923, in Yonkers, New York, made key discoveries about Kuru, a neurodegenerative disease, showing it was infectious and linked to prion proteins.

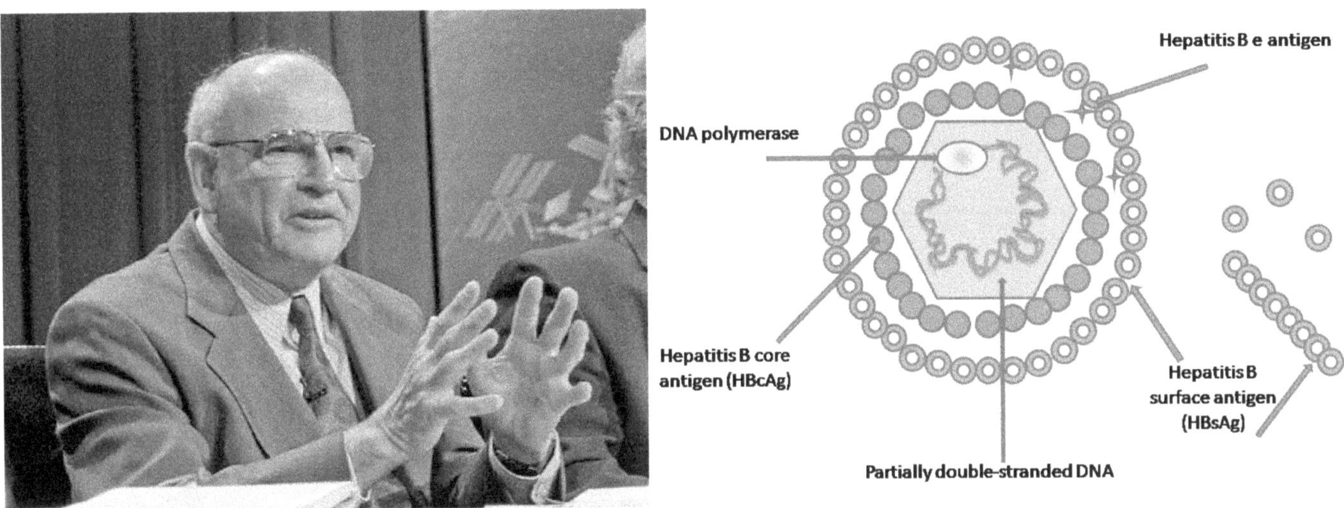

Baruch Blumberg and Hepatris B virus

Snippets

Blumberg's work not only identified the hepatitis B virus but also linked it to liver cancer, prompting the creation of the vaccine, a major step in cancer prevention. Gajdusek's research into kuru opened new paths in understanding prion diseases, which are crucial for neurodegenerative disease research.

Current Implications

The discoveries by Blumberg and Gajdusek have led to significant advances in preventing and treating infectious and prion diseases. Their work laid the foundation for ongoing research in disease transmission, vaccine development, and the study of neurodegenerative conditions.

Impact and Products

Thanks to their efforts, strategies for combating diseases like hepatitis B have been revolutionized, with the vaccine drastically reducing infection rates and liver cancer rate. Gajdusek's findings on kuru have informed research into similar neurodegenerative diseases, enhancing scientific understanding and treatment approaches.

ROGER GUILLEMIN, ANDREW SCHALLY, ROSALYN YALOW
(1977)

Landmark discovery of Radio-immunoassay and peptide hormone production

The Nobel Prize in Medicine in 1977 was awarded jointly to Roger Guillemin and Andrew Schally for their discoveries concerning the peptide hormone production of the brain, and to Rosalyn Yalow for the development of radio-immunoassays of peptide hormones.

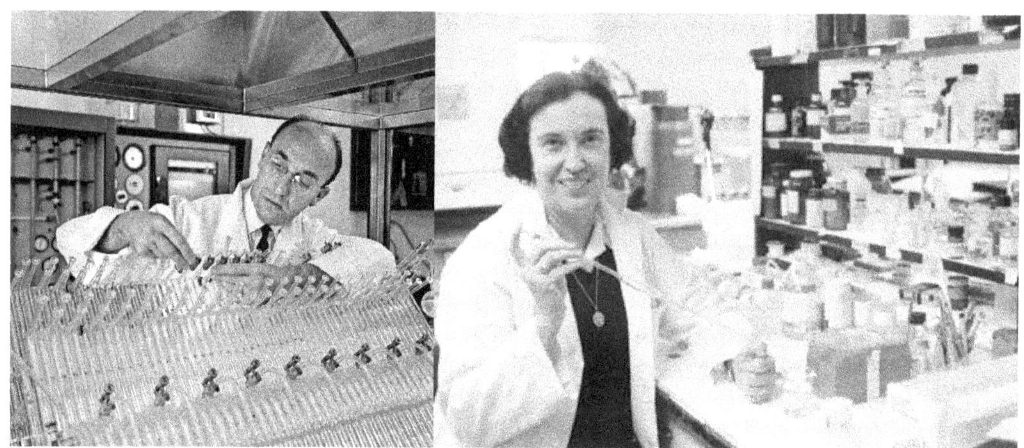
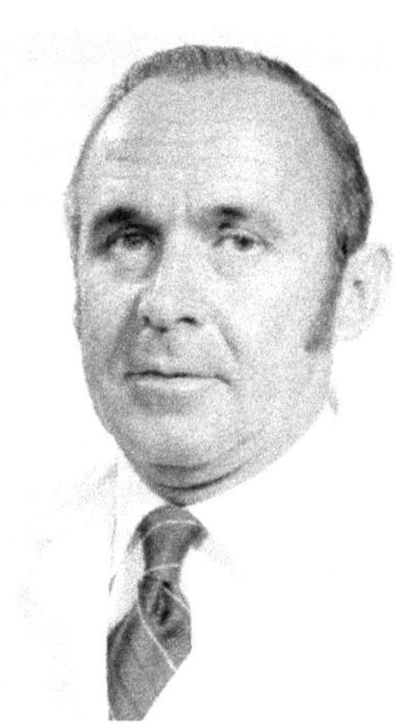

History

Roger Guillemin, born in France in 1924, moved to the United States in the 1950s, where he joined the faculty at Baylor College of Medicine in Houston, Texas. Guillemin's research focused on understanding how the brain controls the pituitary gland's release of hormones, leading to the isolation of several hypothalamic hormones.

Andrew Schally, born in Poland in 1926, also immigrated to the United States where his work paralleled Guillemin's. At the Veterans Administration Hospital in New Orleans, Schally's research led to the discovery of hypothalamic hormones that regulate anterior pituitary function, a groundbreaking achievement in neuroendocrinology.

Rosalyn Yalow, born in New York City in 1921, co-developed the radioimmunoassay (RIA) technique, a breakthrough in medical diagnostics. Her work at the Bronx VA Medical Center revolutionized the measurement of peptide hormones in the blood, providing tools essential for diagnosing various hormonal disorders.

Snippets

Guillemin and Schally's Brain Hormone Discoveries: They independently identified and characterized several key hypothalamic hormones that regulate the anterior pituitary gland, crucial for understanding endocrine system functions.

Yalow's Radioimmunoassay Technique: Developed a groundbreaking method for measuring concentrations of hormones in the blood, significantly advancing diagnostic capabilities in endocrinology and beyond.

Impact on Endocrine Research: Their work collectively ushered in a new era of research on hormonal regulation and interaction within the body, providing a foundation for numerous subsequent discoveries in physiology and medicine.

Applications in Clinical Diagnostics: Yalow's radioimmunoassay technology transformed the ability to diagnose and monitor a wide range of hormonal disorders, making it a staple in medical laboratories worldwide.

Advances in Hormone Therapy: The elucidation of hypothalamic hormones by Guillemin and Schally paved the way for synthetic hormone production and therapies targeting specific endocrine disorders.

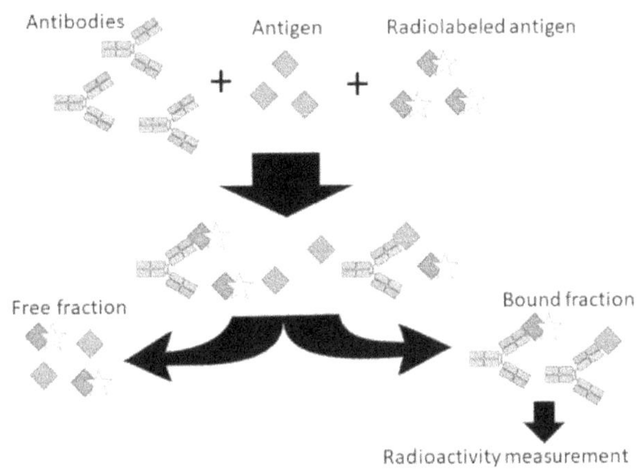

The principle of radio Immuno assay

Early Researchers

Charles Best, often remembered for his co-discovery of insulin, who played a crucial role in the early studies of pancreatic functions and the hormonal regulation of blood sugar. His work was instrumental in identifying the role of insulin in diabetes, setting the stage for future hormonal therapies.

Another notable pioneer is Edgar Allen, whose early work in the 1920s on female reproductive hormones contributed to the identification of estrogen. Alongside Edward Doisy, Allen's efforts in extracting and characterizing estrogen marked significant progress in reproductive endocrinology and women's health.

Ernest Starling, a physiologist who coined the term "hormone," and his colleague William Bayliss, made seminal contributions through their discovery of secretin, the first identified hormone, in 1902. Their work demonstrated the existence of chemical messengers in the body, laying a conceptual foundation for the field of endocrinology.

Additionally, Rosalind Franklin, whose work in X-ray diffraction provided critical insights into the structure of DNA, also contributed to the understanding of viral structures and their interactions with the immune system. While her contributions to genetics are widely acknowledged, her impact on the broader field of biological research, including studies related to cellular and viral mechanisms, underscores the interconnectedness of molecular biology and endocrinology.

Current Implications

Enhanced Diagnostic Techniques: The development of the radioimmunoassay (RIA) by Rosalyn Yalow revolutionized the ability to measure hormones and other substances in the blood with precision. This technique remains foundational in diagnosing various conditions, from hormonal imbalances to infectious diseases, facilitating early and accurate treatment.

Understanding of Neuroendocrine Regulation: The discoveries by Guillemin and Schally regarding brain hormones elucidated the neuroendocrine system's complexity. This has profound implications for understanding diseases like obesity, diabetes, and various psychiatric disorders, which can involve dysregulation of these hormonal pathways.

Advancements in Hormone Therapy: Insights into hormone regulation and action have led to the development of new hormone-based therapies for conditions such as infertility, endocrine cancers, and growth disorders. These therapies can mimic, block, or modify the action of natural hormones to treat diseases more effectively.

Impact on Biotechnology and Pharmaceutical Industries: The isolation and characterization of hormones and the ability to measure them accurately have spurred innovations in biotechnology, leading to the synthesis of hormones for medical use. Pharmaceutical companies continue to develop new drugs targeting hormonal pathways, influenced by the foundational work of these Nobel laureates.

Research in Aging and Metabolic Diseases: Understanding hormonal control mechanisms has implications for research into aging and metabolic diseases. By exploring how hormones influence processes like cell growth, metabolism, and aging, scientists are developing interventions to promote healthy aging and treat metabolic disorders.

Impact and Products

Radioimmunoassay (RIA) Kits: The RIA technique developed by Yalow has been commercialized into various diagnostic kits, allowing for the precise measurement of hormones, vitamins, drugs, and other substances in the blood. These kits are used worldwide in clinical laboratories for diagnosing conditions such as thyroid disorders, fertility issues, and doping in sports.

Hormone Replacement Therapies: The discoveries of Guillemin and Schally regarding the brain's control of hormone production have facilitated the development of synthetic hormones used in hormone replacement therapies (HRT). These therapies are crucial for managing symptoms of menopause, hypothyroidism, and growth hormone deficiencies.

Cancer Treatment Drugs: Insights into hormone regulation and function have led to the creation of drugs that target specific hormonal pathways involved in cancer growth, such as breast and prostate cancers. Therapies that either block the body's production of these hormones or prevent their action on cancer cells are now standard treatments for hormone-sensitive cancers.

Fertility Treatments: The isolation and understanding of gonadotropin-releasing hormone (GnRH) and its analogs have revolutionized fertility treatments. GnRH agonists and antagonists are used in assisted reproductive technologies (ART) to control ovulation and improve the success rates of in vitro fertilization (IVF).

Diagnostic and Research Tools: The principles laid down by these laureates have led to the development of advanced tools and techniques for research, including those that study hormone actions at the molecular level. These tools are instrumental in discovering new therapeutic targets and understanding disease mechanisms.

The impact of their contributions extends beyond these applications, influencing ongoing research in endocrinology, neurobiology, and pharmacology. The work of Guillemin, Schally, and Yalow continues to inspire innovations that enhance our ability to diagnose and treat diseases, showcasing the enduring value of their research in improving human health.

WERNER ARBER DANIEL NATHANS, HAMILTON O. SMITH (1978)

The new age of DNA editing molecular knife

In 1978, Werner Arber, Daniel Nathans, and Hamilton O. Smith were awarded the Nobel Prize in Medicine for their discoveries concerning restriction enzymes and their application to molecular genetics. Their work has significantly influenced the field of genetic engineering.

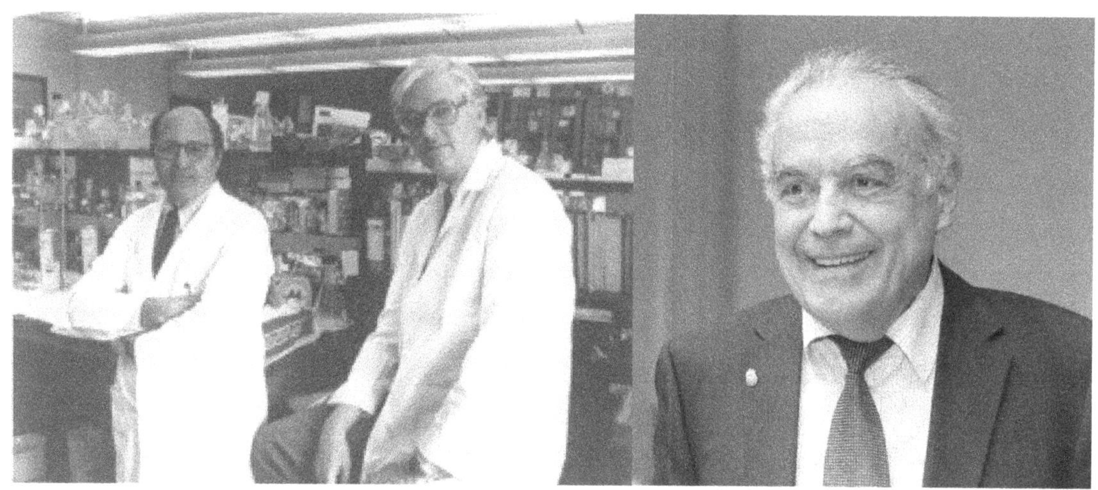

Daniel Nathans   Hamilton Smith   Werner Arber

History

Werner Arber, born on June 3, 1929, in Gränichen, Switzerland, contributed to the discovery and understanding of restriction enzymes, proteins that cut DNA at specific sites. Daniel Nathans, born on October 30, 1928, in Wilmington, Delaware, USA, used these enzymes to map genetic elements of viruses. Hamilton O. Smith, born on August 23, 1931, in New York City, USA, identified the first type II restriction enzyme, which became a fundamental tool in molecular biology.

Snippets

The trio's research led to the recognition that restriction enzymes could act as precise tools for cutting and studying DNA, thereby laying the groundwork for genetic mapping, cloning, and sequencing. Their work has enabled scientists to manipulate genetic material in ways that were previously not possible, opening up new possibilities in research and medicine.

Current Implications

The discoveries by Arber, Nathans, and Smith have had a lasting impact on biotechnology and medicine, facilitating advances in gene therapy, the development of genetically modified organisms, and the study of genetic diseases. Their work on restriction enzymes has been crucial for the Human Genome Project and other genetic research that seeks to understand the blueprint of life.

Impact and Products

Today, the research conducted by them is fundamental to genetic engineering and molecular biology. It has led to practical applications such as the production of insulin and growth hormones through recombinant DNA technology, as well as improved diagnostics and treatments for genetic disorders.

ALLAN CORMACK AND GODFREY HOUNSFIELD (1979)

CT Scan : A glittering crown in medical imaging, a fusion science of computer with X-rays

Allan M. Cormack and Godfrey N. Hounsfield were jointly awarded the Nobel Prize in Medicine in 1979 for the development of computer-assisted tomography, a pivotal advancement in diagnostic medicine.

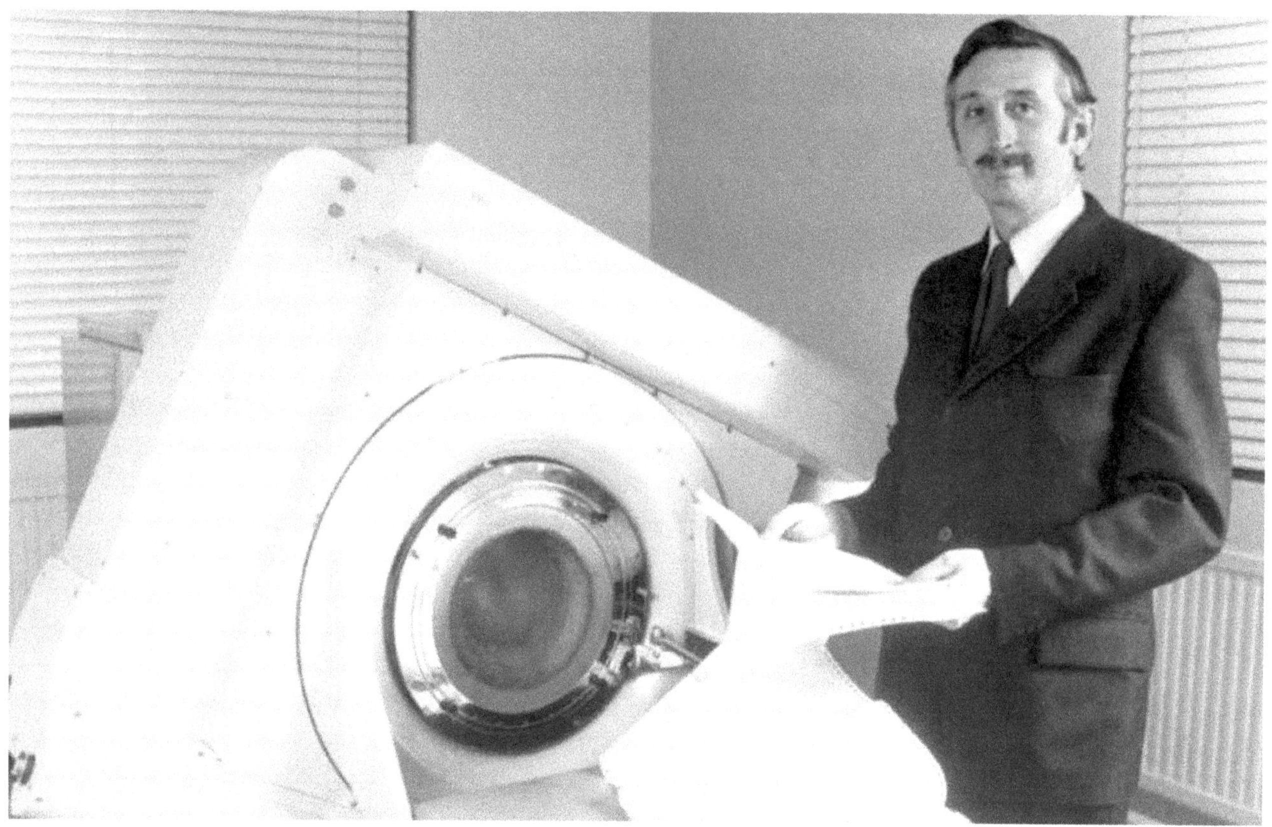

History

Allan MacLeod Cormack was born in Johannesburg, South Africa, in 1924, into a family that had recently emigrated from Scotland. Growing up, Cormack's family moved frequently due to his father's job, but they eventually settled in Cape Town following his father's death. Cormack's academic pursuits began at the University of Cape Town, where, despite initially studying electrical engineering, his interest shifted to physics, spurred by a deep fascination with astronomy learned from the works of Sir Arthur Eddington and Sir James Jeans.

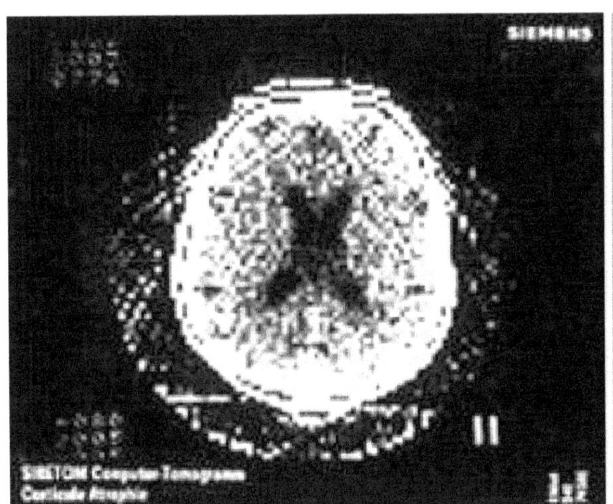
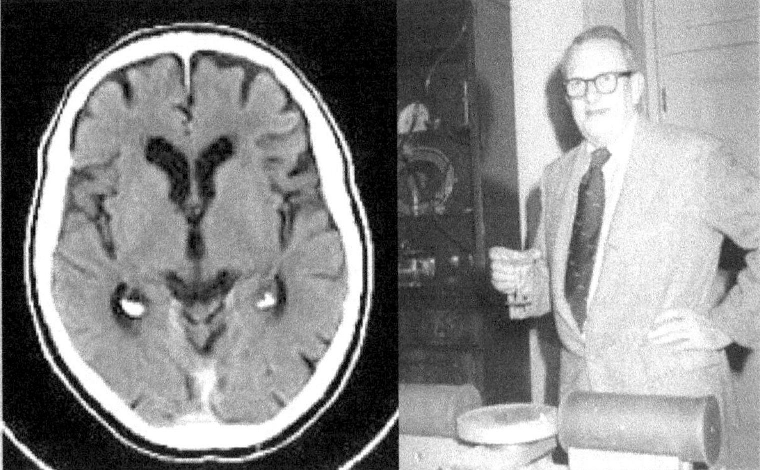

Cormack's academic journey led him to St. John's College, Cambridge, for his research degree, where he worked under Prof. Otto Frisch at the Cavendish Laboratory. Although his initial research focused on nuclear physics, a turn of events, including marriage and financial necessity, brought him back to Cape Town, this time as a lecturer. It was here, somewhat serendipitously, that Cormack's interest in what would later be known as CT scanning began.

Godfrey Newbold Hounsfield, born in Nottinghamshire, England, in 1919, had a quintessential tinkerer's upbringing. His early years on a farm instilled in him a fascination with mechanical and electrical devices, fostering a self-taught ethos that would characterize his approach to problem-solving. Unlike Cormack, Hounsfield's formal education did not spark until his experiences in the Royal Air Force during World War II, where he was introduced to radar technology and radio mechanics.

Hounsfield's academic career was supported by an Air Vice-Marshal who recognized his potential, leading him to Faraday House Electrical Engineering College in London. His career at EMI Laboratories began in the radar and guided weapons department, but his interests quickly turned towards the nascent field of computers.

Hounsfield's transition to medical imaging technology came from his work in pattern recognition and computer technology at EMI. In 1967, the idea of using computer technology to create detailed images of the brain marked the inception of CT technology. Hounsfield's perseverance through technical and conceptual challenges led to the development of the first clinically used CT scanner, a breakthrough in medical diagnostics.

Snippets

The Inception of CT Scanning: Cormack's theoretical work provided the mathematical foundation for CT imaging, despite his focus being largely academic and isolated from practical application. It wasn't until Hounsfield, working independently at EMI Laboratories, applied Cormack's theories to construct the first CT scanner that the practical potential of CT scanning was realized. This convergence of theory and application underscores the serendipitous nature of their joint achievement.

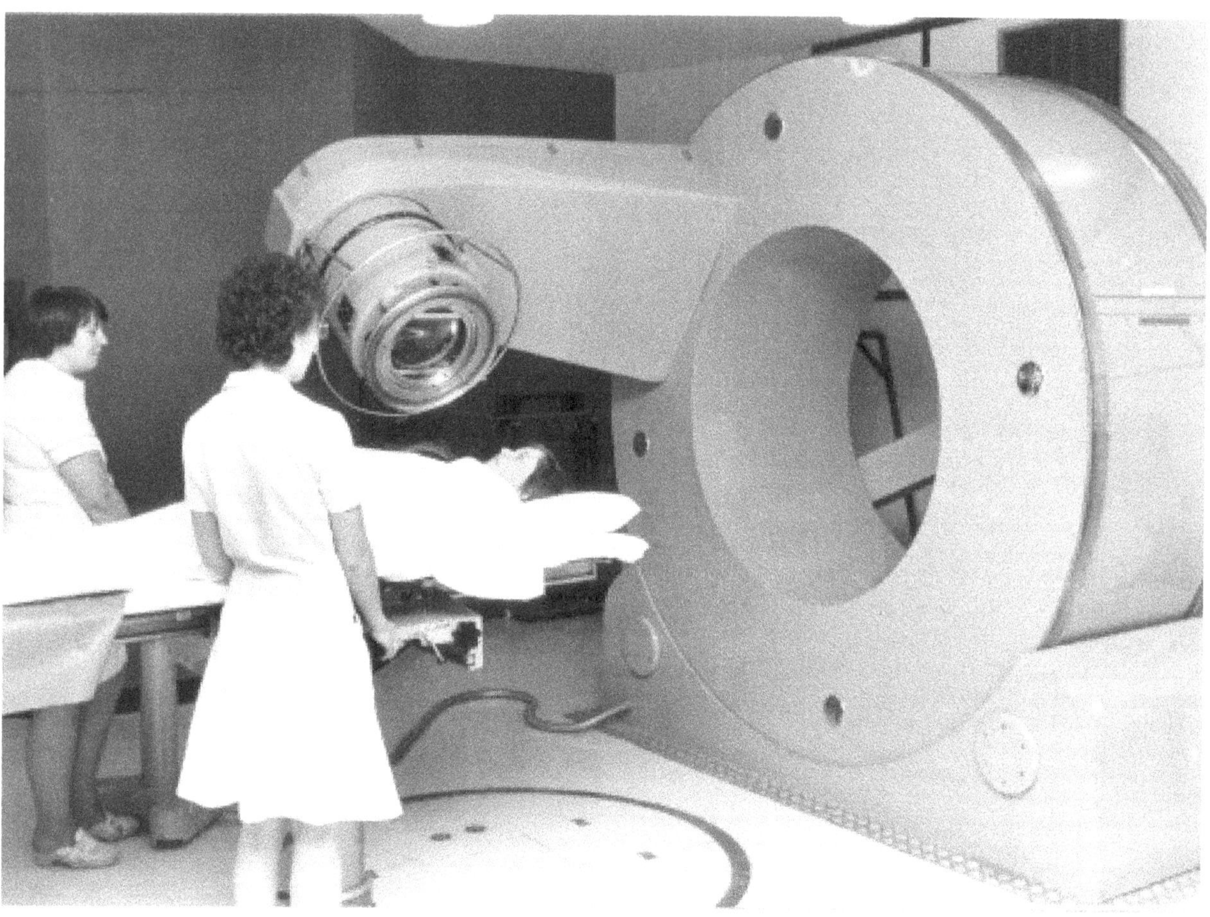

Technical Breakthroughs: Hounsfield's initial idea in 1967 to use computer technology for brain imaging was a radical departure from existing diagnostic methods. His work involved overcoming significant technical challenges, including the development of sensitive enough detectors and computational methods to reconstruct images from multiple x-ray readings. The first clinical brain scanner was completed in 1971, a direct result of Hounsfield's perseverance and innovative thinking.

Global Impact on Medicine: The introduction of CT scanning technology has had a profound and lasting impact on the field of diagnostic medicine. By providing clear, detailed cross-sectional images of the body, CT scans have revolutionized the way diseases are diagnosed, treatments are planned, and surgeries are performed. This technology has become an indispensable tool in hospitals and clinics worldwide, saving countless lives through early detection and precise medical intervention.

Early Researchers

Emil Grubbe: Often considered one of the first medical practitioners to use X-rays for cancer treatment, Grubbe's early exploration into the medical application of radiation paved the way for diagnostic imaging techniques, including CT scanning.

Rosalind Franklin: Known for her crucial contributions to the understanding of DNA structure, Franklin's pioneering work in X-ray crystallography also laid the groundwork for advanced imaging techniques. Her expertise in revealing the detailed structures of biological materials demonstrated the potential of X-ray imaging for medical and scientific research.

Werner Forssmann: Forssmann performed the first human catheterization of the heart, a daring feat that not only advanced cardiac medicine but also exemplified the potential of invasive techniques for diagnostic purposes. His work indirectly highlighted the need for non-invasive diagnostic tools, setting the stage for innovations like CT scanning.

John Wild: A pioneer in the field of ultrasound, Wild's early work in the 1950s demonstrated the use of ultrasound for medical diagnostics. While distinct from CT technology, his contributions to imaging techniques share the spirit of innovation and non-invasive diagnosis that CT scanning embodies.

Current Implications

Early Detection and Diagnosis: CT scans enable the early detection of diseases such as cancer, cardiovascular diseases, and musculoskeletal disorders. This technology allows for the identification of abnormalities before symptoms become apparent, significantly improving patient outcomes.

Improved Treatment Planning: The detailed imagery provided by CT scans aids in precise treatment planning, including surgery and radiation therapy. It helps in determining the size, shape, and location of tumors and other abnormalities, leading to more effective and targeted treatment approaches.

Minimally Invasive Procedures: The use of CT scans has facilitated the development of minimally invasive diagnostic procedures, such as biopsies, reducing the need for exploratory surgeries. This has led to shorter recovery times and less risk for patients.

Emergency Medicine: In emergency settings, CT technology is crucial for quickly assessing injuries from accidents, strokes, and acute illnesses. The speed and accuracy of CT scans enable rapid decision-making and treatment, saving lives in critical situations.

Research and Development: Beyond clinical applications, CT scanning drives advancements in medical research, offering insights into disease mechanisms and the effectiveness of new treatments. It's an invaluable tool in the development of novel therapies and understanding human anatomy.

Personalized Medicine: CT scanning contributes to the evolution of personalized medicine, where treatments can be tailored to the individual characteristics of each patient's condition. By providing detailed internal images, CT scans help in customizing therapeutic approaches to the specific needs of patients.

Impact and Products

Medical Diagnostics and Therapeutics: The advent of CT technology has catalyzed the development of various diagnostic tools and therapeutic devices, particularly those that require precise imaging to function correctly. This includes enhancements in oncology for tumor detection, neurology for brain imaging, and cardiology for heart examinations.

Advanced Imaging Modalities: The principles underlying CT scanning have paved the way for advancements in other imaging modalities, such as positron emission tomography (PET) scans and magnetic resonance imaging (MRI), which offer different kinds of tissue contrast and functional information. Hybrid machines that combine CT with these technologies provide comprehensive diagnostic capabilities.

3D Printing and Modeling: The detailed images produced by CT scans are utilized in 3D printing and modeling, especially in custom medical devices like prosthetics and dental implants. This application extends into reconstructive surgery planning and the customization of implants to fit individual anatomical structures precisely.

Archaeology and Paleontology: CT scans have become an invaluable tool in archaeology and paleontology, allowing researchers to examine the internal structures of ancient artifacts and fossils without the need for physical dissection. This non-invasive method has led to significant discoveries regarding ancient cultures and extinct species.

Security and Inspection: The use of CT technology in security screening, particularly in airports, has significantly improved the detection of prohibited items, including explosives and weapons, inside luggage. This enhancement in security protocols illustrates the technology's impact on public safety.

Art Restoration and Analysis: In the art world, CT scanning offers a non-destructive means to analyze and authenticate paintings, sculptures, and other artworks. It enables experts to examine the layers and materials used, assisting in restoration projects and understanding the techniques of historical artists.

The continuous refinement and adaptation of this technology ensure its enduring relevance and expanding impact on society, from enhancing patient care to advancing scientific research and innovation in numerous industries.

BARUJ BENACERRAF, JEAN DAUSSET, GEORGE SNELL (1980)

Human Leukocyte Antigen (HLA) system that revolutionized transplantation science

In 1980, Baruj Benacerraf, Jean Dausset, and George Snell were awarded the Nobel Prize in Medicine for their discoveries regarding genetically determined structures on the cell surface that regulate immunological reactions. Their work has been crucial in understanding the immune system and has had significant implications for organ transplantation, autoimmune diseases, and more.

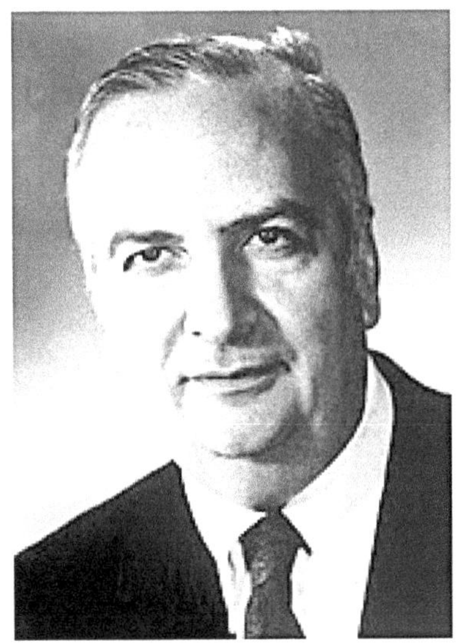

Baruj Benacerraf

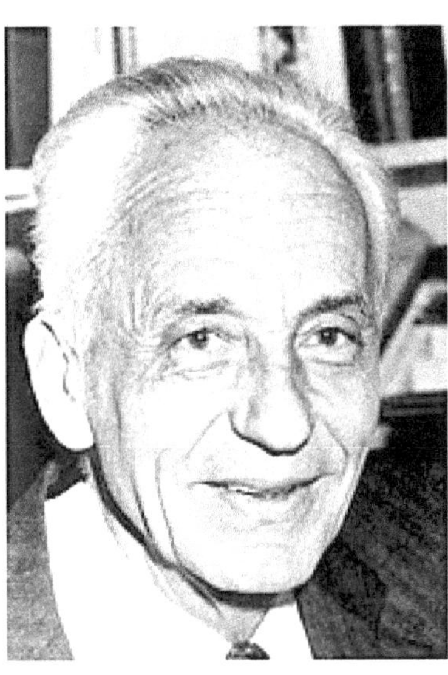

Jean Dausset

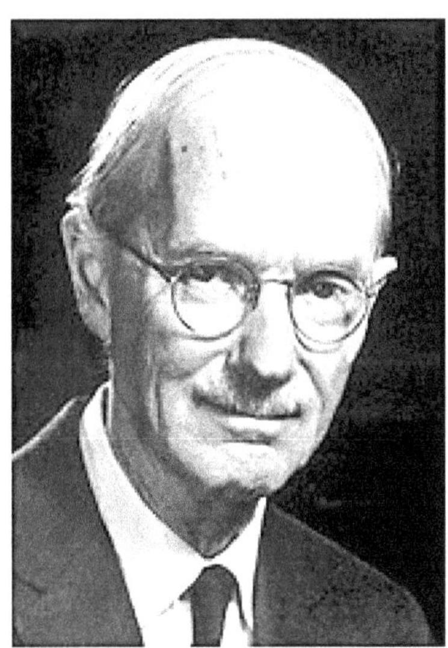

George D. Snell

History

Baruj Benacerraf, born on October 29, 1920, in Caracas, Venezuela, was recognized for his work on immune response genes. Jean Dausset, born on October 19, 1916, in Toulouse, France, discovered the human leukocyte antigen (HLA) system, a key to understanding the immune system's ability to differentiate between self and non-self. George Snell, born on December 19, 1903, in Bradford, Massachusetts, USA, made foundational contributions to the genetics of the immune response, particularly through his work on the major histocompatibility complex (MHC) in mice.

Snippets

The trio's research collectively revealed how the immune system recognizes and reacts to foreign substances. Benacerraf's identification of immune response (Ir) genes provided insights into how genetic variations influence individual immune responses. Dausset's work on the HLA system laid the groundwork for understanding tissue compatibility in organ transplantation. Snell's discoveries on MHC helped explain the genetic basis of immune recognition and rejection.

Current Implications

Their discoveries have transformed medical approaches to treating and managing organ transplants, autoimmune diseases, and understanding cancer immunotherapy. The HLA typing, for instance, is a standard practice in organ transplantation to ensure compatibility between donors and recipients.

Impact and Products

Today, the work of Benacerraf, Dausset, and Snell continues to guide research in immunology, genetics, and medicine. Their contributions have led to improved methods for diagnosing and treating immune-related diseases, significantly impacting patient care and opening new avenues for therapeutic interventions.

ROGER SPERRY, DAVID HUBEL, TORSTEN WIESEL (1981)

The trio brought new insight in the Inter – hemispherical regulatory network of brain

In 1981, Roger Sperry, David Hubel, and Torsten Wiesel were awarded the Nobel Prize in Medicine for their contributions to understanding the nervous system's organization and processing of information. Their work shed light on the brain's visual processing system and the functional specialization of its hemispheres.

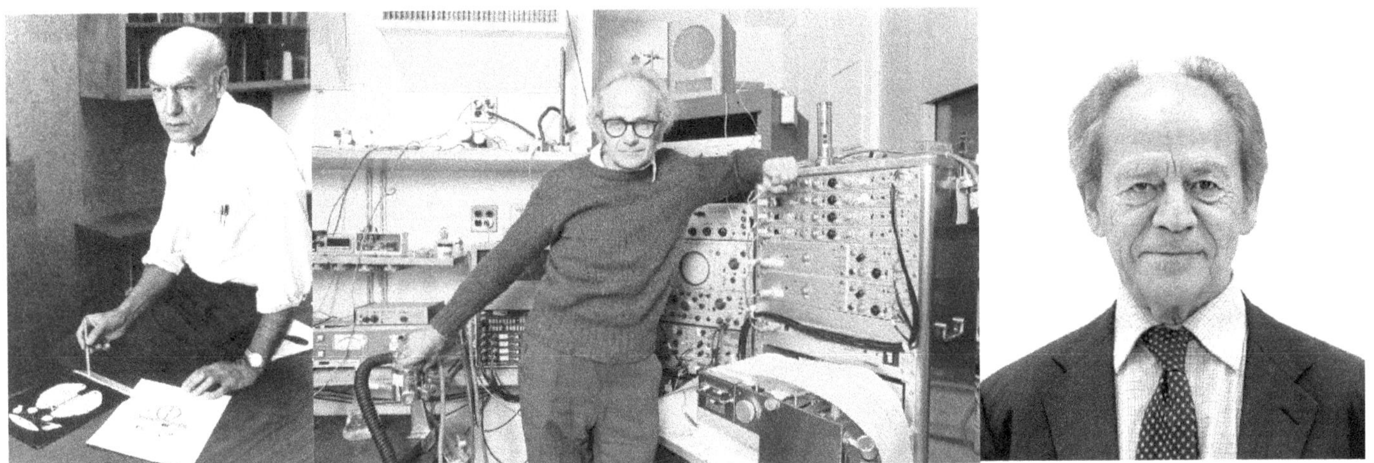

Roger Sperry   David Hubel   Torsten Wiesel

History

Roger Sperry, born August 20, 1913, in Hartford, Connecticut, USA, conducted innovative research on the brain's divided functions, revealing how each hemisphere has specialized tasks. David Hubel, born February 27, 1926, in Windsor, Ontario, Canada, and Torsten Wiesel, born June 3, 1924, in Uppsala, Sweden, collaborated on research that demonstrated how visual information is received and processed in the brain.

Snippets

Sperry's experiments with split-brain patients illustrated the independent functioning of the brain's left and right hemispheres, altering previous notions about brain organization. Hubel and Wiesel's work on the visual cortex of cats and monkeys revealed how the brain interprets visual signals, identifying the critical role of specific neurons in processing visual stimuli such as light, shapes, and movement.

Current Implications

Their discoveries have deep implications for neuroscience, psychology, and medicine, enhancing the understanding of brain injuries, developmental disorders, and the rehabilitation of brain function. The research has influenced teaching methods for individuals with brain damage and expanded knowledge on sensory perception and consciousness.

Impact and Products

The work of Sperry, Hubel, and Wiesel has been pivotal in neuroscience, paving the way for advanced research on brain function and perception. Their findings have contributed to developing therapeutic strategies for neurological disorders and improving educational approaches for people with cognitive impairments due to brain injuries.

SUNE BERGSTRÖM, BENGT SAMUELSSON, JOHN VANE (1982)

*The crucial discovery of Prostaglandins, the magical molecules that regulate
body homeostasis*

The 1982 Nobel Prize in Medicine was awarded to Sune K. Bergström, Bengt I. Samuelsson, and John R. Vane for their groundbreaking discoveries concerning prostaglandins and related biologically active substances. Their research unveiled the crucial roles these substances play in various physiological processes within the body.

History

Sune K. Bergström: Bergström's journey began in Stockholm, Sweden, where his early interest in biochemistry at the Karolinska Institutet set the stage for his pioneering work on prostaglandins. Over the decades, his career saw him transition from research fellowships in London and the United States to esteemed academic positions in Sweden, including the chairmanship at the Nobel Foundation and the rector ship at the Karolinska Institutet. His dedication to uncovering the biochemical secrets of the body laid a crucial foundation for the field.

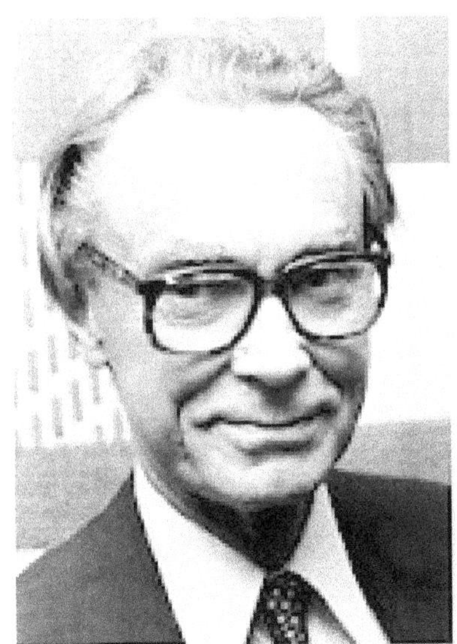
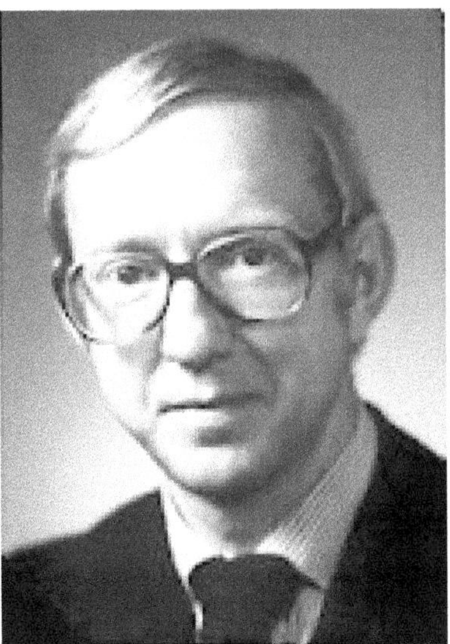
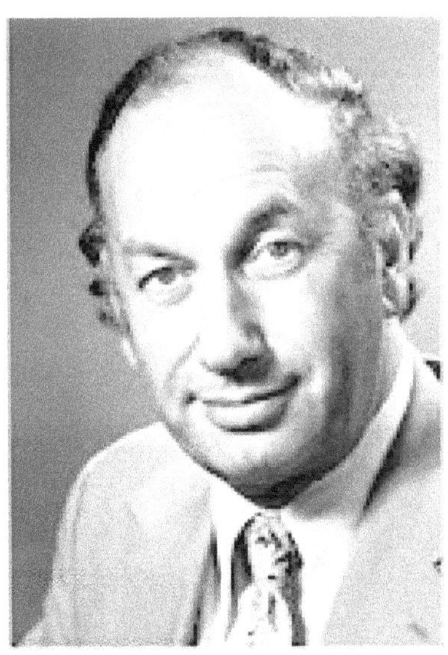

Sune K. Bergström   Bengt I. Samuelsson   John R. Vane

Bengt I. Samuelsson: Samuelsson's story also unfolds in Sweden, where his fascination with biochemistry led him from the University of Lund to the Karolinska Institutet. His doctoral work under Bergström's guidance and subsequent research, notably on cholesterol metabolism and later on prostaglandins and their derivatives like thromboxanes and leukotrienes, positioned him at the forefront of biochemical research. Samuelsson's findings have vast implications, extending into clinical areas such as thrombosis, inflammation, and allergy.

John R. Vane: Vane's contribution came from across the North Sea, in the United Kingdom, where his work at The Wellcome Research Laboratories unveiled the mechanisms by which prostaglandins influence vascular function and platelet aggregation. His discovery of prostacyclin and its effects, along with the revelation of how drugs like aspirin inhibit prostaglandin synthesis, brought to light the integral role of these substances in managing pain and inflammation. Vane's research bridged the gap between basic pharmacology and clinical medicine, providing a scientific basis for the therapeutic use of non-steroidal anti-inflammatory drugs (NSAIDs).

Snippets

Prostaglandins Unveiled: They found out that our body produces substances called prostaglandins, which act a bit like hormones. These substances play a key role in managing pain, inflammation, and even the healing process of our stomach lining. It's fascinating how our body has its own natural way of dealing with these issues.

Aspirin's Action Explained: John R. Vane showed the world how aspirin works. It turns out, aspirin stops the production of certain prostaglandins that cause pain and swelling. So, when we take aspirin for a headache or sore muscles, we're actually interfering with our body's prostaglandin production.

From Laboratory to Medicine Cabinet: The work of these three scientists has led to the development of many medicines we use today to control pain and inflammation. It's a direct link from their research in the lab to the relief we get from a simple pill.

A Balancing Act: These discoveries also highlighted the balance our body maintains through prostaglandins. For example, certain prostaglandins can cause inflammation, which is part of our body's defense mechanism, while others help heal our stomach lining or keep our blood flowing smoothly.

Early Researchers

Ulf von Euler, a Swedish physiologist who, in the 1930s, discovered a substance in human semen that he named "prostaglandin" due to its origin in the prostate gland. Von Euler's initial identification and description of prostaglandins sparked interest in these compounds, setting the stage for the detailed investigations that would follow.

Another significant figure in the history of hormone research is Derek Barton, a British chemist whose work on the conformation of steroid molecules provided crucial insights into how molecular shape affects biological activity. While Barton's primary contributions were in the field of organic chemistry, his theories on conformation and function significantly influenced the understanding of hormonal activity at the molecular level.

E.J. Corey, an American chemist, also contributed substantially to the field through his development of retrosynthetic analysis, a method that revolutionized the synthesis of complex organic molecules. Corey's work facilitated the synthesis of prostaglandins, enabling researchers to study these compounds in greater detail and understand their roles in physiological and pathological processes.

Current Implications

Treatment of Inflammatory Conditions: Understanding the role of prostaglandins in inflammation has led to the development and refinement of anti-inflammatory medications. Today, NSAIDs (Non-Steroidal Anti-Inflammatory Drugs), which include aspirin, ibuprofen, and newer selective inhibitors, are widely used to treat conditions ranging from mild headaches to chronic arthritic pain.

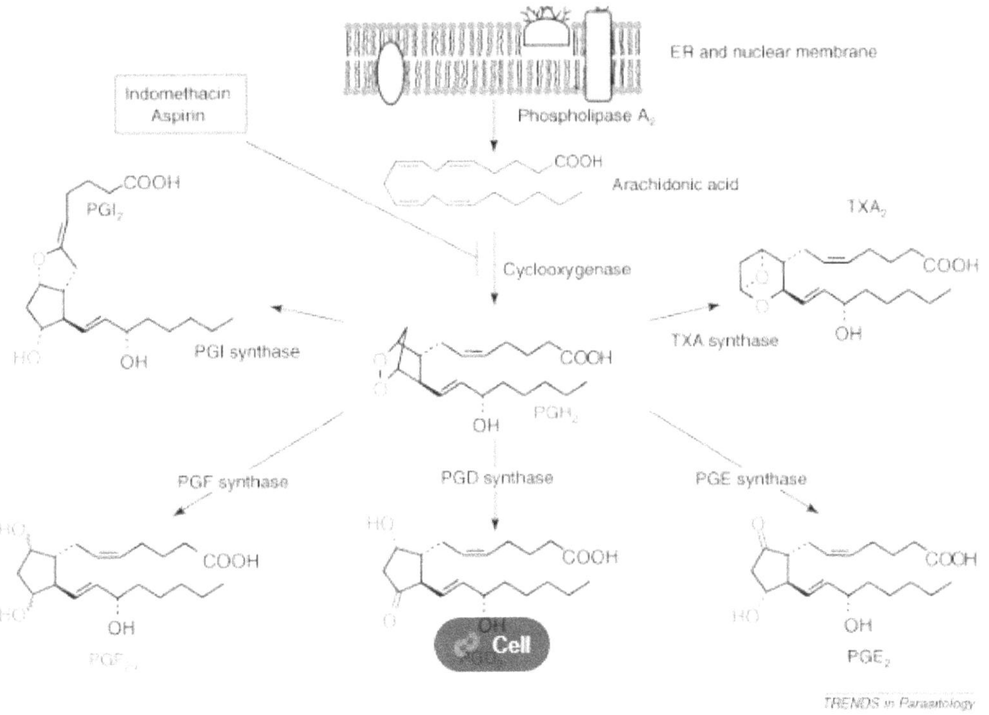

Management of Cardiovascular Diseases: The role of prostaglandins in blood flow and clotting has informed treatments for heart disease. Drugs that mimic the action of beneficial prostaglandins or inhibit harmful ones are used to manage conditions such as hypertension and reduce the risk of heart attacks.

Advances in Pain Relief: The mechanism by which prostaglandins contribute to pain sensation has been targeted by pharmaceuticals to develop more effective pain relievers. This understanding helps in designing drugs that can block the pain at its source more efficiently.

Understanding of Disease Mechanisms: Beyond their immediate applications in treatment, the pathways involving prostaglandins are studied in relation to a variety of diseases. This research helps in understanding the mechanisms behind conditions like cancer, asthma, and neurodegenerative diseases, opening up possibilities for new therapeutic approaches.

Reproductive Health: Prostaglandins play a significant role in childbirth by inducing labor. This has led to the use of prostaglandin analogs in medical procedures to induce labor in pregnant women safely.

Gastrointestinal Health: The protective effects of certain prostaglandins on the stomach lining have informed treatments for peptic ulcers and gastritis. Medications that enhance the production of these protective prostaglandins can prevent and treat these conditions more effectively.

Impact and Products

Development of NSAIDs: Their findings underpin the mechanism of action for non-steroidal anti-inflammatory drugs (NSAIDs), including aspirin, ibuprofen, and naproxen. These drugs are widely used to reduce inflammation, relieve pain, and lower fevers, impacting the everyday health management of millions worldwide.

Cardiovascular Treatments: The discovery of prostacyclin by John R. Vane and its role in inhibiting platelet aggregation has informed the development of drugs that prevent blood clots, reducing the risk of heart attacks and strokes. This has significant implications for the treatment and management of cardiovascular diseases.

Treatment of Gastric Ulcers: The understanding that certain prostaglandins protect the stomach lining has led to the use of prostaglandin analogs in treating and preventing gastric ulcers. These drugs help reduce the stomach acid's damaging effects, promoting healing in patients with peptic ulcer disease.

Reproductive Health: Prostaglandins are used in obstetrics to induce labor and manage complications of pregnancy, representing a critical application in reproductive health. Prostaglandin analogs facilitate labor and are used in certain procedures related to pregnancy termination and the management of miscarriages.

Research on Inflammatory Diseases: The role of prostaglandins in inflammation has spurred ongoing research into treatments for chronic inflammatory diseases such as rheumatoid arthritis, osteoarthritis, and more. This research aims to develop more targeted therapies that can manage inflammation without the side effects associated with some current treatments.

Asthma and Allergy Medications: The identification of leukotrienes, substances related to prostaglandins, has led to the development of specific inhibitors used in treating asthma and allergic rhinitis. These drugs help control asthma symptoms and allergic responses by targeting the pathways that lead to inflammation and constriction of airways.

The work of Bergström, Samuelsson, and Vane has not only expanded our knowledge of human biology but also led to practical applications that improve patient care across multiple fields of medicine. The ongoing development of drugs targeting prostaglandin pathways continues to offer promising avenues for new treatments, showcasing the lasting impact of their Nobel Prize-winning discoveries.

BARBARA McCLINTOCK (1983)

This famous American women's concept of Jumping genes was prodigious

In 1983, Barbara McClintock was awarded the Nobel Prize in Medicine for her discovery of mobile genetic elements, known as "jumping genes," in corn. This groundbreaking work demonstrated that genes can move between different locations on the chromosome, a finding that revolutionized our understanding of genetic regulation and mutation.

History

Born on June 16, 1902, in Hartford, Connecticut, McClintock pursued her passion for science and genetics at Cornell University. There, she specialized in cytogenetics, the study of chromosomes, and conducted most of her Nobel Prize-winning research. Her work on the genetics of maize led her to discover transposable elements during the 1940s and 1950s, a concept ahead of its time.

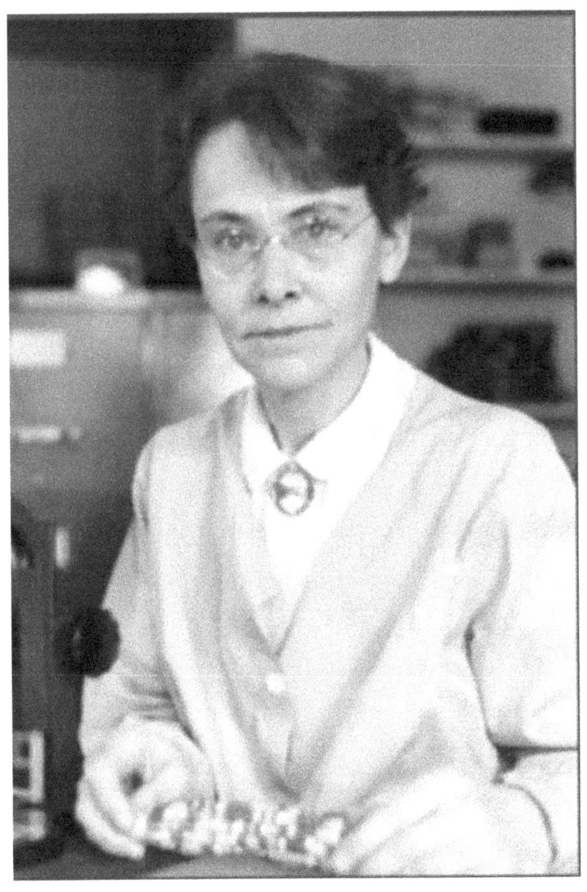

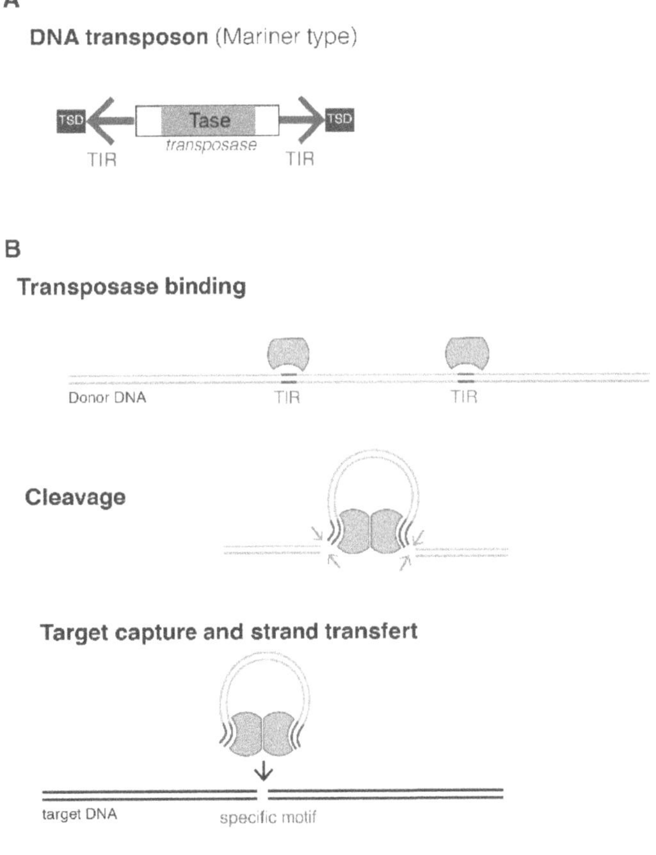

Snippets

McClintock's research showed that genetic elements could "jump" from one chromosome location to another, affecting the genetic traits of corn. This explained the unusual patterns of coloration in maize kernels and provided insights into mechanisms of genetic diversity and evolution. Despite initial skepticism, her findings were later recognized as a fundamental mechanism of genetic change.

Current Implications

McClintock's discoveries have far-reaching implications in biology and medicine, influencing fields such as genetic engineering, cancer research, and the study of evolutionary biology. Understanding how genes move within the genome has shed light on genetic mutations and the development of diseases.

Impact and Products

Barbara McClintock's legacy extends beyond her Nobel Prize, influencing contemporary research in genetics and genomics. Her work on jumping genes has paved the way for advancements in gene therapy, the development of genetically modified organisms (GMOs), and the exploration of genetic regulation mechanisms.

NIELS JERNE, GEORGES KÖHLER, AND CÉSAR MILSTEIN (1984)

One of the top discovery of this century: Mono clonal antibody

Niels Jerne, Georges Köhler, and César Milstein were awarded the Nobel Prize in Medicine in 1984. They were recognized for theories concerning the specificity in development and control of the immune system and the discovery of the principle for production of monoclonal antibodies

History

Niels Jerne was born on December 23, 1911, in London, United Kingdom, into a Danish-British family. He spent much of his career in Europe, contributing significant theories to the field of immunology before his death on October 7, 1994, in Castillon-du-Gard, France.

Georges Köhler, a key figure in the development of monoclonal antibody technology, was born on April 17, 1946, in Munich, Germany. His collaboration with César Milstein at the Basel Institute for Immunology in Switzerland led to groundbreaking work that would earn them the Nobel Prize. Köhler passed away on March 1, 1995, in Freiburg im Breisgau, Germany.

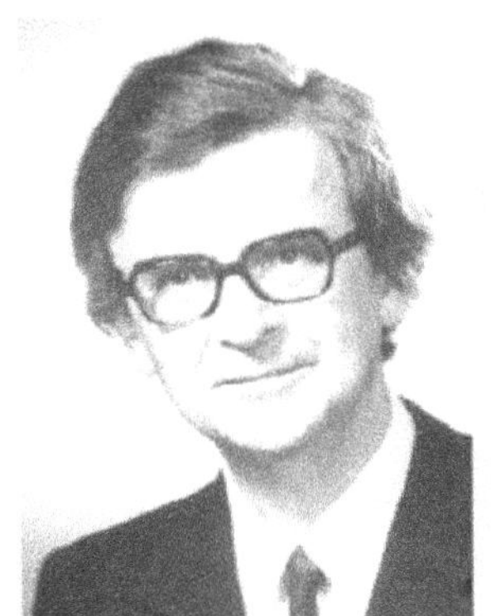

Niels Jerne

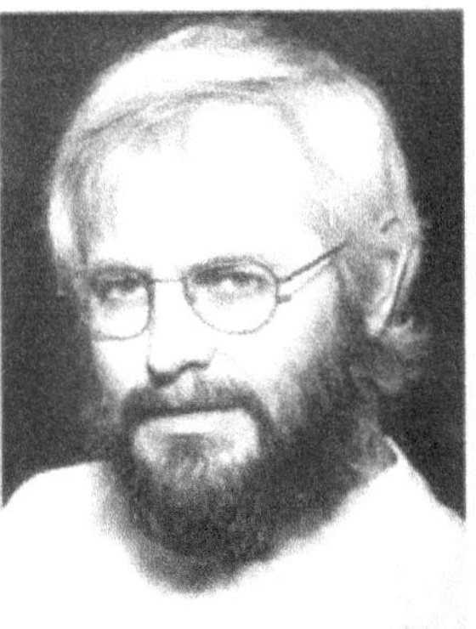

Georges Köhler

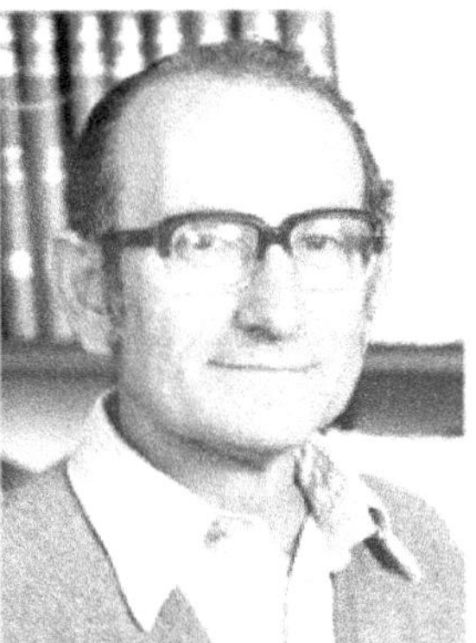

César Milstein

César Milstein was born on October 8, 1927, in Bahía Blanca, Argentina. He moved to the United Kingdom for his research, where he made significant discoveries in the field of immunology alongside Georges Köhler. Milstein died on March 24, 2002, in Cambridge, England.

Their contributions to understanding how the immune system works and their development of a method to produce monoclonal antibodies, a breakthrough with profound implications for both diagnostic and therapeutic applications.

Snippets

Jerne's Immune System Theories: Niels Jerne introduced groundbreaking theories about how our immune system recognizes and fights off invaders. His work, particularly the network theory, provided a novel understanding of the immune response, suggesting a complex interaction among antibodies.

Birth of Monoclonal Antibodies: In 1975, Köhler and Milstein's development of the hybridoma technique marked a significant leap in biomedical research. This method allowed for the production of monoclonal antibodies, which are identical antibodies that target a specific antigen, revolutionizing medical diagnostics and treatments.

Diverse Applications: The trio's contributions have paved the way for the use of monoclonal antibodies in a wide range of applications, from the treatment of chronic diseases like cancer and autoimmune disorders to the detection of pathogens in diagnostic tests.

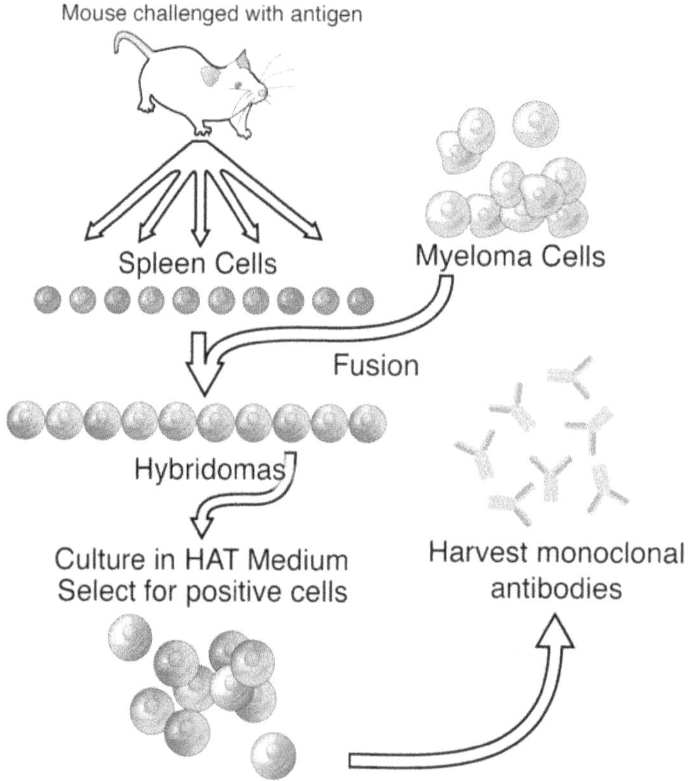

A Global Impact: Their research underscored the importance of international collaboration in science, with Jerne's Danish-British background, Köhler's German roots, and Milstein's Argentine-British heritage coming together to achieve a milestone in immunology.

Early Researchers

Paul Ehrlich laid foundational concepts of the immune system in the late 19th and early 20th centuries, introducing ideas such as the side-chain theory which prefigured the concept of antibodies. Another key figure, Macfarlane Burnet, formulated the clonal selection theory in the 1950s, proposing that each lymphocyte makes a single type of antibody, a concept that underpins much of today's understanding of the immune response.

Additionally, the work of Michael Heidelberger and Edward Kendall in the early to mid-20th century on identifying antibodies as proteins and characterizing their roles in the immune response provided crucial biochemical insights that set the stage for the later development of hybridoma technology.

Moreover, the discovery of the structure of antibodies by Rodney Porter and Gerald Edelman in the 1960s, for which they received the Nobel Prize, was another significant milestone that enabled further advances in the field.

Current Implications

Medical Treatments and Therapeutics: Monoclonal antibodies have become a cornerstone in treating a range of diseases, including various types of cancer, autoimmune diseases, and infectious diseases. They offer targeted therapy by recognizing and binding to specific cells, minimizing damage to healthy cells and reducing side effects compared to traditional treatments.

Diagnostics: The ability to produce antibodies that precisely target specific antigens has revolutionized diagnostic tests. Monoclonal antibodies are used in tests for numerous conditions, from infectious diseases like COVID-19 and HIV to cancer markers, providing high specificity and sensitivity.

Research and Discovery: In scientific research, monoclonal antibodies are invaluable tools for identifying and studying the role of specific proteins in health and disease. They facilitate the exploration of cellular processes at a molecular level, advancing our understanding of biology and pathology.

Vaccine Development: The specificity of monoclonal antibodies has also been harnessed in designing vaccines and studying immune responses. They are used to identify and neutralize specific pathogens, aiding in the development of effective vaccines.

Autoimmune Diseases and Transplantation: Treatments developed from monoclonal antibodies have improved the management of autoimmune diseases by targeting overactive immune responses. Additionally, they are used to prevent the rejection of transplanted organs by suppressing certain immune functions.

Impact and Products

Cancer Therapy: Monoclonal antibodies have become a mainstay in oncology, with products designed to target specific cancer cells without harming healthy tissue. Examples include rituximab for non-Hodgkin's lymphoma and trastuzumab for HER2-positive breast cancer, which specifically target cancer cells, leading to improved survival rates.

Autoimmune Diseases: The development of monoclonal antibodies has led to breakthrough treatments for autoimmune conditions such as rheumatoid arthritis and multiple sclerosis. Adalimumab and infliximab are examples of antibodies that inhibit tumor necrosis factor-alpha (TNF-α), a cytokine involved in systemic inflammation, providing relief to millions of patients worldwide.

Chronic Inflammatory Diseases: Treatments for conditions like Crohn's disease and ulcerative colitis have benefited from monoclonal antibody therapies, which help manage inflammation and reduce flare-ups.

Cardiovascular Risk Management: Monoclonal antibodies targeting cholesterol, such as PCSK9 inhibitors, have been developed to help reduce the risk of cardiovascular disease in patients who are statin-intolerant or require additional lipid-lowering beyond what statins can provide.

Infectious Diseases: The fight against infectious diseases has seen the advent of monoclonal antibodies designed to neutralize pathogens. This includes treatments for conditions ranging from RSV (respiratory syncytial virus) in infants to emergency therapies for diseases like Ebola.

The ongoing research and innovation in monoclonal antibody technology promise to deliver even more targeted, effective treatments across a broad spectrum of diseases, underscoring the lasting legacy of Jerne, Köhler, and Milstein's seminal work.

MICHAEL BROWN AND JOSEPH GOLDSTEIN (1985)

Defined the key elements in lipid metabolism and LDL receptor physiology

Michael Brown and Joseph Goldstein were awarded the Nobel Prize in Medicine in 1985 for their pioneering work on the regulation of cholesterol metabolism. Their discoveries laid the groundwork for understanding how cholesterol levels are controlled in the body and led to significant advancements in the treatment of high cholesterol and related cardiovascular diseases

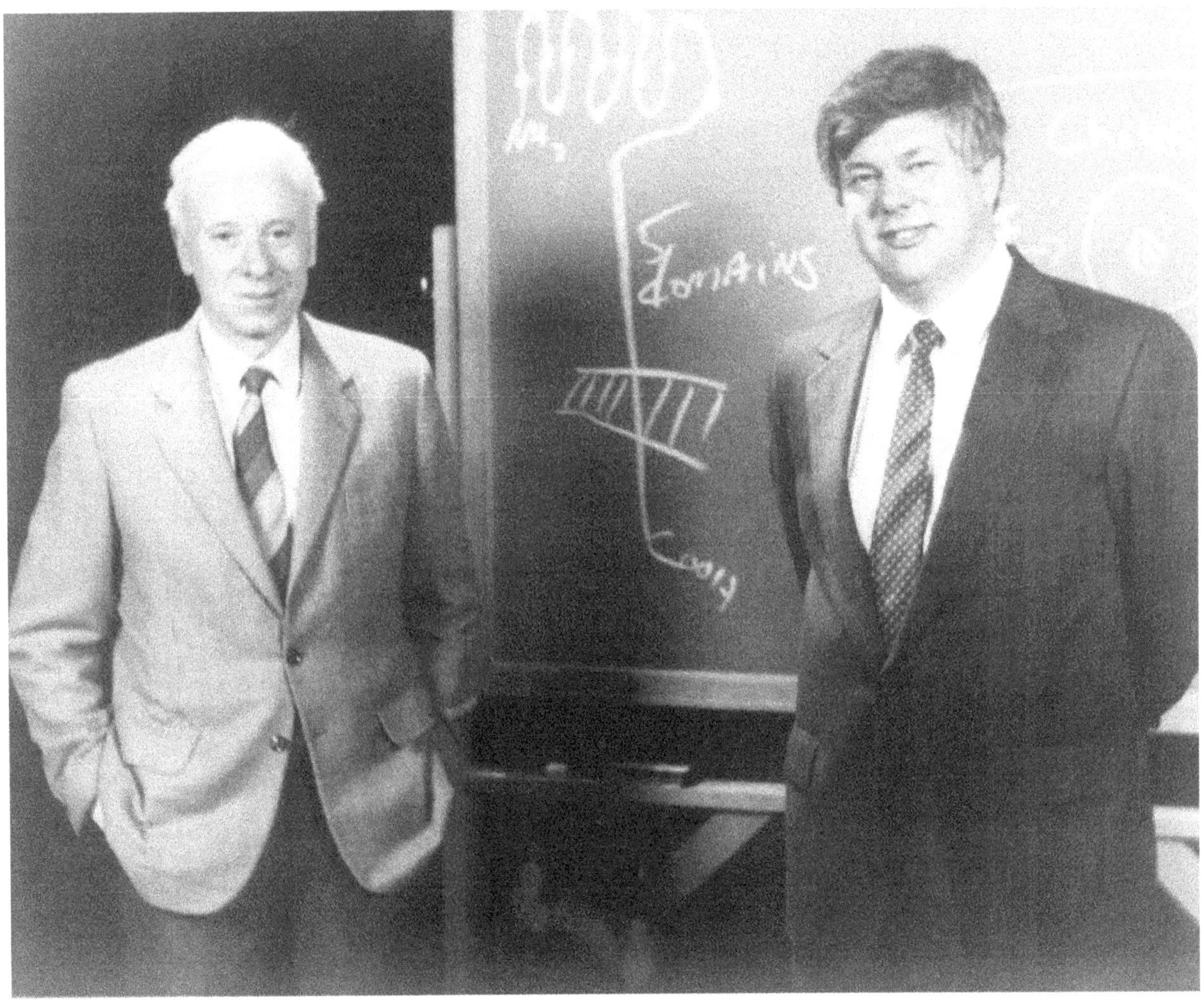

History

Michael S. Brown was born on April 13, 1941, in Brooklyn, New York. He spent his childhood in a suburb of Philadelphia after moving there at the age of 11. Brown's early interests in science were sparked by amateur radio, a hobby through which he learned the scientific method by building and troubleshooting his own radio transmitters and receivers. Despite financial challenges, Brown's intellectual curiosity and ambition were evident from a young age, leading him to pursue a career in medicine and research, inspired by his mother's encouragement and his own desire to rise to the challenges posed by his environment.

Joseph L. Goldstein, on the other hand, showcased his exceptional medical intellect early in his career, which caught the attention of Michael Brown during their training. Goldstein, whose precise birth details were not highlighted in the provided sources, demonstrated a deep understanding of medical science and a knack for critical clinical assessments, traits that would define his illustrious career in genetics and biochemistry alongside Brown.

Their partnership began fortuitously when they were both assigned to Massachusetts General Hospital for their medical internships. Despite initial skepticism from Brown about Goldstein, who came from a less known Texas medical school, their collaboration quickly flourished after Goldstein's accurate prediction about a patient's imminent health decline. This incident marked the beginning of a lifelong collaboration and friendship between the two.

Snippets

Discovery of LDL Receptors: Brown and Goldstein's most notable discovery was the identification of the low-density lipoprotein (LDL) receptor, which plays a crucial role in the regulation of cholesterol in the bloodstream. This breakthrough explained how cells maintain cholesterol balance and what goes awry in hypercholesterolemia.

Impact on Heart Disease Understanding: Their work provided a molecular understanding of how high levels of LDL cholesterol contribute to heart disease, fundamentally changing the medical community's approach to preventing and treating cardiovascular conditions.

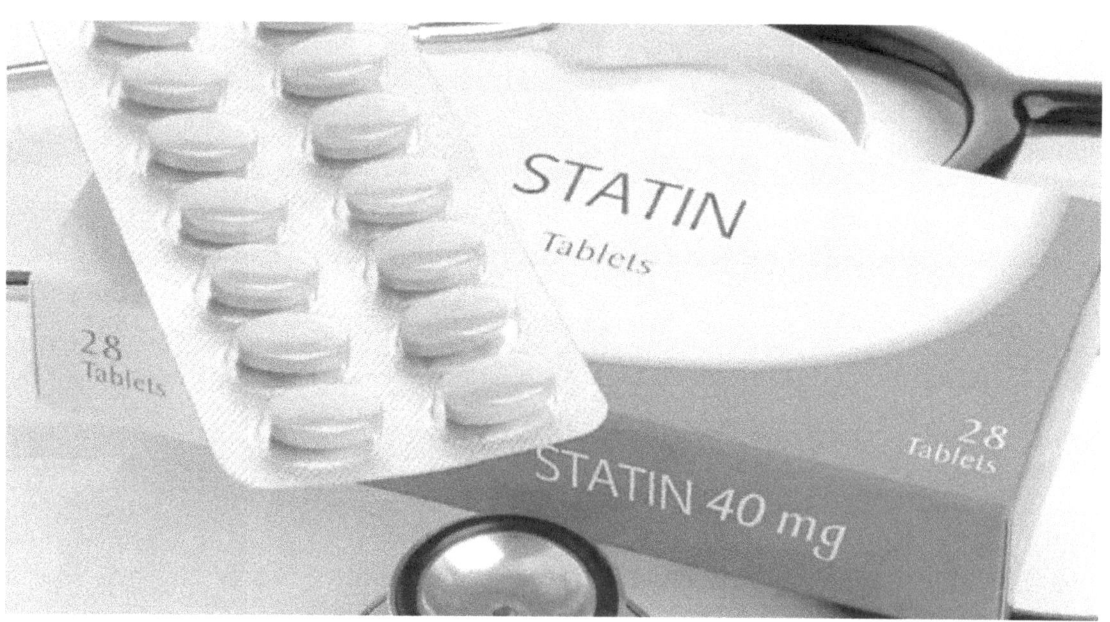

Familial Hypercholesterolemia Research: By studying individuals with familial hypercholesterolemia, a genetic condition leading to high cholesterol levels, they illuminated how a lack of functional LDL receptors results in cholesterol buildup in the blood, increasing heart disease risk.

Foundation for Statins Development: The elucidation of cholesterol metabolism laid the groundwork for the development of statins, drugs that lower cholesterol by inhibiting its production in the liver. Statins have become one of the most significant advances in cardiovascular disease prevention.

Further Research and PCSK9 Inhibitors: Building on their initial discoveries, subsequent research at UT Southwestern led to the identification of PCSK9 as another key player in cholesterol regulation. This has resulted in a new class of drugs, PCSK9 inhibitors, offering additional treatment options for patients with high cholesterol.

Early Researchers

Among these pioneers, researchers like Gerty Cori and Carl Cori come to mind, who elucidated the mechanism of catalytic conversion of glycogen, setting the stage for understanding complex biochemical pathways, including those involving cholesterol. Their Nobel Prize in 1947, while recognized for their work on glycogen, also indirectly spotlighted the importance of metabolic regulation, a theme central to Brown and Goldstein's later work.

Another notable figure is Nikolai Anitschkow, who, in the early 20th century, demonstrated the role of cholesterol in the development of atherosclerosis through his experiments with rabbits, a controversial idea at the time but one that is foundational to current understandings of heart disease.

Also deserving mention is John Gofman, whose research in the 1950s and 60s on lipoproteins helped to further unravel the complex relationship between cholesterol fractions and cardiovascular disease, reinforcing the concept that not all cholesterol is equal in its effects on health.

Current Implications

Revolutionizing Cholesterol Management: The discoveries by Brown and Goldstein have fundamentally changed the approach to managing cholesterol, highlighting the critical role of LDL receptors in cardiovascular health.

Widespread Use of Statins: Statins, developed based on their research, have become one of the most commonly prescribed medications worldwide, significantly reducing the incidence of heart attacks and strokes by lowering LDL cholesterol levels.

New Treatment Options: The understanding of cholesterol metabolism has also led to the development of PCSK9 inhibitors, a newer class of drugs that further reduce LDL cholesterol levels, offering options for patients who do not respond well to statins.

Impact on Public Health Guidelines: Their work has influenced dietary and public health guidelines aimed at reducing cardiovascular disease risk, emphasizing the importance of managing cholesterol levels through diet, exercise, and medication.

Continuing Research and Innovation: The foundational knowledge established by Brown and Goldstein's research continues to inspire ongoing studies into the genetic and molecular underpinnings of cholesterol metabolism, paving the way for future therapeutic innovations.

Impact and Products

Widespread Use of Statins: The discoveries by Brown and Goldstein directly led to the development and widespread adoption of statins, such as Lovastatin, Simvastatin, and Atorvastatin. These drugs are now foundational in the treatment of high cholesterol, representing one of the most significant advances in preventing cardiovascular diseases.

New Class of Cholesterol-lowering Drugs: Building on their work, further research into cholesterol metabolism facilitated the development of PCSK9 inhibitors, such as Alirocumab and Evolocumab. These drugs offer an alternative for patients who do not respond adequately to statins, marking another leap forward in cardiovascular disease treatment.

Influence on Dietary Guidelines: The understanding of cholesterol metabolism and its impact on heart disease has also informed dietary guidelines worldwide. Recommendations for reducing saturated fat intake and emphasizing fruits, vegetables, and whole grains in the diet are partly based on the foundational work of Brown and Goldstein.

Public Health Policies: Their research has influenced public health policies aimed at reducing cardiovascular disease rates. Screening for high cholesterol levels and early intervention strategies are now standard parts of preventive healthcare, thanks in part to their discoveries.

Educational Impact: Beyond direct medical applications, their work has shaped the education of countless medical professionals, biochemists, and researchers. The mechanisms of cholesterol metabolism and the clinical application of statins are now essential components of medical and bioscience curricula.

Economic Influence: The development of statins and PCSK9 inhibitors has had significant economic impacts, creating a multibillion-dollar market for cholesterol-lowering medications. This market continues to evolve as new drugs and treatments are developed based on the foundational understanding of cholesterol regulation discovered by Brown and Goldstein.

Their work not only changed the landscape of cardiovascular disease treatment but also laid the groundwork for ongoing advancements in the field.

STANLEY COHEN AND RITA LEVI-MONTALCINI (1986)

Emergence of new concept of growth factor in cellular biology

In 1986, Stanley Cohen and Rita Levi-Montalcini were awarded the Nobel Prize in Medicine for their discovery of growth factors, shedding light on how cells grow and develop. This work has significantly influenced the fields of developmental biology and cancer research.

History

Stanley Cohen, born November 17, 1922, in Brooklyn, New York, USA, and Rita Levi-Montalcini, born April 22, 1909, in Turin, Italy, conducted pioneering research that unveiled the complex mechanisms governing cellular growth and development. Their collaborative efforts have been fundamental in understanding the physiological processes that control cell and organ growth.

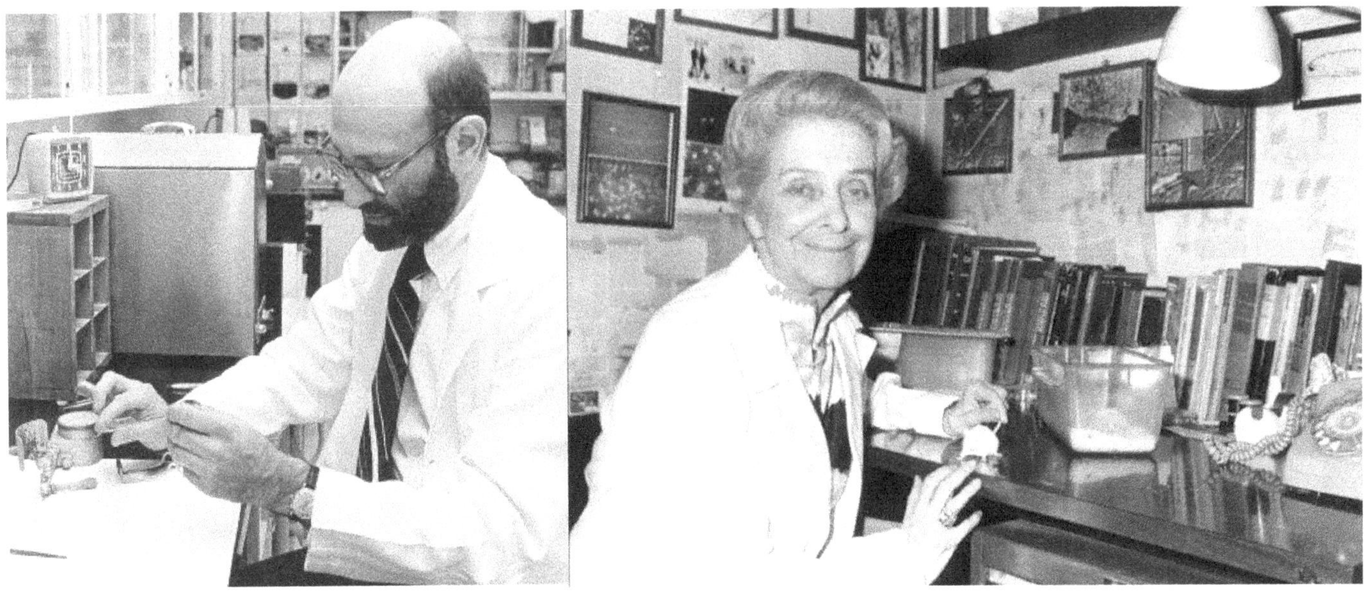

Snippets

Levi-Montalcini's research led to the identification of nerve growth factor (NGF), a protein that plays a crucial role in the growth and maintenance of nerve cells. Cohen, building on this work, discovered epidermal growth factor (EGF), which stimulates cell growth and differentiation by binding to its specific receptor on the cell surface. These discoveries have opened new pathways in the study of cellular biology and the treatment of diseases.

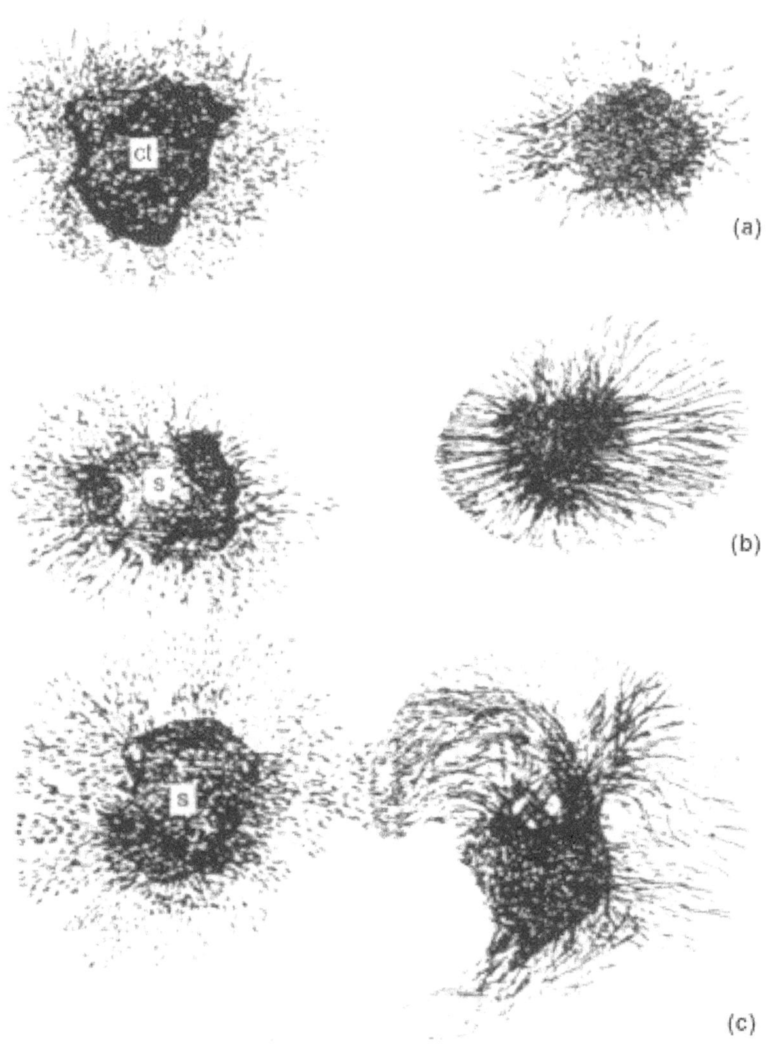

The nerve growth factor discovered by Cohen and Rita Levi

Current Implications

The work of Cohen and Levi-Montalcini has far-reaching implications, especially in medical research and treatment strategies. Understanding growth factors has advanced our knowledge of wound healing, embryonic development, and the pathology of diseases such as cancer. Their discoveries have led to innovative treatments that target growth factors and their receptors in various diseases.

Impact and Products

The identification of NGF and EGF has revolutionized the field of biomedicine, providing key insights into cell biology and offering new approaches to disease treatment and prevention. Their research has laid the groundwork for developing therapeutic agents that modulate the activity of growth factors, which is crucial for treating conditions like cancer and neurodegenerative diseases.

SUSUMU TONEGAWA (1987)

Sowed the seeds of recombinant molecular technology that started a new era of pharmacotherapy

In 1987, Susumu Tonegawa was honored with the Nobel Prize in Medicine for his seminal discovery of the genetic principle for generation of antibody diversity.

History

Born on September 5, 1939, in Nagoya, Japan, Tonegawa embarked on his scientific journey with studies in molecular biology at the University of California at San Diego, where he received his Ph.D. in 1968. His postdoctoral work included significant research at the Salk Institute under Dr. Renato Dulbecco.

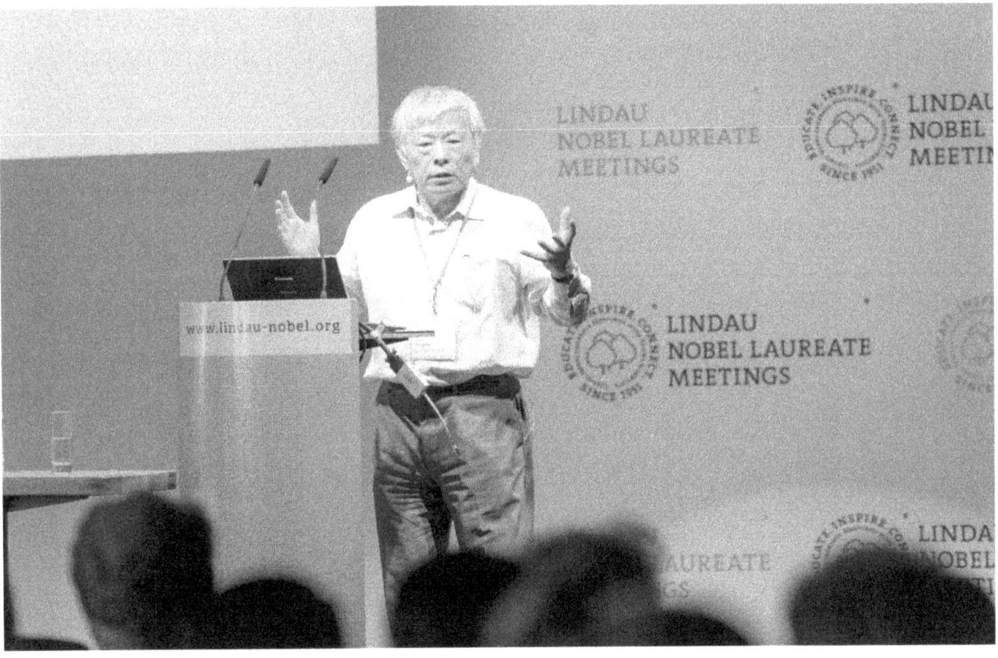

Tonegawa's career took a pivotal turn when he transitioned to the Basel Institute for Immunology in Switzerland, where his research into immunology began to flourish.

Snippets

Tonegawa's work showed that antibody diversity results from the rearrangement of gene segments in B cells during their development. This process, known as somatic recombination, allows for the production of hundreds of millions of different antibodies, far surpassing the number of genes in the human genome. His discovery of a transcriptional enhancer element associated with the antibody gene complex in 1983 marked the first identification of such cellular enhancers, further cementing his role as a pioneer in genetic research.

Current Implications

The implications of Tonegawa's discoveries extend far beyond the realm of immunology, influencing the fields of genetics, biotechnology, and therapeutic development. His findings laid the foundation for the development of monoclonal antibody therapies, which have become vital in the treatment of cancer, autoimmune diseases, and other conditions. Moreover, Tonegawa's subsequent transition to neuroscience research has led to significant contributions in understanding memory formation, demonstrating the versatility and impact of his scientific pursuits.

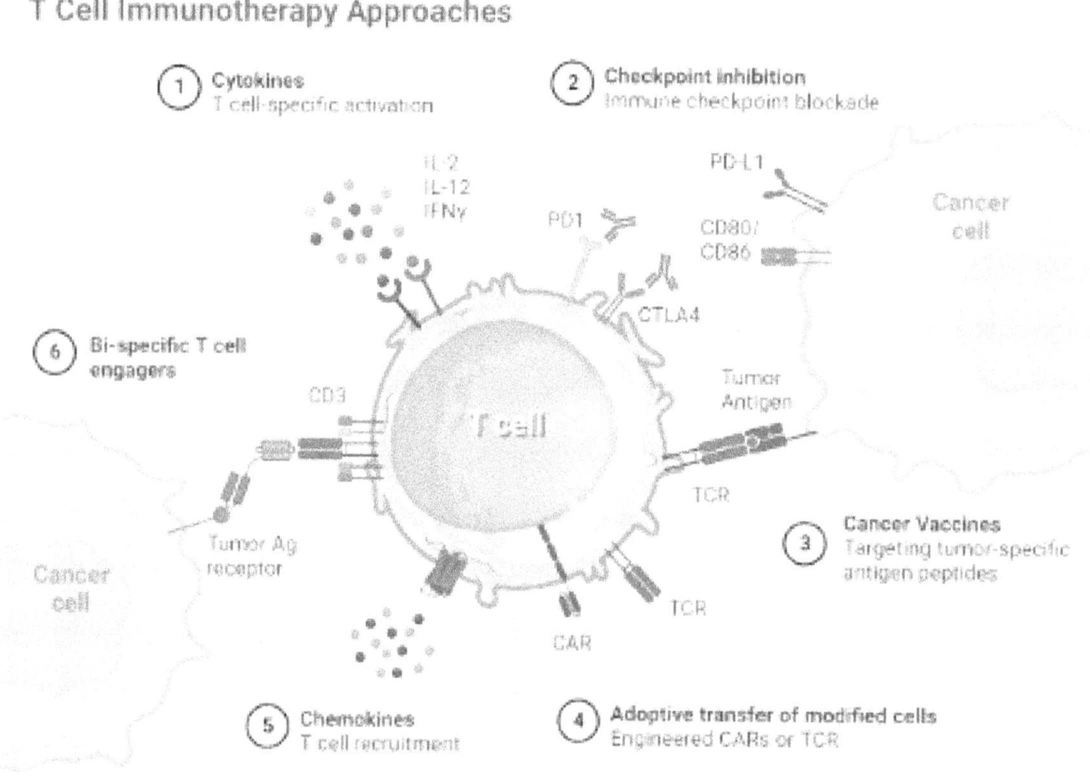

Impact and Products

Tonegawa's legacy is evident in the ongoing research and development of new immunotherapies and in the neuroscience field's exploration of memory and brain disorders. His pioneering work not only resolved a fundamental question of biology but also opened new pathways for medical advancements, highlighting the interconnectedness of genetic research and human health.

JAMES BLACK, GERTRUDE ELION, GEORGE HITCHINGS
(1988)

Award winning drug inventions, including the famous Beta-Blockers

In 1988, the Nobel Prize in Medicine was jointly awarded to Sir James W. Black, Gertrude B. Elion, and George H. Hitchings for their pioneering work on important principles for drug treatment, which fundamentally changed the approach to developing new medicines.

History

Sir James W. Black was born on June 14, 1924, in Uddingston, Scotland. His profound contributions to pharmacology include the development of propranolol, a beta-blocker used to treat heart disease, and cimetidine, a medication for peptic ulcers. His innovative approach to drug discovery, focusing on understanding fundamental mechanisms of disease rather than the traditional trial-and-error method, revolutionized the field of medicine.

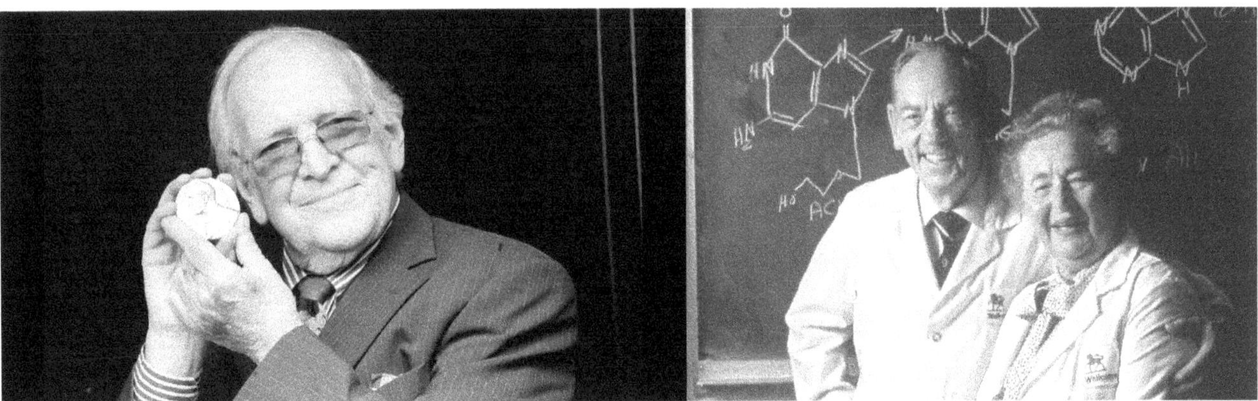

Gertrude B. Elion was born on January 23, 1918, in New York City, USA. Facing significant obstacles in her early career due to gender discrimination, Elion overcame these challenges to make seminal contributions to pharmacology. Her work, in partnership with George H. Hitchings, led to the development of several key drugs, including those for leukemia (mercaptopurine) and the antiviral acyclovir. Her dedication to science was driven by personal loss and a deep desire to contribute to the field of medicine.

George H. Hitchings, born in 1905 in Hoquiam, Washington, USA, worked closely with Gertrude Elion. Together, they developed a novel approach to drug development that targeted the biochemical pathways involved in disease processes. This method led to the discovery and development of drugs with specific mechanisms of action, significantly advancing the treatment of diseases such as leukemia, malaria, and viral infections.

Snippets

James Black's Development of Beta Blockers and Anti-ulcer Drugs:

- Invented propranolol, the first clinically significant beta-blocker for heart disease treatment.
- Developed cimetidine, a revolutionary drug for treating peptic ulcers, significantly impacting gastrointestinal medicine.

Gertrude Elion and George Hitchings' Drug Development Innovations:

- Pioneered a novel approach to drug design, focusing on biochemical pathways to develop drugs with specific targets.
- Their work led to the creation of mercaptopurine and thioguanine for leukemia treatment, paving the way for chemotherapy.
- Developed acyclovir, one of the first antiviral drugs, marking a milestone in the treatment of viral infections.

Collaborative Achievements in Pharmacology:

- Elion and Hitchings' partnership exemplified the power of collaborative research in drug discovery, leading to significant advances in treating various diseases.
- Their approach laid the groundwork for the rational design of drugs, a methodology that has since become a cornerstone of pharmaceutical development.

Early Researchers

Alexander Fleming, is best known for his discovery of penicillin in 1928. While not directly in the field of synthetic drug development, Fleming's breakthrough introduced the world to the potential of natural compounds in treating bacterial infections, inspiring further research into antibiotics and eventually leading to the broader field of antimicrobial therapy.

Johannes Abel, working in the early 20th century, was one of the first to purify hormones and study their effects on the body, contributing to our understanding of biological signaling mechanisms that modern pharmacologists exploit to design drugs that can mimic or inhibit these natural processes.

Current Implications

Advancement in Drug Design and Development: Their pioneering approach to drug development, focusing on understanding the biochemical mechanisms underlying diseases, has become a standard in the pharmaceutical industry. This rational drug design approach enables more efficient and targeted therapies, reducing the time and cost associated with drug discovery.

Impact on Personalized Medicine: The specificity of drug action discovered through their research has paved the way for personalized medicine. By targeting specific molecular pathways, treatments can now be tailored to individual patients' genetic profiles, increasing effectiveness and minimizing side effects.

Foundation for Modern Pharmacotherapy: The drugs developed by Black, Elion, and Hitchings—such as beta-blockers, anti-leukemia drugs, and antivirals—are cornerstones of modern therapy for a wide range of diseases. Their work continues to inspire new generations of drugs that build on these foundational treatments.

Educational Influence: Their research has significantly impacted medical and pharmacological education, embedding the principles of rational drug design and the importance of understanding disease mechanisms at a molecular level into the curriculum of medical and pharmaceutical sciences.

Global Health Impact: The availability of effective treatments for previously difficult-to-manage conditions, like heart disease, leukemia, and viral infections, has had a global health impact. These advancements have contributed to increased life expectancy and improved quality of life for millions around the world.

Inspiration for Future Research: The success of Black, Elion, and Hitchings has inspired countless researchers to explore novel therapeutic targets and innovative drug discovery methods. Their legacy is evident in the ongoing research aimed at tackling some of the most challenging diseases facing humanity today.

Impact and Products

Beta-blockers, such as Propranolol: Introduced by James Black, beta-blockers have become a cornerstone in treating heart disease, hypertension, and anxiety. Propranolol, in particular, has revolutionized the management of angina pectoris and irregular heart rhythms, illustrating the practical applications of understanding specific biological targets in drug development.

Cimetidine (Tagamet): Another of Black's contributions, cimetidine was the first of the H2-receptor antagonists used to treat peptic ulcers. By reducing stomach acid production, it has provided relief for millions of people suffering from ulcers and gastroesophageal reflux disease (GERD), showcasing the benefits of targeted therapy at the molecular level.

Mercaptopurine and Thioguanine: Developed by Elion and Hitchings, these drugs were among the first to treat leukemia by interfering with DNA synthesis in cancer cells, offering a new lease on life for patients with this previously untreatable condition. Their work in purine metabolism has opened doors to developing other anticancer therapies.

Acyclovir (Zovirax): Another significant contribution from Elion and Hitchings, acyclovir was among the first antiviral drugs to effectively treat herpes simplex virus infections. It marked a pivotal shift in treating viral diseases, moving from symptomatic treatment to directly targeting the viral replication process.

Allopurinol: Although not mentioned earlier, allopurinol is another crucial drug developed from the collaborative work of Elion and Hitchings. It is used to treat gout and kidney stones by reducing uric acid production, demonstrating the versatility and impact of their research on purine metabolism on a range of diseases.

Their contributions extend beyond these individual drugs, influencing drug development processes, inspiring new pharmacological strategies, and fundamentally changing how diseases are treated. Their legacy continues in the form of improved healthcare outcomes, a better understanding of disease mechanisms, and the ongoing development of new drugs that follow in the footsteps of their pioneering work.

J. MICHAEL BISHOP AND HAROLD VARMUS (1989)

Discovery of Oncogenes and the secret pathway of Virus, Gene & Cancer interaction

In 1989, the Nobel Prize in Medicine was awarded to J. Michael Bishop and Harold E. Varmus for their revolutionary discovery of the cellular origin of retroviral oncogenes. This discovery was pivotal in the field of cancer research, providing crucial insights into how cancers develop from changes in normal cellular genes.

History

J. Michael Bishop, born on February 22, 1936, in York, Pennsylvania, USA, and Harold E. Varmus, born on December 18, 1939, in Oceanside, New York, USA, embarked on careers that would lead them to uncover some of the fundamental mechanisms by which cancer arises. Their collaboration at the University of California, San Francisco (UCSF), where they both worked, was instrumental in identifying and understanding oncogenes, genes that can lead to cancer when mutated or expressed at high levels.

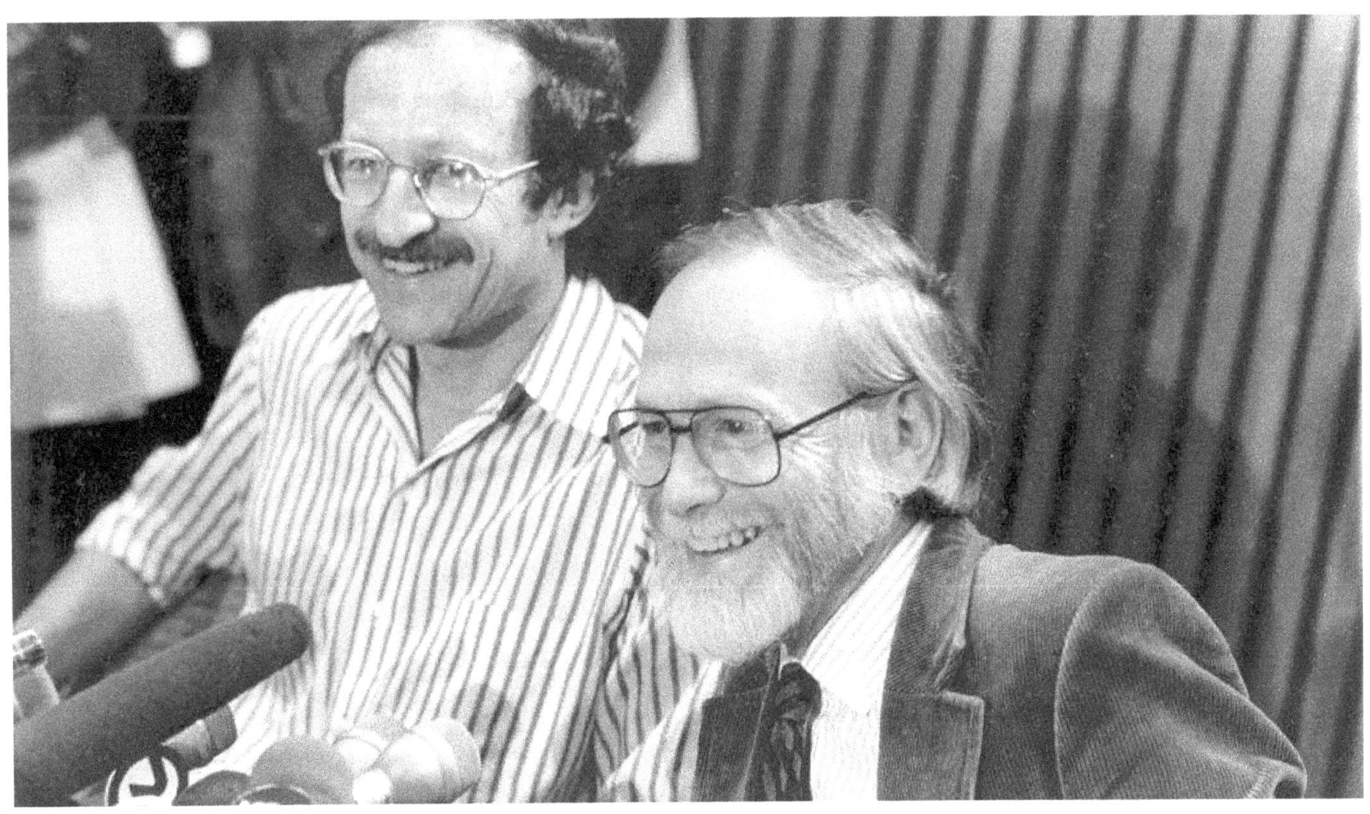

Snippets

The partnership between Bishop and Varmus led to the identification of a cellular gene (c-Src) that gave rise to the v-Src oncogene of Rous sarcoma virus. This landmark finding showed that normal cellular genes (proto-oncogenes) could become oncogenes, contributing to cancer when their functions are altered. Their work fundamentally changed the understanding of cancer, showing it can arise from the mutation of genes that are normally involved in cell growth and regulation.

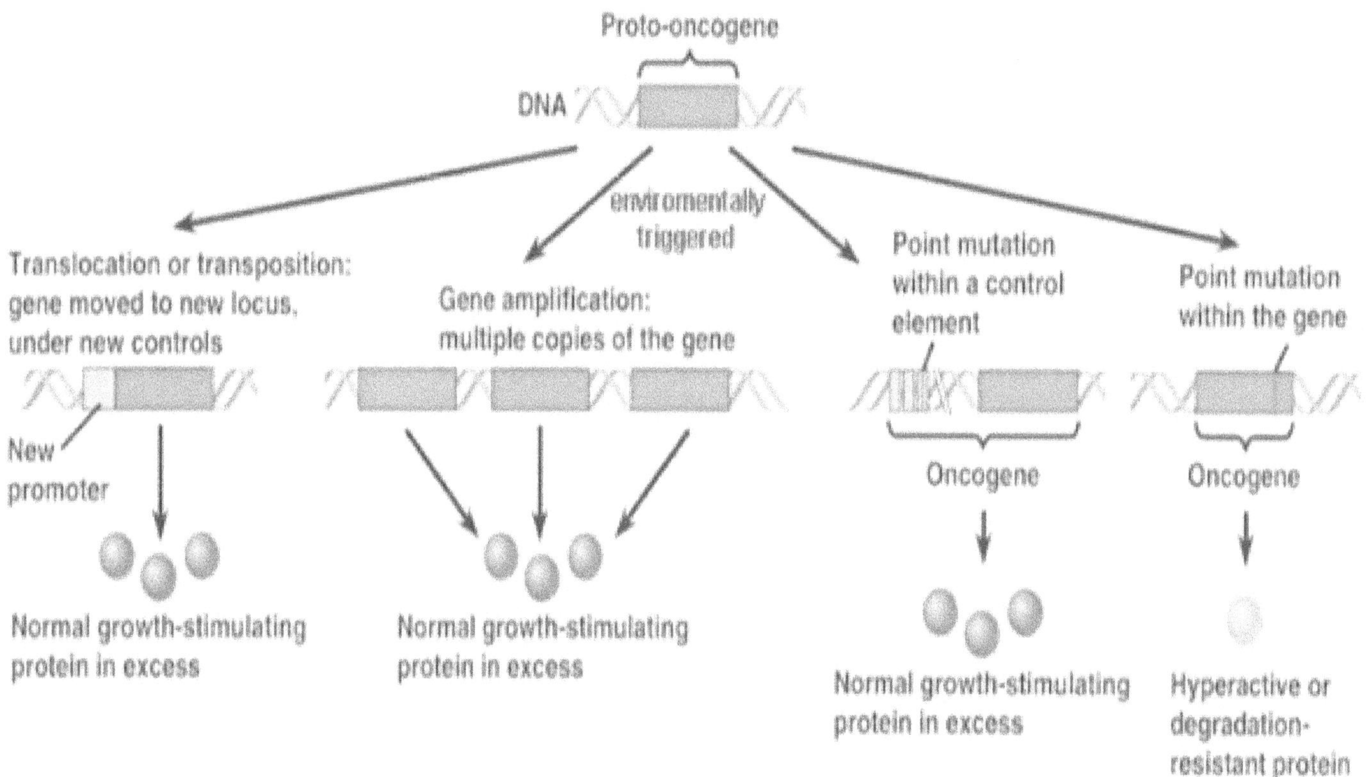

Current Implications

The implications of Bishop and Varmus discovery are vast and ongoing. Their work laid the groundwork for the identification of numerous proto-oncogenes and understanding their role in various cancers. This has paved the way for targeted cancer therapies that aim to specifically inhibit the function of oncogenes. Today, research into oncogenes and tumor suppressor genes continues to be a cornerstone of cancer biology, with direct impacts on the development of new diagnostic methods and treatments.

Impact and Products

The discovery by Bishop and Varmus has had a lasting impact on the field of medical research, particularly in the study and treatment of cancer. Their findings have not only enriched the scientific understanding of the genetic basis of cancer but also have opened new avenues for the development of targeted therapies. This work exemplifies how fundamental research can lead to practical applications that improve human health and combat disease.

JOSEPH MURRAY AND E. DONNALL THOMAS (1990)

The genius minds who made human organ transplantation a reality

In 1990, Joseph Murray and E. Donnall Thomas were jointly awarded the Nobel Prize in Medicine for their seminal discoveries concerning organ and cell transplantation in treating human diseases

History

Joseph E. Murray was born on April 1, 1919, in Milford, Massachusetts, USA. His medical journey began with his education at Harvard Medical School, leading to his historic performance of the first successful human kidney transplant between identical twins in 1954 at the Peter Bent Brigham Hospital in Boston.

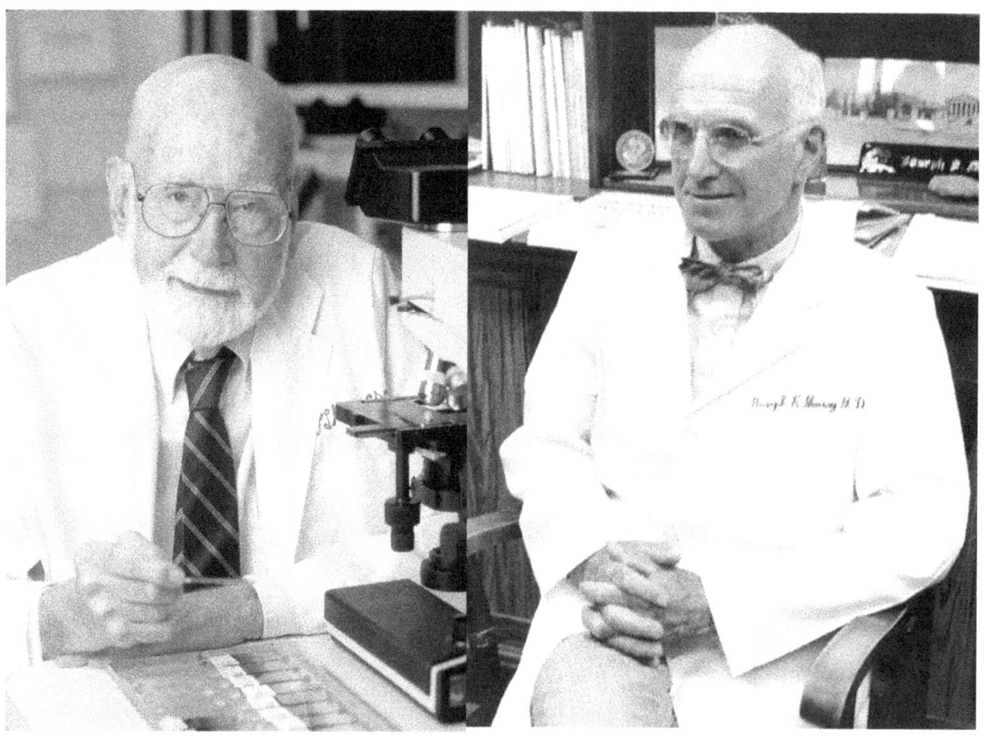

This groundbreaking operation demonstrated that organ transplants were possible, a monumental step forward in medical science. Murray's work extended beyond kidney transplants to include significant contributions to the development of immunosuppressive drugs to prevent organ rejection, enhancing the success rates of transplant surgeries. His dedication to the field was recognized through numerous awards and honors, reflecting his status as a trailblazer in transplant surgery.

E. Donnall Thomas, born in Mart, Texas, entered Harvard Medical School in 1943 and graduated with his M.D. in 1946. His medical career was diverse, including an internship, a year of hematology training, two years in the army, and a postdoctoral year at MIT, among other experiences. Thomas's work focused on bone marrow and its role in treating leukemia and other blood disorders. His development of bone marrow transplantation has fundamentally changed the treatment of hematologic malignancies, making previously incurable diseases treatable. Thomas's passion for improving patient outcomes through research in hematology and transplantation led to numerous accolades throughout his career, highlighting his significant contributions to medical science and patient care.

Snippets

Joseph E. Murray's Pioneering Work in Organ Transplantation:

- Performed the first successful human kidney transplant between identical twins in 1954, proving the feasibility of organ transplants.
- Developed methods to manage organ rejection, including the use of immunosuppressive drugs, significantly improving transplant success rates.

E. Donnall Thomas's Development of Bone Marrow Transplantation:

- Focused on bone marrow's role in treating leukemia and other blood disorders, establishing bone marrow transplantation as a viable treatment.
- His work has been crucial in making previously incurable diseases treatable, dramatically changing the prognosis for patients with hematologic malignancies.

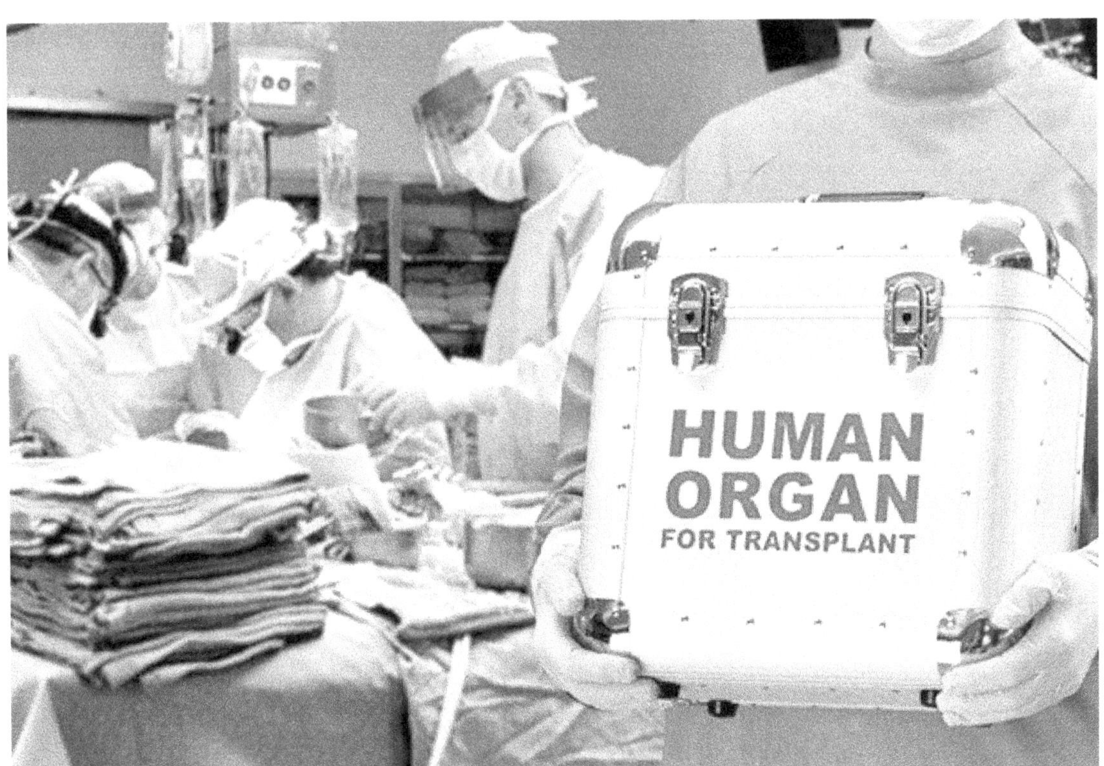

Early Researchers

Dr. George H. Whipple, whose work on liver regeneration in the 1920s contributed to the understanding of the liver's remarkable ability to regenerate, hinting at the possibilities of organ recovery and setting a precedent for organ transplantation research.

Dr. Peter Medawar's work in the 1940s and 1950s on skin grafts and acquired immunological tolerance provided essential insights into the rejection of transplanted tissues, directly informing strategies to manage organ rejection.

Dr. Jean Dausset's discovery of the human leukocyte antigen (HLA) system in 1958 revolutionized the field of transplantation by allowing for the matching of donors and recipients based on their HLA types, thereby reducing the risk of organ rejection.

In hematology, Dr. Karl Landsteiner's identification of blood groups in the early 20th century was crucial for the development of safe blood transfusions, a principle that underpins the success of bone marrow transplants.

Dr. Sydney Farber is often hailed as the father of modern chemotherapy for his work in the 1940s on antifolates, which paved the way for the use of chemical agents to treat cancer, including leukemias treatable by bone marrow transplantation.

Current Implications

Advancement in Transplantation Medicine: Their pioneering efforts have significantly advanced organ and bone marrow transplantation techniques, leading to improved survival rates for patients with end-stage organ failure and hematological malignancies. The developments in immunosuppressive therapy and graft-versus-host disease management, based on their discoveries, have become foundational in transplant medicine.

Broader Applications in Regenerative Medicine: The principles established by Murray and Thomas have paved the way for regenerative medicine, including stem cell research and tissue engineering. This area of medicine aims to regenerate damaged tissues and organs in the body, offering potential cures for diseases that are currently considered incurable.

Ethical and Policy Developments: Their work has also led to significant ethical, legal, and policy developments regarding organ donation and transplantation. The need for ethical guidelines and policies to manage organ donation and allocation has become increasingly important as transplantation has become more common.

Global Impact on Health Care: The advancements in transplantation have had a global impact, with organ and bone marrow transplants now performed worldwide. This has led to international collaborations and the establishment of global networks and registries to facilitate organ sharing and match donors with recipients more effectively.

Inspiration for Future Generations: The achievements of Murray and Thomas continue to inspire medical professionals and researchers to pursue innovations in treating diseases and improving patient care. Their legacy encourages ongoing research in transplantation immunology, genetics, and the development of new therapeutic strategies to combat rejection and enhance the success of transplants.

Impact and Products

Widely Adopted Transplantation Protocols: The surgical techniques and post-operative care protocols developed by Murray for organ transplantation have become standard practices worldwide. These protocols have been refined over the years but remain rooted in his original methodologies, ensuring high success rates for organ transplants.

Bone Marrow Transplantation as Standard Care: The techniques pioneered by Thomas for bone marrow transplantation have been adopted globally and are now standard treatment for various blood disorders, including leukemias, lymphomas, and aplastic anemia. This approach has saved countless lives and is continually being improved upon to enhance patient outcomes.

Immunosuppressive Drug Regimens: The development and optimization of immunosuppressive drug regimens to prevent organ rejection were directly influenced by Murray's work. These regimens are essential for the success of organ transplants and have evolved to balance efficacy with minimizing side effects for transplant recipients.

Expansion of Hematopoietic Stem Cell Research: Thomas's work in bone marrow transplantation laid the groundwork for the expansion of hematopoietic stem cell research, leading to innovations in treating a wide range of diseases. This research continues to explore the potential of stem cells in regenerating damaged tissues and treating autoimmune diseases.

Ethical Frameworks and Donor Networks: The successes achieved by Murray and Thomas have necessitated the development of ethical frameworks and organized donor networks to manage organ and bone marrow donations. These systems ensure that transplants are carried out ethically and efficiently, maximizing the life-saving potential of available organs and tissues.

The improved survival rates and quality of life for transplant recipients and patients with blood cancers are a testament to the enduring significance of Murray and Thomas's contributions to medicine.

ERWIN NEHER AND BERT SAKMANN (1991)

A new Impetus in neurophysiology with patch clamp technique for Interrogating Ion channels

In 1991, Erwin Neher and Bert Sakmann were awarded the Nobel Prize in Medicine for their pioneering discoveries concerning the function of single ion channels in cells. Their work provided profound insights into the fundamental mechanisms by which cells regulate vital functions such as the heartbeat, nerve signal transmission, and the release of neurotransmitters.

History

Erwin Neher, born on March 20, 1944, in Landsberg, Germany, and Bert Sakmann, born on June 12, 1942, in Stuttgart, Germany, developed the patch-clamp technique, a revolutionary method that allows for the recording of ionic currents through individual ion channels in the cell membrane. This technique enabled them to study the electrical properties of cells in unprecedented detail.

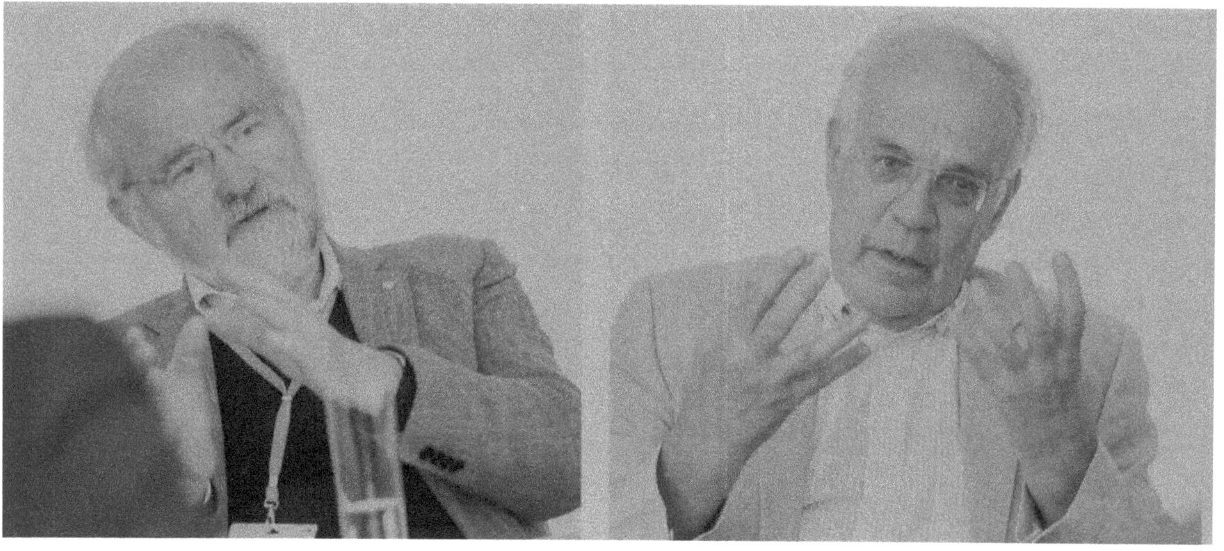

Snippets

The significance of Neher and Sakmann's work cannot be overstated; ion channels are crucial for the electrical activities of cells, and their discoveries have had a wide-ranging impact on biomedical research. By using the patch-clamp technique, they were able to observe how ion channels open and close in response to changes in voltage across the cell membrane, a process essential for the propagation of nerve impulses and muscle contraction.

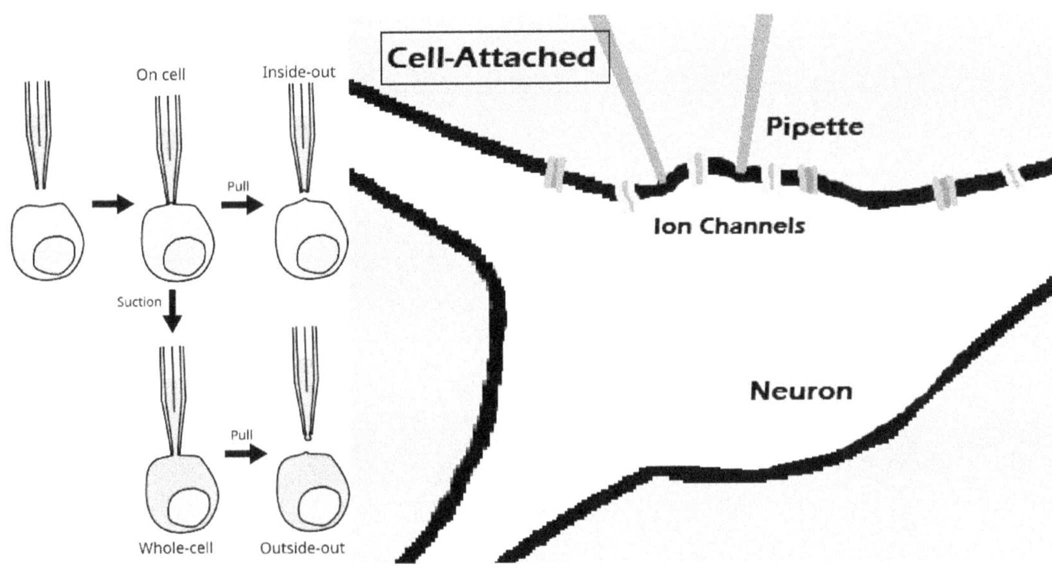

Current Implications

The insights gained from Neher and Sakmann's research have paved the way for the development of new medical therapies for a variety of diseases, including heart arrhythmias, neurological disorders, and diabetes. Their work has also influenced research in pharmacology, where understanding ion channel function is crucial for drug development.

Impact and Products

The legacy of Neher and Sakmann's work continues to influence the fields of cellular physiology, neuroscience, and pharmacology. The patch-clamp technique remains a fundamental tool in biomedical research, enabling scientists to explore the electrical properties of cells and the role of ion channels in health and disease.

EDMOND FISCHER AND EDWIN KREBS (1992)

Segregating the life sustaining Intracellular enzyme system called phosphorylation

In 1992, Edmond H. Fischer and Edwin G. Krebs were awarded the Nobel Prize in Medicine for their pioneering discoveries concerning reversible protein phosphorylation as a biological regulatory mechanism.

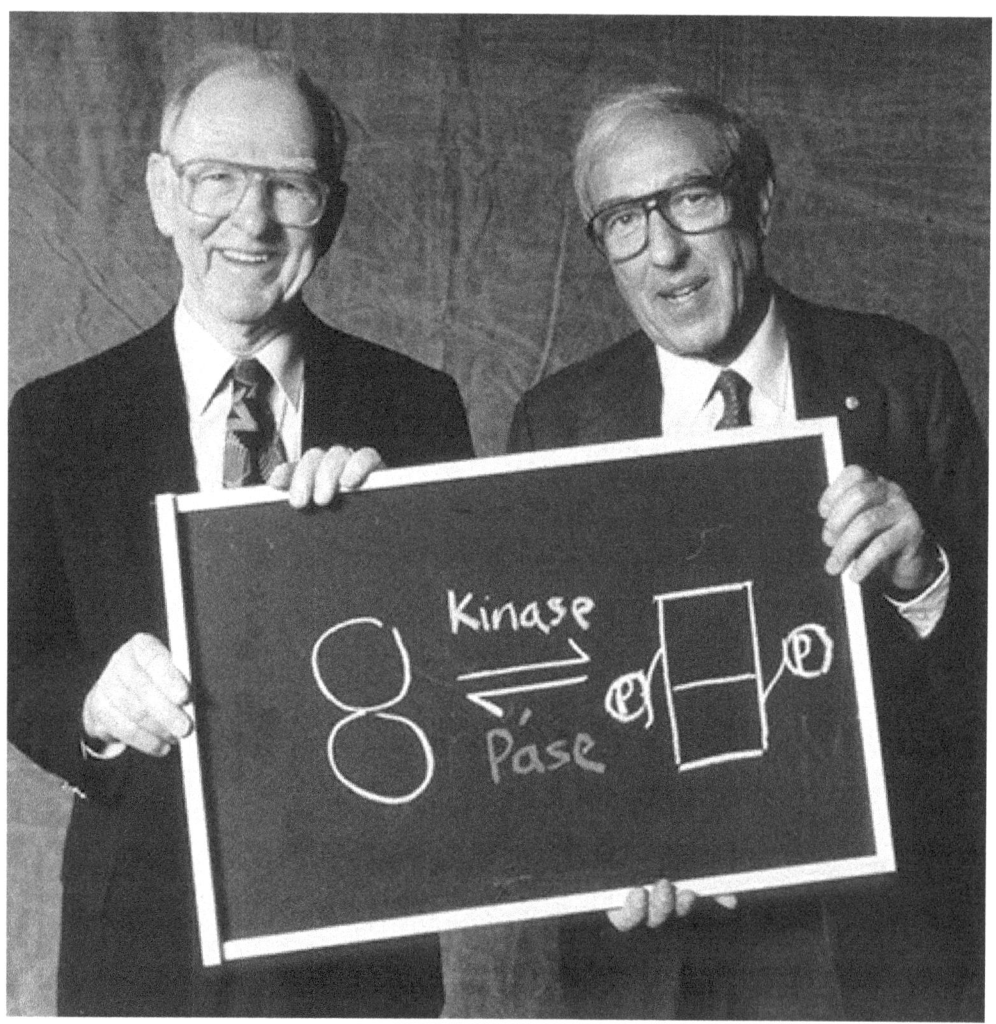

Edwin G. Krebs and Edmond H. Fischer

Their research provided crucial insights into the dynamic regulation of cellular activities, a fundamental aspect of biochemistry and cell biology that impacts our understanding of health and disease.

History

Edmond H. Fischer, born on April 6, 1920, in Shanghai, China, and Edwin G. Krebs, born on June 6, 1918, in Lansing, Iowa, USA, embarked on a collaboration that would fundamentally change our understanding of how cells regulate various biochemical processes. Fischer and Krebs's work highlighted the reversible addition of phosphate groups to proteins as a way of activating or deactivating their functions, an essential mechanism for controlling cellular processes.

Snippets

Their groundbreaking work in the mid-20th century led to the identification of protein kinases and phosphatases, enzymes responsible for the addition and removal of phosphate groups, respectively. This discovery shed light on the regulatory pathways governing various physiological processes, including muscle contraction, glycogen metabolism, and cell division, marking a significant advancement in the field of molecular biology and opening new avenues for therapeutic intervention.

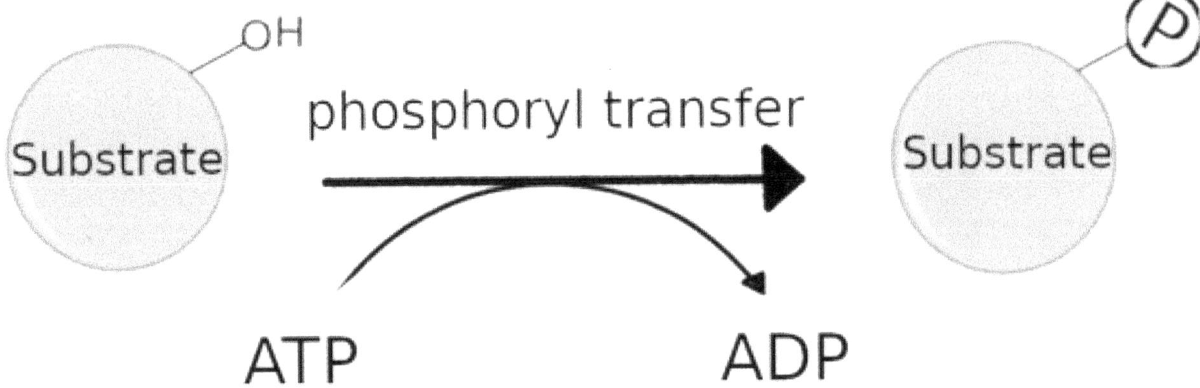

Current Implications

The discovery of reversible protein phosphorylation by Fischer and Krebs has had profound implications for biomedical research, particularly in understanding diseases such as cancer, diabetes, and neurodegenerative disorders. By elucidating how cells transmit signals and regulate their internal environment, their work has paved the way for the development of targeted therapies that modulate these signaling pathways for disease treatment and prevention.

Impact and Products

Their findings on protein phosphorylation have become a cornerstone of modern biological research, contributing to the development of drugs that target specific enzymes within signaling pathways, offering hope for treatments that are more effective and with fewer side effects. The enduring impact of their discovery continues to inspire scientific exploration into the molecular mechanisms of life and disease.

RICHARD ROBERTS AND PHILLIP SHARP (1993)

The iconic invention of Split Genes that led to unlimited innovations in gene therapy

In 1993, Richard J. Roberts and Phillip A. Sharp were jointly awarded the Nobel Prize in Medicine for their discovery of "split genes," fundamentally changing our understanding of gene structure.

History

Richard J. Roberts, born on September 6, 1943, in Derby, England, and Phillip A. Sharp, born on June 6, 1944, in Falmouth, Kentucky, USA, conducted parallel research that led to the groundbreaking discovery of split genes in the late 1970s. Roberts worked at the Cold Spring Harbor Laboratory, while Sharp conducted his research at the Massachusetts Institute of Technology (MIT). Their independent findings showed that genes could be segmented, with non-coding introns interrupting the coding regions or exons within a gene.

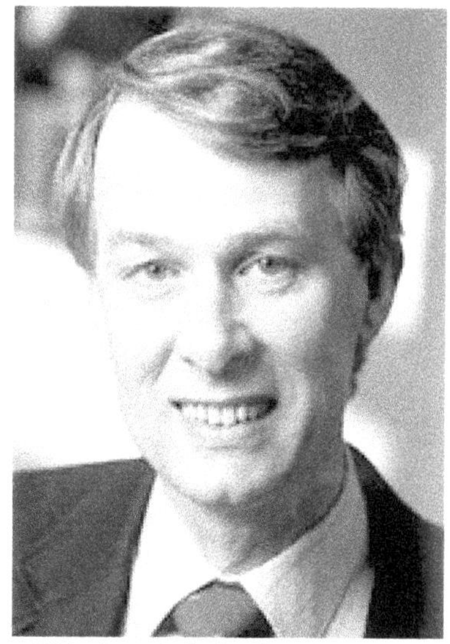

Richard J. Roberts
(1943 -)

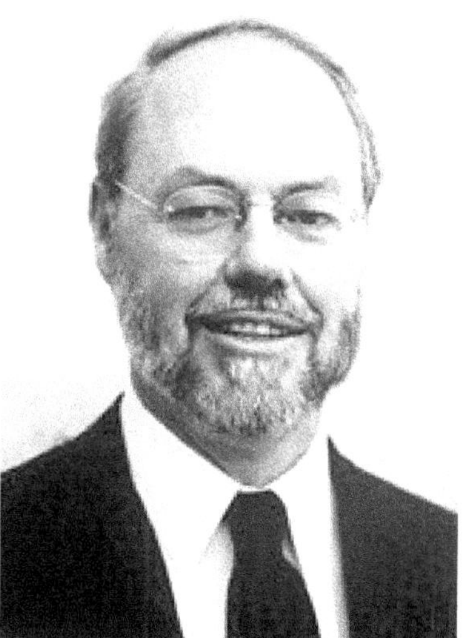

Phillip A. Sharp
(1944 -)

Snippets

Their discovery was initially made while studying the adenovirus, leading to the realization that the genetic information within these genes was not contiguous. The implications of this finding were vast, indicating that the splicing of RNA is a critical process that allows for the removal of introns, joining of exons, and the creation of a functional mRNA sequence that could be translated into proteins. This process, known as splicing, added a new layer of complexity to gene expression and regulation in higher organisms.

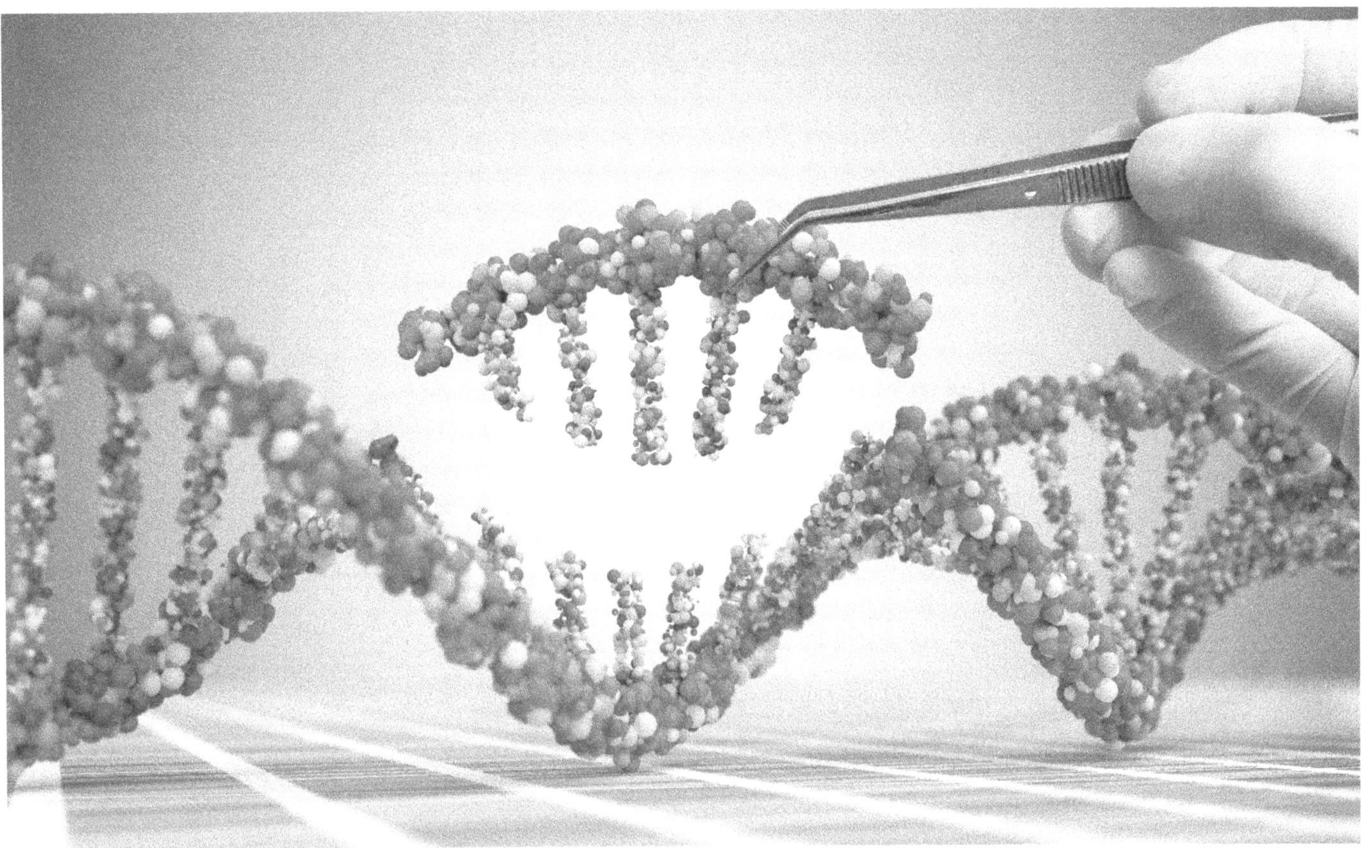

Current Implications

The elucidation of split genes and RNA splicing has significantly impacted our understanding of genetic diversity and the regulatory mechanisms of gene expression. It introduced the concept of alternative splicing, which allows for multiple proteins to be produced from a single gene, influencing development, physiology, and the adaptation of organisms. Furthermore, this discovery has been instrumental in biotechnology and medicine, contributing to advances in gene therapy, understanding genetic diseases, and the development of new therapeutic approaches.

Impact and Products

The work of Roberts and Sharp has had lasting effects across various fields, from basic research in molecular genetics to practical applications in biotechnology and medicine. Their discovery has facilitated the development of novel diagnostic and therapeutic strategies, including the manipulation of splicing patterns to treat diseases. It has also enhanced our comprehension of evolutionary biology, demonstrating how gene arrangements can drive the evolution of complex organisms by rearranging functional domains within proteins.

ALFRED GILMAN AND MARTIN RODBELL (1994)

The discovery of G-protein complex led us to a new glorious phase in molecular biology

In 1994, Alfred G. Gilman and Martin Rodbell were awarded the Nobel Prize in Medicine for their discovery of G-proteins and their role in signal transduction in cells.

History

Alfred Gilman, born on July 1, 1941, in New Haven, Connecticut, came from a family deeply rooted in the scientific community. His father was a renowned pharmacologist, co-author of a classic pharmacology textbook. Gilman's academic journey led him to significant discoveries in cell signaling. Martin Rodbell, born on December 1, 1925, in Baltimore, Maryland, expressed early interests that spanned from French literature to the sciences, ultimately leading him to a career in biochemistry and molecular biology.

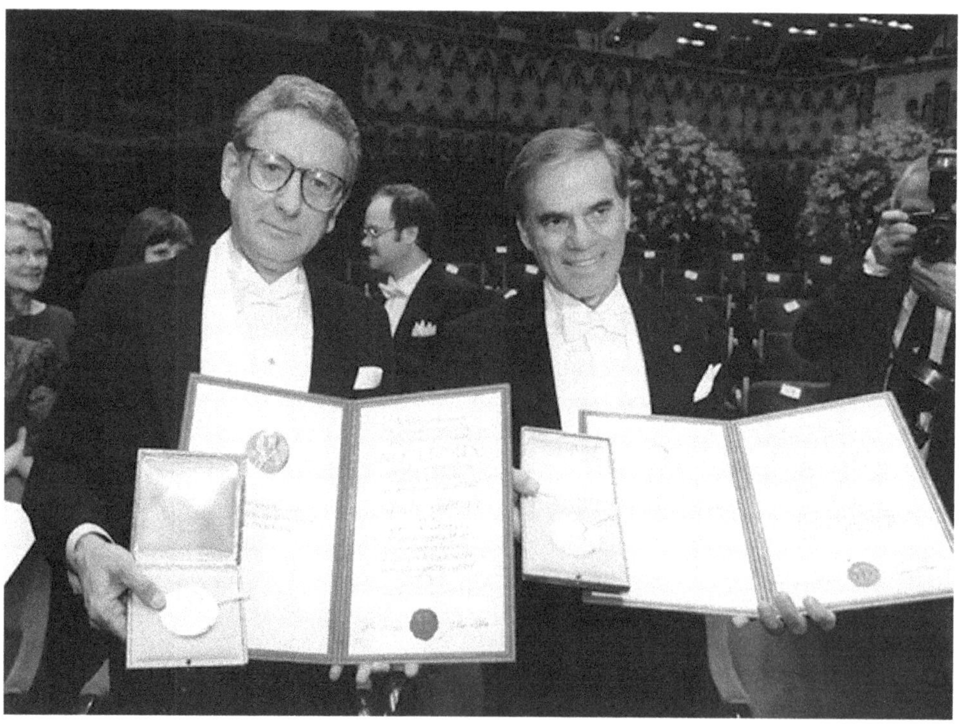

Snippets

Gilman's work highlighted the critical intermediary role of G proteins in the cell's ability to process external signals through receptors on its surface, initiating internal actions. Rodbell's earlier work in the 1960s identified GTP's role in cell signaling, laying the groundwork for understanding the dynamic process of signal transduction. Together, their discoveries unveiled the complex mechanisms by which cells communicate, significantly advancing the field of cellular biology.

Current Implication

The discovery of G-proteins revolutionized the understanding of cellular signal transduction. It provided insight into how cells respond to a variety of signals, from hormones to neurotransmitters, affecting nearly every aspect of cell physiology. This knowledge has shown the way for research into the molecular mechanisms underlying numerous diseases, including c ancer, diabetes, and heart disease, and has informed the development of targeted therapies.

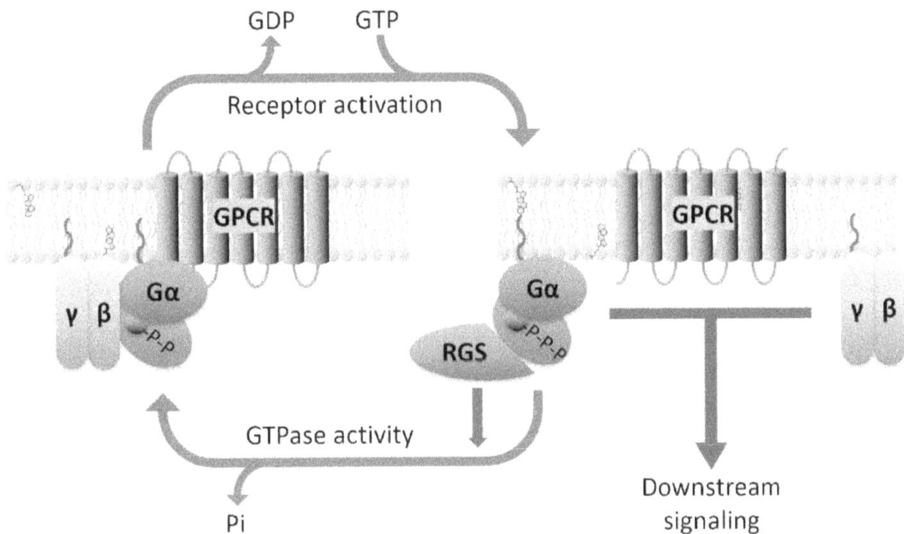

Impact and Products

The work of Gilman and Rodbell has had a lasting impact on biomedical research and pharmaceutical development. By elucidating the role of G-proteins in signal transduction, their discoveries have contributed to the development of drugs targeting specific pathways involved in disease processes. Their legacy continues to influence new generations of scientists in the exploration of cellular signaling pathways and the development of novel therapeutic strategies.

EDWARD B. LEWIS, CHRISTIANE N, VOLHARD, ERIC F. WIESCHAUS (1995)

Distinguished discovery in the embryonal genetics and early morphogenesis of organisms

In 1995, Edward B. Lewis, Christiane Nüsslein-Volhard, and Eric F. Wieschaus were awarded the Nobel Prize in Medicine for their discoveries concerning the genetic control of early embryonic development.

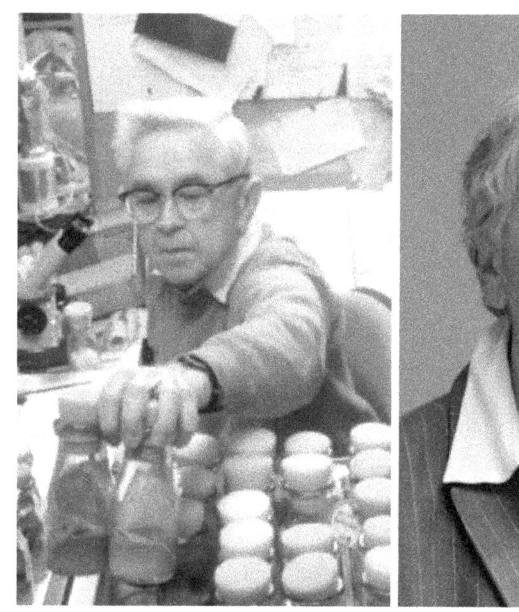

Edward B. Lewis

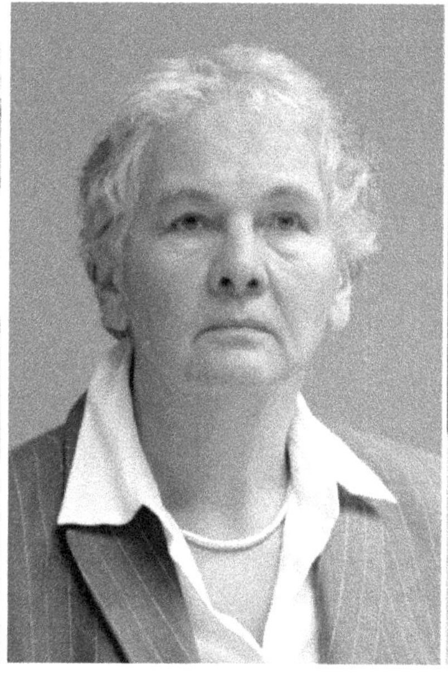

Christiane Nüsslein-Volhard

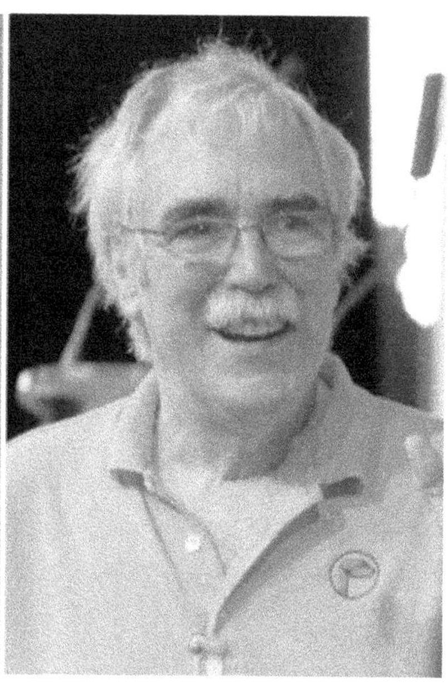

Eric F. Wieschaus

History

Edward B. Lewis (May 20, 1918 – July 21, 2004) was an American geneticist who spent much of his career at the California Institute of Technology. Lewis's research into the bithorax complex in Drosophila provided insights into the role of genes in segment development and the organization of the body plan of the fruit fly.

Christiane Nüsslein-Volhard (born October 20, 1942) is a German biologist recognized for her work on genetic mutations affecting the development of fruit fly embryos. In the late 1970s and early 1980s, alongside Wieschaus, she conducted a series of pioneering experiments that led to the identification of key genes responsible for the segmentation and patterning of the Drosophila embryo.

Eric F. Wieschaus (born June 8, 1947) is an American developmental biologist who collaborated closely with Nüsslein-Volhard on the landmark genetic screens that identified mutations affecting embryonic development in fruit flies. Their collaborative work was crucial in understanding the genetic basis of morphogenesis—the process by which an organism takes shape during early embryonic development.

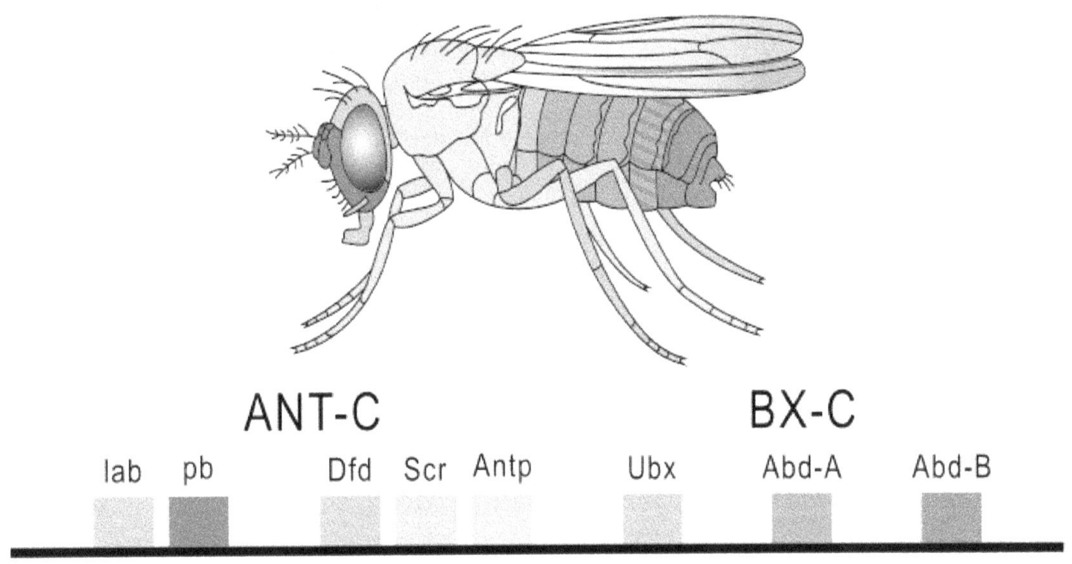

Homeobox gene expression in *Drosophila melanogaster*

Snippets

Edward B. Lewis's Contributions:

- Discovered the bithorax complex in Drosophila, revealing how genes control the development of the body plan.
- His work elucidated the concept of "homeotic" genes, which are responsible for the correct placement of body segments.

Christiane Nüsslein-Volhard's Groundbreaking Work:

- Led a comprehensive genetic screen in Drosophila that identified key genes responsible for embryonic development.
- Her research highlighted the genetic mechanisms of segmentation and axis formation in the early embryo.

Eric F. Wieschaus's Role in Developmental Genetics:

- Collaborated with Nüsslein-Volhard in pioneering genetic screenings, identifying mutations that affect embryonic development.
- Contributed significantly to our understanding of morphogenesis, the biological process that causes an organism to develop its shape.

Early Researchers

Thomas Hunt Morgan, whose early 20th-century work with Drosophila melanogaster established the fruit fly as an essential model organism for genetics. Morgan's discovery of the white-eyed mutant fly and his subsequent mapping of the Drosophila chromosome provided the first solid proof that genes are located on chromosomes, setting the stage for future genetic discoveries.

Nettie Stevens and Edmund Beecher Wilson independently discovered the sex chromosomes, a pivotal advancement in understanding genetic determination of sex. Their work in the early 1900s challenged existing theories and demonstrated that sex is inherited through specific chromosome configurations.

Another unsung hero, Reginald Punnett, co-developer of the Punnett square, contributed significantly to the field of genetic linkage and inheritance patterns. His collaboration with William Bateson helped popularize the Mendelian approach to genetics in the early 20th century.

Alfred Sturtevant, a student of Morgan, created the first genetic map of a chromosome, illustrating the linear arrangement of genes. This breakthrough concept of gene linkage and recombination frequency as a mapping tool was fundamental for the later detailed genetic studies, including those of Lewis, Nüsslein-Volhard, and Wieschaus.

Current Implications

Genetic and Congenital Disorders: The trio's research into the genetic basis of development has significantly advanced our understanding of congenital disorders. By identifying the genes responsible for embryonic development, scientists can better understand genetic mutations that lead to developmental abnormalities in humans. This knowledge is crucial for developing targeted gene therapies and diagnostic tools for congenital disorders.

Cancer Research: Their work has also informed cancer research, as many of the fundamental processes involved in embryonic development, such as cell growth and division, are often hijacked in cancer. Understanding these processes at a genetic level allows for the development of more effective cancer treatments targeting these pathways.

Stem Cell Research and Regenerative Medicine: Insights into embryonic development and cell differentiation have fueled advances in stem cell research and regenerative medicine. Knowledge of how specific genes control the development of tissues and organs in the embryo is being applied to generate tissue and organ systems from pluripotent stem cells for therapeutic purposes.

Evolutionary Developmental Biology (Evo-Devo): The trio's discoveries have also had a profound impact on the field of evolutionary developmental biology, which explores how changes in developmental processes lead to the evolution of new forms. The conservation of developmental genes across species highlights the shared genetic heritage among all living organisms and provides insights into the mechanisms of evolutionary change.

Drug Development: Understanding the genetic control of development has implications for drug development, particularly in identifying potential targets for drug action in developmental pathways that may be dysregulated in disease conditions.

Impact and Products

Genetic Screening Technologies: Their work has contributed to the development of genetic screening methods that can identify mutations in embryos. This has applications in agriculture for breeding programs and in medicine for prenatal diagnostics.

Model Organisms in Research: The extensive use of Drosophila in their research has reinforced the importance of model organisms in biological research, leading to refined techniques for genetic manipulation and analysis that are now applied across various species, including mice, zebrafish, and even human cell lines.

Educational Resources: The clarity and accessibility of the genetic principles uncovered by their research have enriched educational materials in genetics and developmental biology. This includes textbooks, online courses, and laboratory protocols that train the next generation of scientists.

Biotechnology Applications: Insights from their discoveries have been applied in biotechnology, particularly in the development of drugs targeting specific genetic pathways implicated in diseases. The understanding of gene function and regulation is crucial for designing gene therapies and other genomic medicines.

Software and Computational Tools: The need to analyze complex genetic interactions and developmental pathways has spurred the development of sophisticated bioinformatics tools and software. These tools are used for mapping gene networks, predicting gene function, and understanding the genetic basis of diseases.

The trio's discoveries have had a lasting impact, setting the stage for innovations in genetic research, medical diagnostics, and treatment strategies, thus underscoring the transformative power of basic scientific research.

PETER C. DOHERTY AND ROLF M. ZINKERNAGEL (1996)

MHC restriction phenomenon: The secret commands of Immune system to target viruses

In 1996, Peter C. Doherty and Rolf M. Zinkernagel received the Nobel Prize in Medicine for their discovery clarifying how the immune system identifies and destroys virus-infected cells. Their research revealed that T-cells require recognition of both viral antigens and self molecules from the major histocompatibility complex (MHC) on the surface of infected cells, a mechanism known as "MHC restriction."

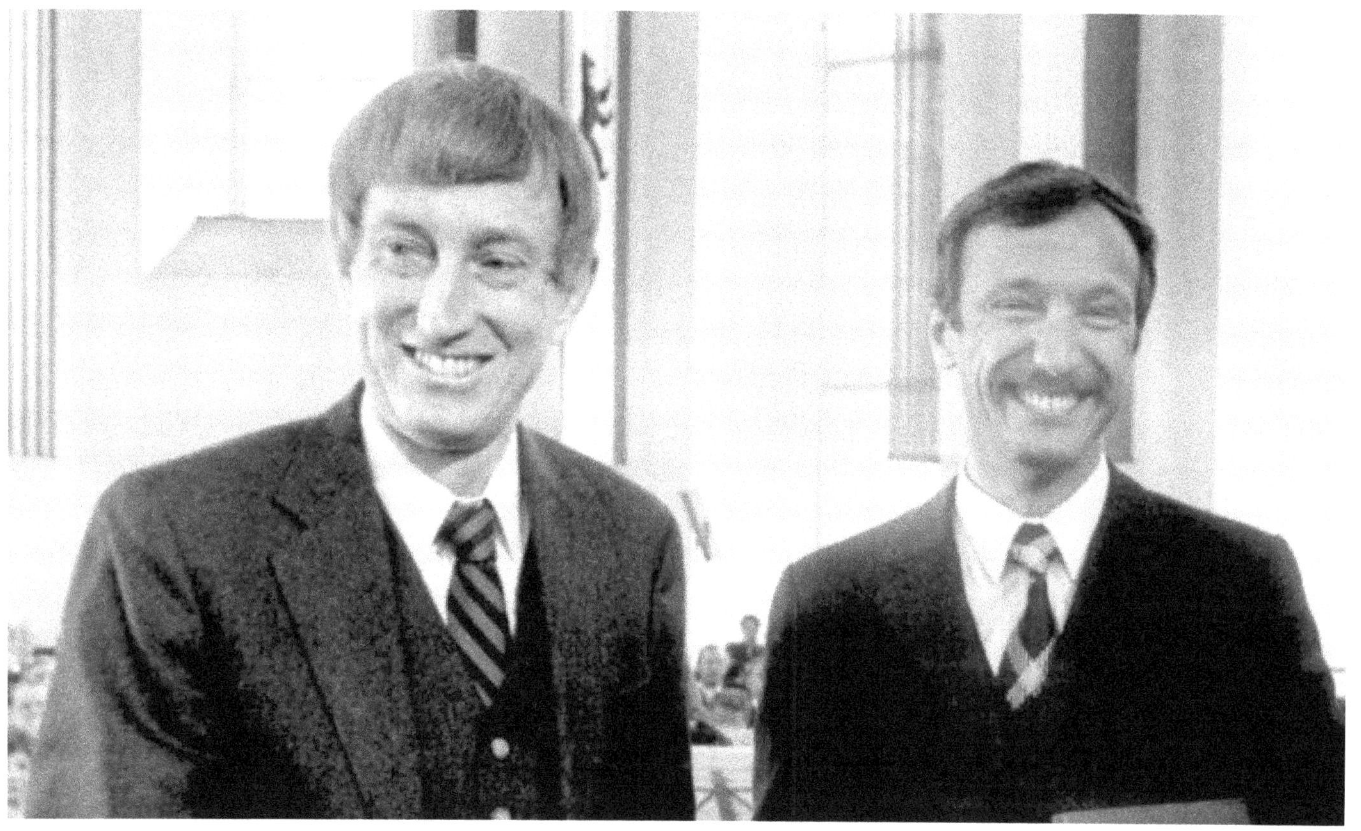

History

Peter C. Doherty, born on October 15, 1940, in Brisbane, Australia, and Rolf M. Zinkernagel, born on January 6, 1944, in Basel, Switzerland, made their groundbreaking discovery in the early 1970s. Their work significantly altered the understanding of immune system specificity and the fundamental mechanisms of cellular immunity.

Snippets

Their collaborative research demonstrated the immune system's precision in targeting virus-infected cells. They showed that T-cells can only eliminate infected cells by recognizing both viral antigens and specific MHC molecules, highlighting a dual recognition system essential for the immune response.

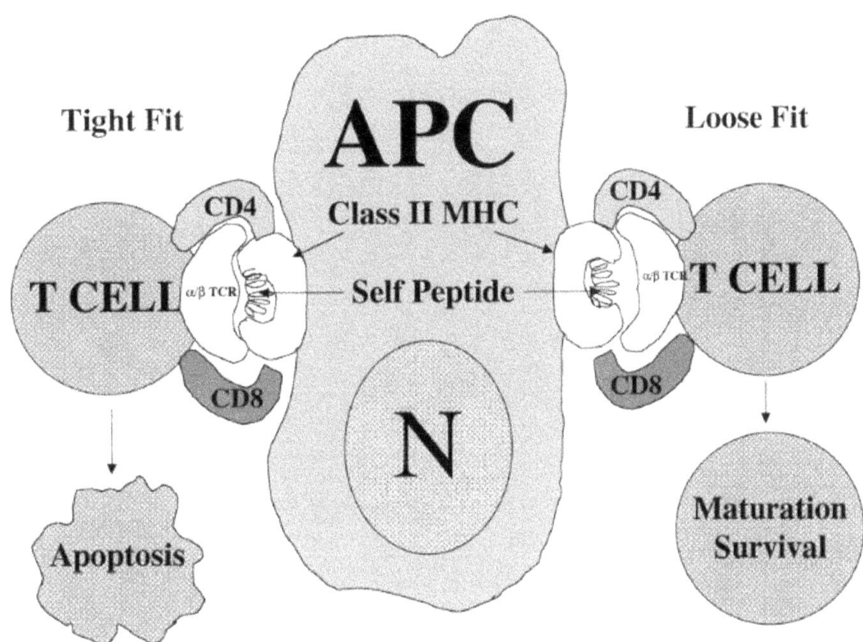

Current Implications

The discovery has significant implications for medical research and treatment strategies. It has been crucial in the development of vaccines, understanding autoimmune diseases, and improving organ transplant outcomes. Furthermore, it has opened avenues for new therapeutic approaches in treating infectious diseases and cancer by targeting specific immune response mechanisms.

Impact and Products

The contributions of Doherty and Zinkernagel have been transformative, influencing both theoretical and applied immunology. Their findings have facilitated advancements in manipulating the immune system to better fight diseases, leading to innovative treatments and preventive measures against various conditions.

STANLEY B. PRUSINER (1997)

The ubiquitous discovery of Prion disease of proteins, that mimics a virus

In 1997, Stanley B. Prusiner was awarded the Nobel Prize in Medicine for his discovery of prions, infectious proteins that challenged established scientific doctrines about pathogens. Prusiner's work demonstrated that prions, distinct from bacteria, viruses, and other known infectious agents, cause a variety of neurodegenerative diseases by misfolding normal cellular proteins.

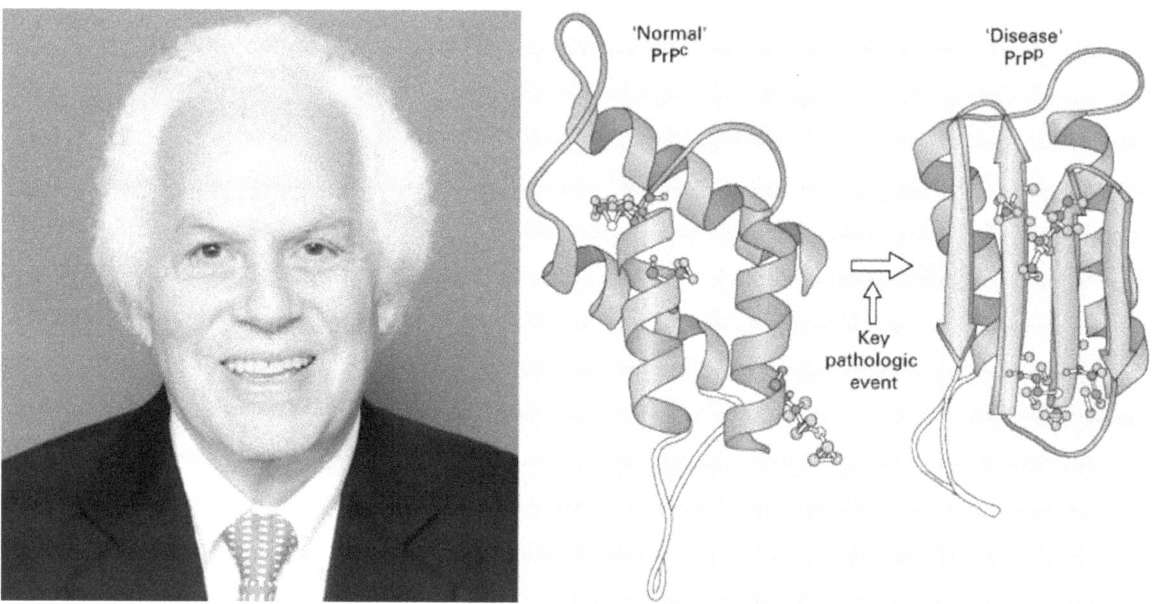

History

Stanley B. Prusiner, born on May 28, 1942, in Des Moines, Iowa, pursued his education at the University of Pennsylvania, where he earned both his Bachelor of Arts degree in chemistry and his M.D. His early career, including a significant period at the National Institutes of Health, honed his interest in neurology and biochemistry. Prusiner's curiosity in neurodegenerative diseases intensified during his residency at the University of California, San Francisco (UCSF), leading to his lifelong research into prions.

Snippets

Prusiner's hypothesis of prions emerged from studying diseases like scrapie in sheep and Creutzfeldt-Jakob Disease (CJD) in humans. He proposed that these diseases stemmed from proteins capable of replicating themselves without nucleic acids, an idea initially met with skepticism. Over time, his theory gained acceptance, significantly altering our understanding of how certain diseases deteriorate the nervous system.

Current Implications

The concept of prions has far-reaching implications in medical research, especially in understanding and treating neurodegenerative diseases. Prusiner's discovery paved the way for exploring novel therapeutic strategies against conditions previously thought untreatable, such as Alzheimer's disease and CJD. His work continues to inspire research into the molecular mechanisms of neurodegeneration and potential interventions.

Impact and Products

Stanley B. Prusiner's identification of prions as a new biological principle of infection has transformed the fields of neurology, biochemistry, and infectious diseases. His pioneering research has not only expanded the scientific community's understanding of pathogenic mechanisms but also highlighted the complexity of protein folding and its implications for health and disease. Prusiner's work underscores the importance of challenging established scientific beliefs and the potential for groundbreaking discoveries in uncharted territories of biomedical research.

ROBERT F. FURCHGOTT, LOUIS J. IGNARRO, FERID MURAD (1998)

Another mega moment in vascular biology. The discovery of Nitric oxide with a strange connect with Nobel's dynamite

In 1998, the Nobel Prize in Medicine was awarded to Robert F. Furchgott, Louis J. Ignarro, and Ferid Murad for their groundbreaking discoveries concerning nitric oxide as a signaling molecule in the cardiovascular system. Their work revealed how nitric oxide plays a critical role in various physiological processes, especially in regulating blood pressure and blood flow within the cardiovascular system.

History

Robert F. Furchgott (June 4, 1916 – May 19, 2009) was born in Charleston, South Carolina. He embarked on his significant scientific journey after studying chemistry at the University of North Carolina at Chapel Hill and earning his Ph.D. from Northwestern University in Illinois. Furchgott's career included impactful work at Cornell University, Washington University in St. Louis, and, notably, at the State University of New York in Brooklyn, where he made his landmark discovery about the endothelium's role in vascular relaxation.

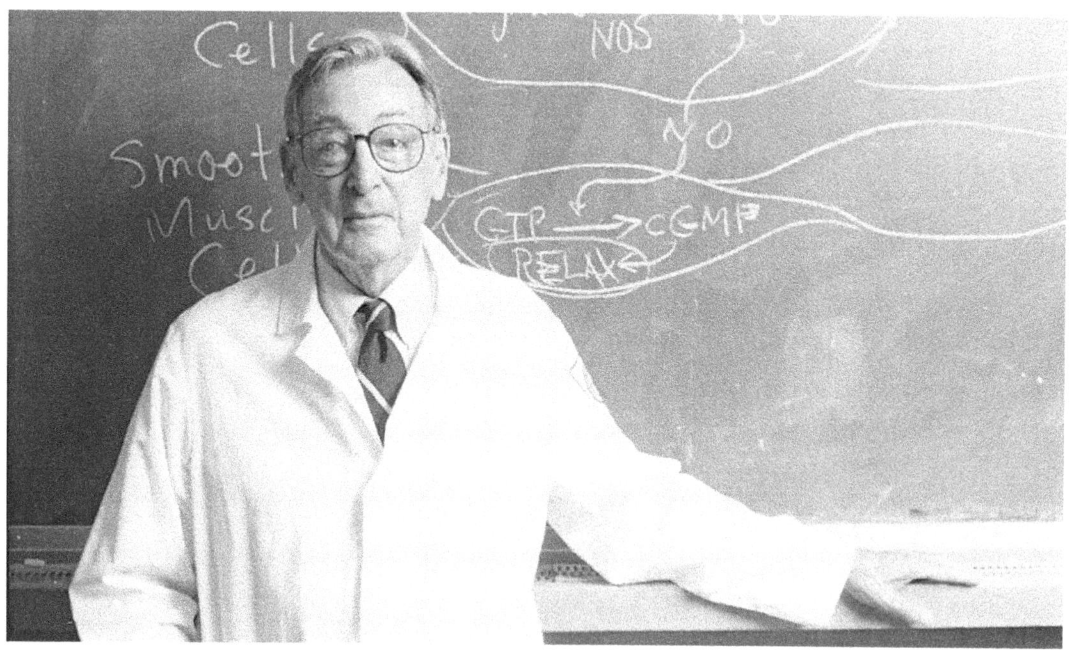

Robert F. Furchgott

Louis J. Ignarro (born May 31, 1941, in Brooklyn, New York) made his mark in the field through his research after moving from Tulane University to UCLA School of Medicine in 1985. His work on nitric oxide and the cardiovascular system has led to significant medical advancements, including the development of drugs to treat heart disease and erectile dysfunction. Beyond his scientific contributions, Ignarro has also been involved in nutritional supplement development, advocatin g for cardiovascular health.

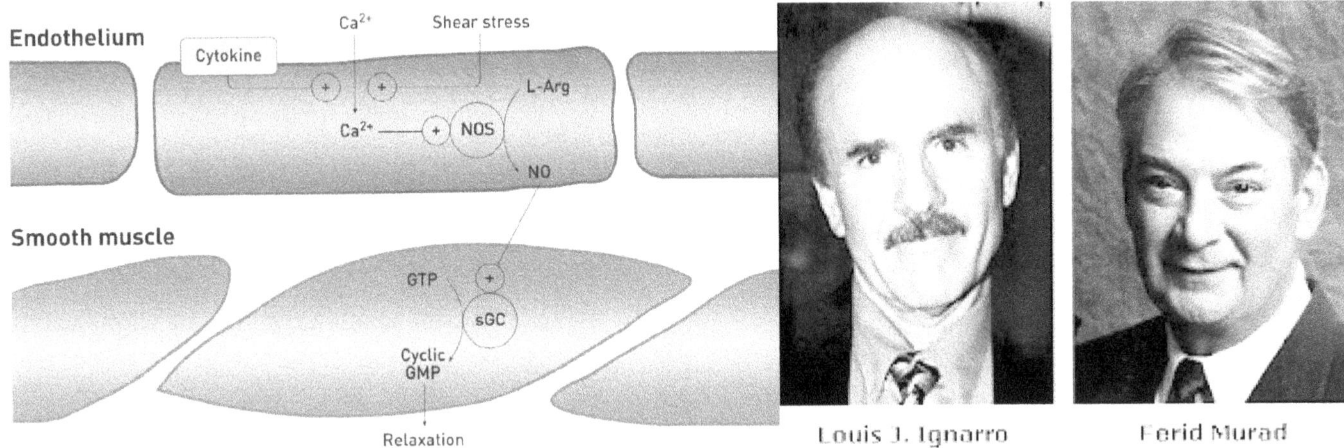

Ferid Murad (September 14, 1936 – September 4, 2023) was born in Whiting, Indiana, and played a foundational role in identifying nitric oxide's mechanism of action within the body. His career was marked by significant research that demonstrated nitroglycerin and related vasodilating drugs work by releasing nitric oxide, a discovery that bridged gaps in our understanding of cardiovascular signaling pathways. Murad's work has been recognized by numerous awards and honors, underlining his influence on modern pharmacology.

Snippets

Robert F. Furchgott's Discovery of EDRF: Furchgott's experiment in 1980 revealed that the endothelium was crucial for blood vessels' ability to relax, leading to the identification of EDRF, later known to be nitric oxide.

Louis J. Ignarro's Role in Identifying Nitric Oxide: Working independently yet concurrently with Furchgott, Ignarro's research led to the discovery that EDRF was indeed nitric oxide, a groundbreaking revelation that highlighted nitric oxide's role as a signaling molecule in the cardiovascular system.

Ferid Murad's Mechanistic Insights: Murad's early work demonstrated that nitroglycerin and similar drugs induce vasodilation through the release of nitric oxide, setting the stage for understanding NO's critical signaling role within the body.

Early Researchers

Sir Henry Hallett Dale: A British pharmacologist who, in the early 20th century, conducted pioneering work on acetylcholine as a neurotransmitter, Dale's research into the chemical transmission of nerve impulses laid foundational knowledge for understanding how signaling molecules could affect vascular tone and blood pressure.

Otto Loewi: Awarded the Nobel Prize in Medicine in 1936 alongside Dale, Loewi's discovery of the chemical transmission of nerve impulses further elucidated the role of neurotransmitters in the autonomic nervous system, setting the stage for the later discovery of nitric oxide as a crucial signaling molecule in various physiological processes.

Salvador Moncada: A pharmacologist and researcher whose work in the 1980s contributed significantly to understanding nitric oxide's biological roles. Although not awarded the Nobel Prize with Furchgott, Ignarro, and Murad, Moncada's research was instrumental in the identification of nitric oxide as a significant biological mediator.

Alfred Gilman and Martin Rodbell: Their discovery of G-proteins and the role these proteins play in signal transduction earned them the Nobel Prize in Medicine in 1994. This discovery is closely related to how nitric oxide functions within cells to induce effects such as vasodilation.

Alfred Nobel : Strangely, Nobel's experiments with nitroglycerine converted it into a explosive dynamite,

Current Implications

Treatment of Cardiovascular Diseases: The understanding of nitric oxide's role in vasodilation and blood pressure regulation has led to the development of innovative treatments for cardiovascular diseases. Medications that influence the nitric oxide pathway are now standard in treating conditions such as hypertension and heart failure.

Erectile Dysfunction Treatments: The research into nitric oxide has directly contributed to the development of phosphodiesterase type 5 (PDE5) inhibitors, such as sildenafil (Viagra), which are used to treat erectile dysfunction. These drugs work by enhancing the effects of nitric oxide, improving blood flow to certain areas of the body.

Advancements in Pharmacology: The elucidation of the nitric oxide signaling pathway has spurred further research into its role across different physiological systems. This has broadened the pharmacological approaches to a range of diseases, including the development of drugs that modulate the NO pathway for therapeutic purposes.

Understanding of Immune System Function: Nitric oxide is also implicated in the functioning of the immune system, where it plays a role in defending against pathogens. This has implications for developing therapies targeting NO signaling in conditions of immune dysfunction.

Insights into Neurological Diseases: The role of nitric oxide in neurotransmission and neurodegeneration opens up potential therapeutic strategies for neurological conditions such as Alzheimer's disease, highlighting the broad implications of NO research beyond cardiovascular health.

Impact and Products

Impact on Medical Research and Treatment

- **Cardiovascular Health:** Understanding nitric oxide's role has revolutionized the approach to treating cardiovascular diseases, leading to the development of new therapies that target the nitric oxide pathway to improve blood flow and reduce blood pressure.
- **Drug Development:** The elucidation of nitric oxide's signaling mechanisms has facilitated the creation of drugs aimed at enhancing or mimicking its action, particularly for conditions like hypertension and heart failure.
- **Erectile Dysfunction Treatments:** Perhaps the most well-known application of their research is the development of phosphodiesterase type 5 (PDE5) inhibitors, such as Viagra (sildenafil), which improve erectile function by enhancing nitric oxide signaling pathways.

Products Derived from Nitric Oxide Research

Pharmaceuticals: Beyond PDE5 inhibitors, the understanding of nitric oxide signaling has led to the exploration of novel therapeutic agents that could leverage nitric oxide for various indications, including wound healing, treatment of diabetic complications, and more.

Nutritional Supplements: The research has spurred the development of dietary supplements designed to boost nitric oxide levels in the body, purported to support cardiovascular health, enhance athletic performance, and improve vascular function.

Broader Scientific and Health-Related Implications

Research Methodologies: Their work has also contributed to advancements in research methodologies, including the development of nitric oxide donors and inhibitors, which are used in laboratory research to elucidate the role of nitric oxide in various biological processes.

Public Health Initiatives: Knowledge about the importance of nitric oxide in cardiovascular health has influenced public health initiatives focused on lifestyle changes that can naturally boost nitric oxide levels, such as dietary modifications, exercise, and smoking cessation.

The research by Furchgott, Ignarro, and Murad has not only expanded our understanding of cellular signaling and cardiovascular physiology but also paved the way for innovative treatments that have significantly impacted patient care. Their legacy is evident in the ongoing research into nitric oxide and its applications across various fields of medicine and health sciences.

GÜNTER BLOBEL (1999)

Insights into Independent protein behavior

A true Nobel connect 999, Günter Blobel was awarded the Nobel Prize in Medicine for his discovery that proteins have intrinsic signals that govern their transport and localization within the cell, a fundamental mechanism known as "protein targeting."

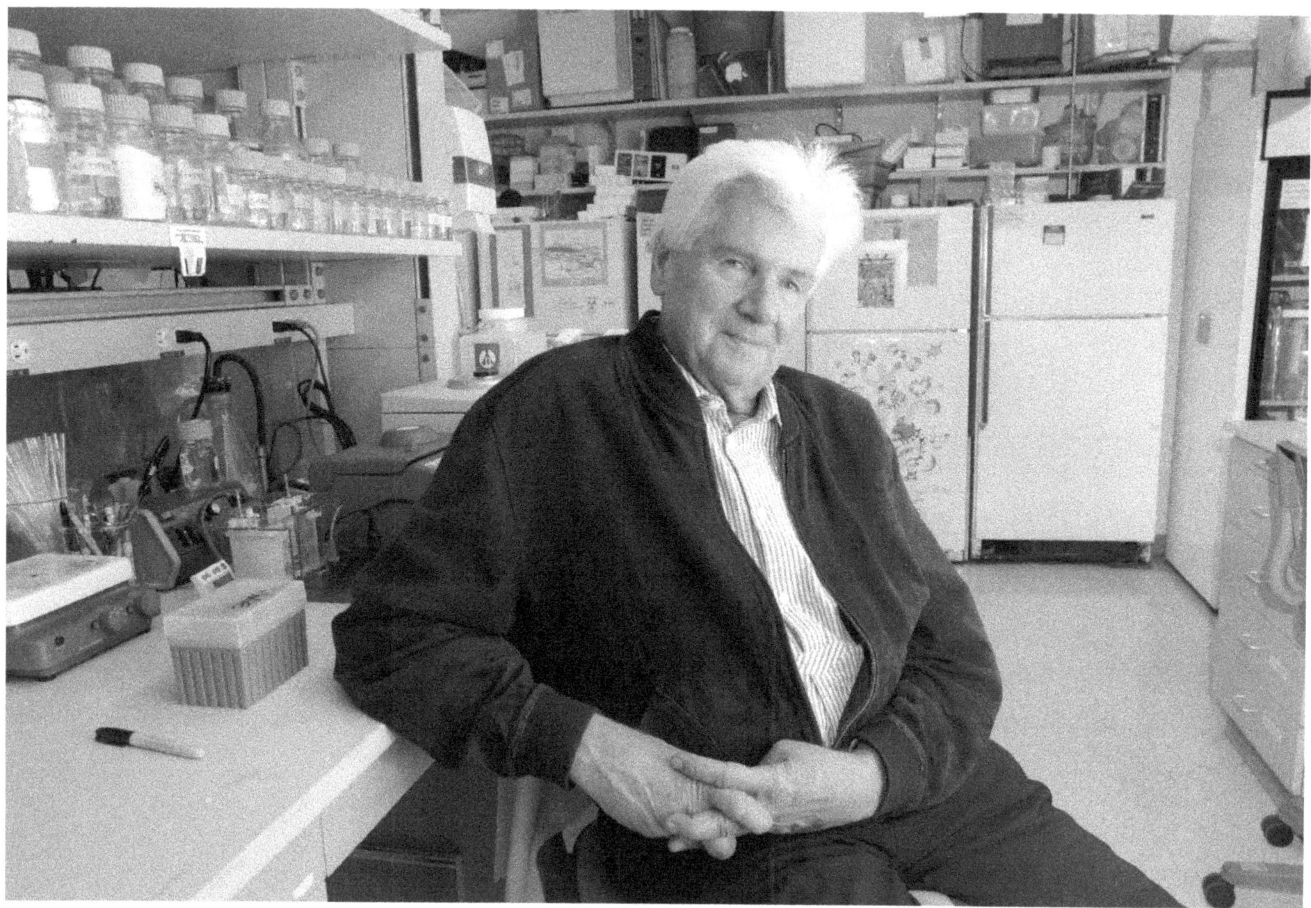

History

Günter Blobel was born on May 21, 1936, in Waltersdorf, Silesia (now Niegosławice, Poland) and faced the upheavals of World War II during his childhood. After moving to the United States for higher education, he earned a Ph.D. in oncology from the University of Wisconsin in 1967. Blobel's postdoctoral work at Rockefeller University under George Palade laid the groundwork for his future discoveries in cell biology.

Snippets

Blobel's seminal work revolved around the hypothesis that proteins contain built-in signals that direct their movement and positioning within a cell. This concept, initially met with skepticism, was eventually proven through his innovative research, fundamentally altering our understanding of how cellular processes are organized and executed.

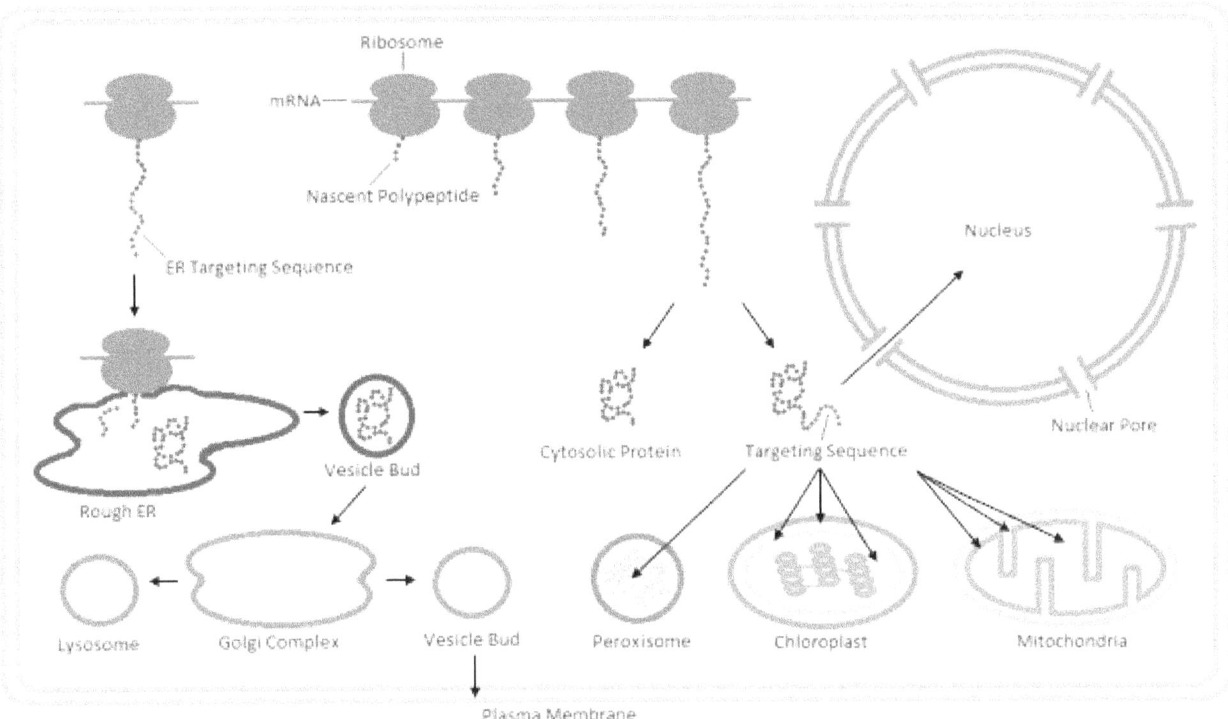

Current Implications

The principle of protein targeting has vast implications across biology and medicine, influencing our understanding of disease mechanisms and the development of new therapeutic strategies. Blobel's work has led to insights into genetic disorders and diseases caused by misdirected proteins, providing a basis for targeted drug delivery systems and molecular biology techniques.

Impact and Products

Blobel's contributions have extended beyond the laboratory to his philanthropic efforts, notably in the restoration of Dresden, Germany, demonstrating a commitment to both scientific and cultural reconstruction. His legacy in cell biology continues to inspire research into cellular mechanisms and the treatment of diseases related to protein misfolding and mislocalization.

ARVID CARLSSON, PAUL GREENGARD, AND ERIC KANDEL (2000)

Refined the science of neurotransmitters with a major Impact in neuropsychiatric therapeutics

In 2000, Arvid Carlsson, Paul Greengard, and Eric Kandel were collectively honored with the Nobel Prize in Medicine for their pioneering work in signal transduction in the nervous system, particularly their research into how neurotransmitters function in the brain.

History

Arvid Carlsson, born on January 25, 1923, in Uppsala, Sweden, was instrumental in recognizing dopamine as a major neurotransmitter, significantly impacting Parkinson's disease treatment. Paul Greengard, born in New York City in 1925, elaborated on the intracellular signaling pathways activated by neurotransmitters. Eric Kandel, born on November 7, 1929, in Vienna, Austria, was celebrated for his work on the biochemical foundations of memory storage in neurons.

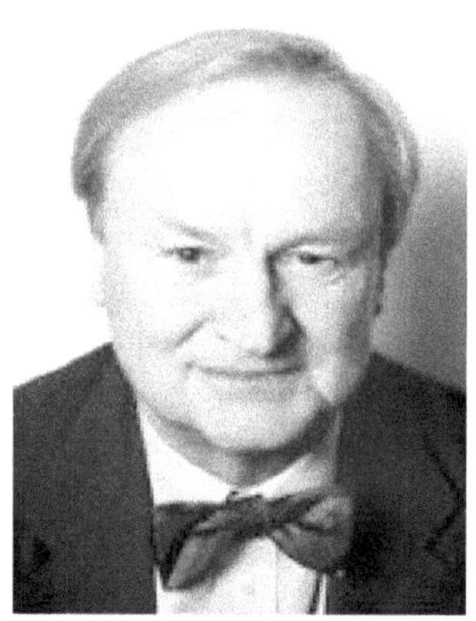

Arvid Carlsson
Prize share: 1/3

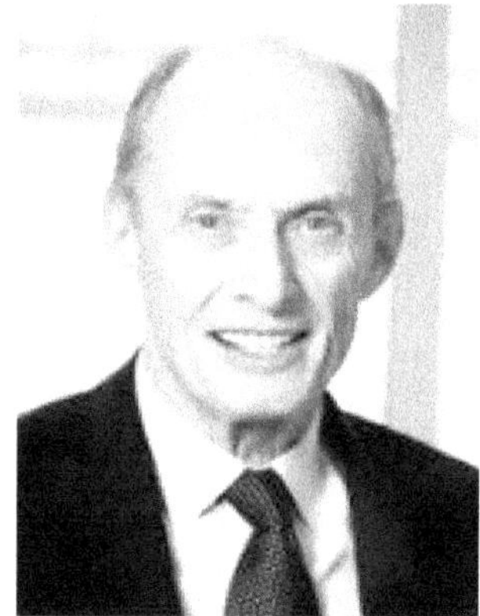

Paul Greengard
Prize share: 1/3

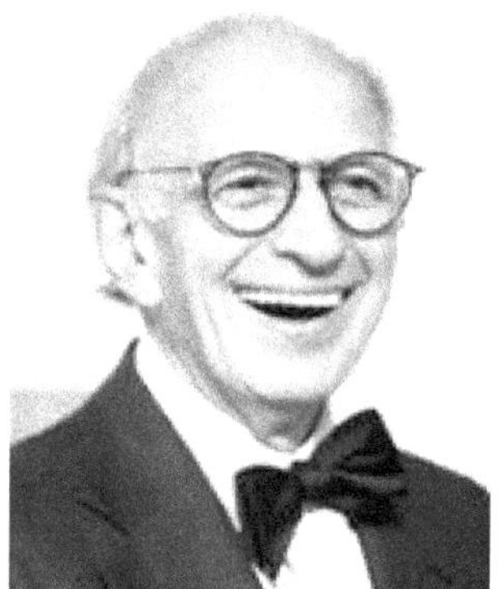

Eric R. Kandel
Prize share: 1/3

Snippets

Carlsson's discovery that dopamine served as a neurotransmitter in the brain led to the use of L-dopa in treating Parkinson's disease, drastically improving the quality of life for those affected. Greengard's research revealed how dopamine and other neurotransmitters affect the neuron's function through second messenger systems, contributing significantly to understanding neurological disorders.

Kandel's studies on the sea slug Aplysia and later on mice demonstrated that changes in the strength of synaptic connections underlie the formation of memories.

Current Implications

The trio's combined efforts have laid the groundwork for modern neuroscience, offering insights into the treatment of neurological disorders, the development of drugs targeting specific pathways in the brain, and our understanding of the cellular basis of learning and memory. Their work has direct implications for treating various conditions, from Parkinson's disease and schizophrenia to understanding the aging process and potential interventions for memory loss.

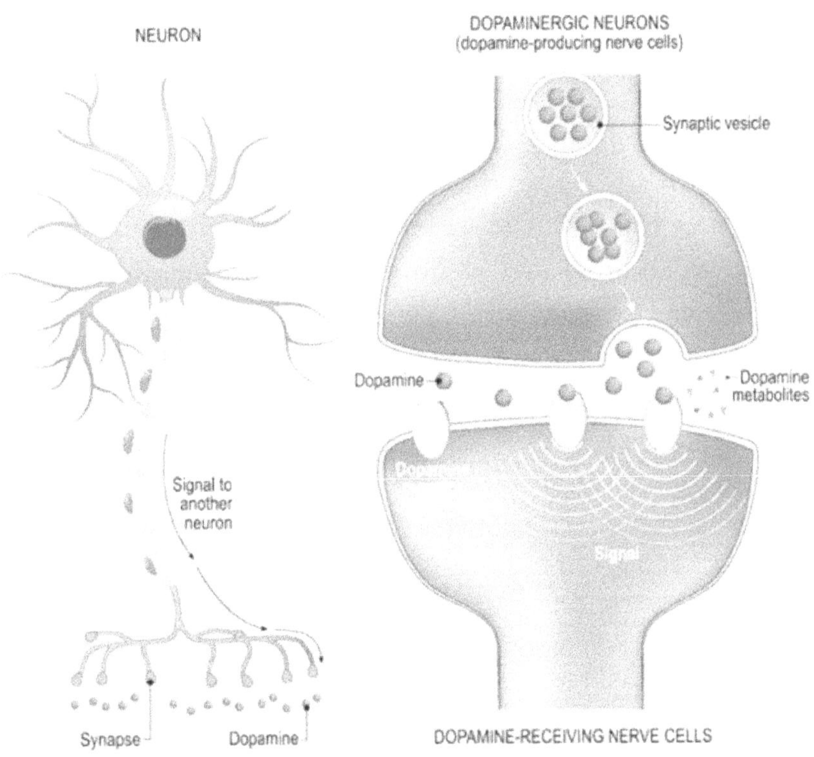

The Dopaminergic receptor Interface

Impact and Products

Carlsson, Greengard, and Kandel's discoveries are vast, affecting both theoretical and applied neuroscience. Their research has not only advanced our understanding of the brain's functioning at a molecular level but also paved the way for effective treatments for several brain disorders, enhancing the therapeutic arsenal available to neurology and psychiatry.

LELAND H. HARTWELL, TIM HUNT, AND PAUL M. NURSE (2001)

Defining the life cycle of a cell, another major moment in human biology

In 2001, Leland H. Hartwell, Tim Hunt, and Paul M. Nurse were awarded the Nobel Prize in Medicine for their discoveries concerning key regulators of the cell cycle, a fundamental process in cellular organization and division.

History

Leland H. Hartwell, born on October 30, 1939, in Los Angeles, California, utilized baker's yeast in the late 1960s to study cell growth and division, identifying over 100 genes involved in cell cycle control. Paul M. Nurse, born on January 25, 1949, in Norwich, Norfolk, England, focused on the gene cdc2, which he discovered in yeast and later found a human equivalent, revealing its role as a master switch in cell cycle control. Tim Hunt, born on February 19, 1943, in Neston, Cheshire, England, identified cyclins, proteins crucial to the cell cycle's progression.

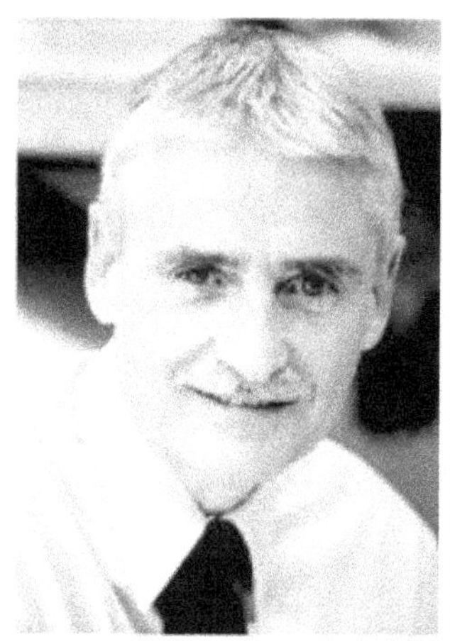
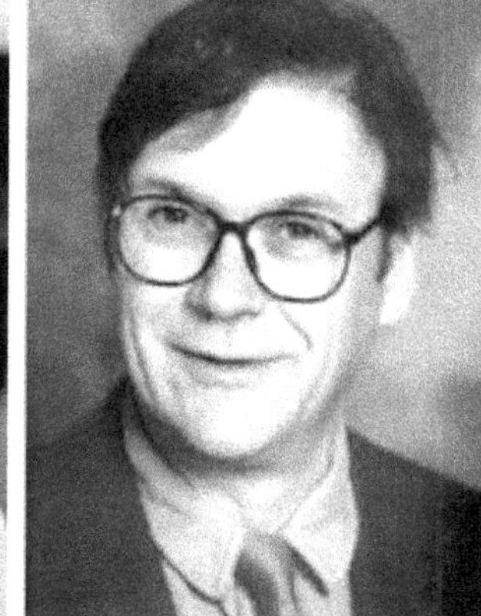
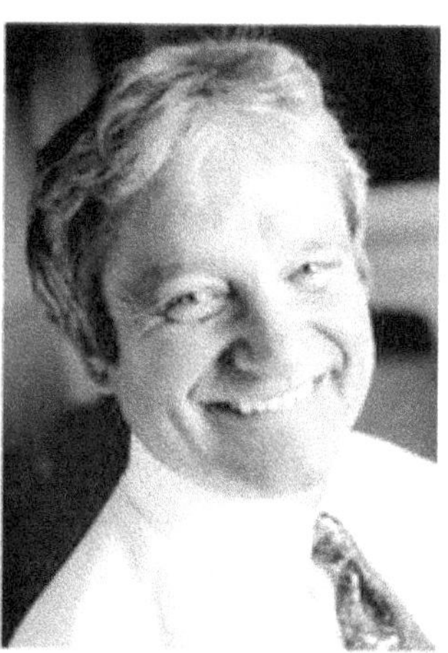

Leland H. Hartwell   Tim Hunt   Sir Paul M. Nurse

Snippets

Leland H. Hartwell's work at the University of Washington and later at the Fred Hutchinson Cancer Research Center in Seattle contributed significantly to understanding cancer and other diseases related to cell cycle dysregulation. Paul M. Nurse's leadership roles at Cancer Research UK and the Francis Crick Institute highlight his significant contributions to cancer research and molecular biology. Tim Hunt's discovery that cyclins bind to and activate cyclin-dependent kinases has been vital in understanding cell division and has implications for cancer research.

Current Implications

The collective work of Hartwell, Hunt, and Nurse has profoundly impacted the biological and medical sciences, particularly in understanding how cells duplicate and divide, which is crucial for the development of treatments for diseases like cancer. Their discoveries have paved the way for new therapeutic strategies targeting the cell cycle in cancerous cells.

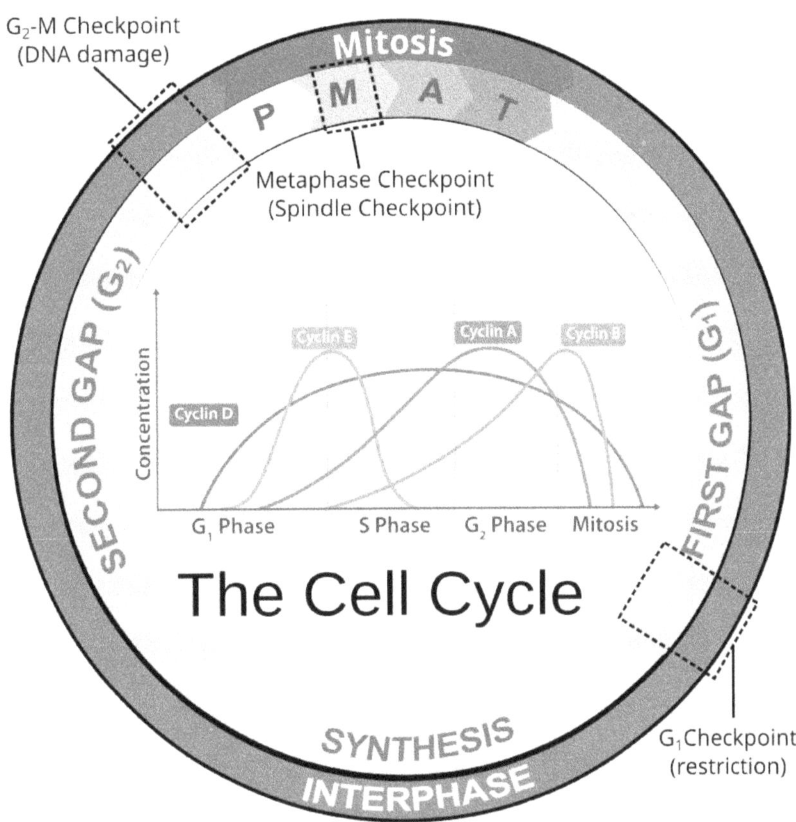

Impact and Products

Their research has fundamentally changed the way scientists view the cell cycle, contributing to a deeper understanding of cellular processes and the development of cancer. The work of these three laureates continues to inspire ongoing research into cell biology, genetics, and the development of new cancer treatments, underscoring the importance of basic scientific research in advancing medical knowledge and treatment strategies.

SYDNEY BRENNER H. ROBERT HORVITZ, JOHN E. SULSTON (2002)

Apoptosis and programmed cell death. While others were researching life, this trio was looking other way.

In 2002, Sydney Brenner, H. Robert Horvitz, and John E. Sulston were recognized with the Nobel Prize in Medicine for their groundbreaking research on the genetic regulation of organ dev elopment and programmed cell death, using the model organism Caenorhabditis elegans.

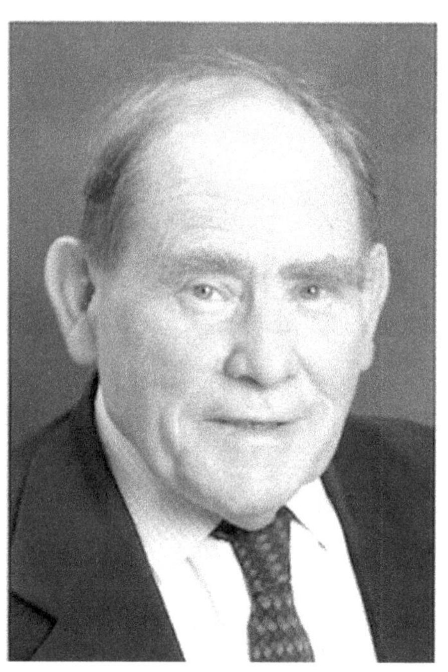 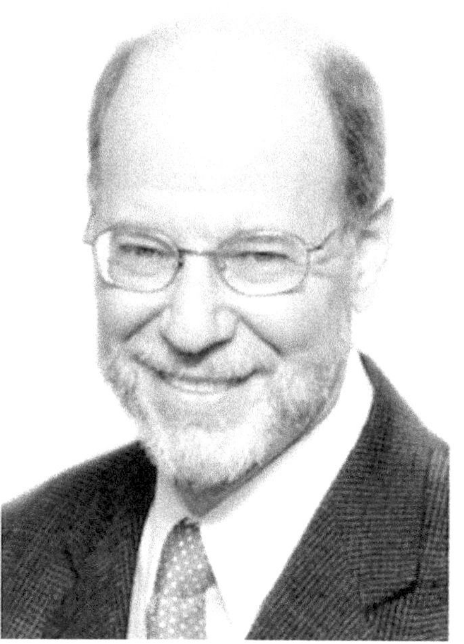 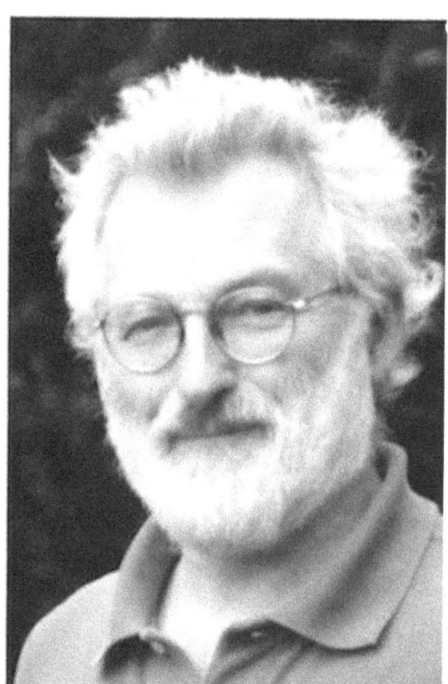

History

Sydney Brenner, born on January 13, 1927, in Germiston, South Africa, and died on April 5, 2019, in Singapore, was a pioneering figure in establishing C. elegans as a model organism for genetic research. H. Robert Horvitz, born on May 8, 1947, in Chicago, Illinois, USA, expanded upon Brenner's work, discovering and characterizing the genes involved in the apoptosis pathway in C. elegans. John E. Sulston, playing a crucial role alongside Brenner and Horvitz, mapped the entire cell lineage of C. elegans and contributed significantly to understanding how genes control cell death and differentiation during development.

Snippets

Their collective research highlighted the importance of programmed cell death (apoptosis) as a normal part of organism development and maintenance. Brenner's pioneering use of C. elegans paved the way for future genetic studies, while Horvitz identified key genes that control the cell death mechanism. Sulston's work in tracing the cell lineage of C. elegans was instrumental in understanding the development and functioning of tissues.

Current Implications

The trio's discoveries have profound implications across biology and medicine, offering insights into the mechanisms of diseases, including cancer, where the process of cell death is often disrupted. Their work laid the foundation for the development of new therapeutic strategies targeting the pathways involved in cell growth and death.

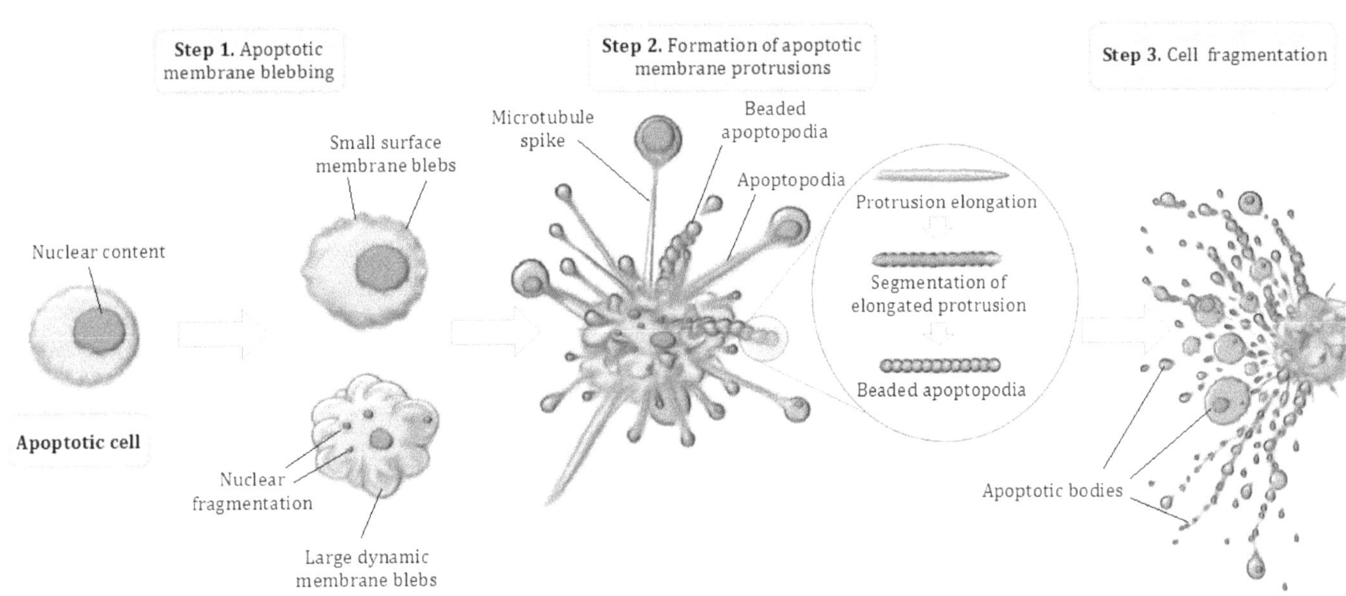

The process of Apoptosis

Impact and Products

Brenner, Horvitz, and Sulston's research was huge, influencing both the theoretical framework of developmental biology and practical approaches to disease treatment and prevention. Their work on programmed cell death remains crucial for the ongoing development of medical research, providing a deeper understanding of cellular processes that are fundamental to life.

PAUL LAUTERBUR AND SIR PETER MANSFIELD (2003)

Magnetic resonance Imaging : One more monumental moment in medical Imaging

Paul Lauterbur and Sir Peter Mansfield were awarded the 2003 Nobel Prize in Medicine for their groundbreaking work on Magnetic Resonance Imaging (MRI), a technique that has revolutionized medical diagnostics by providing detailed images of the body's internal structures without the need for invasive procedures.

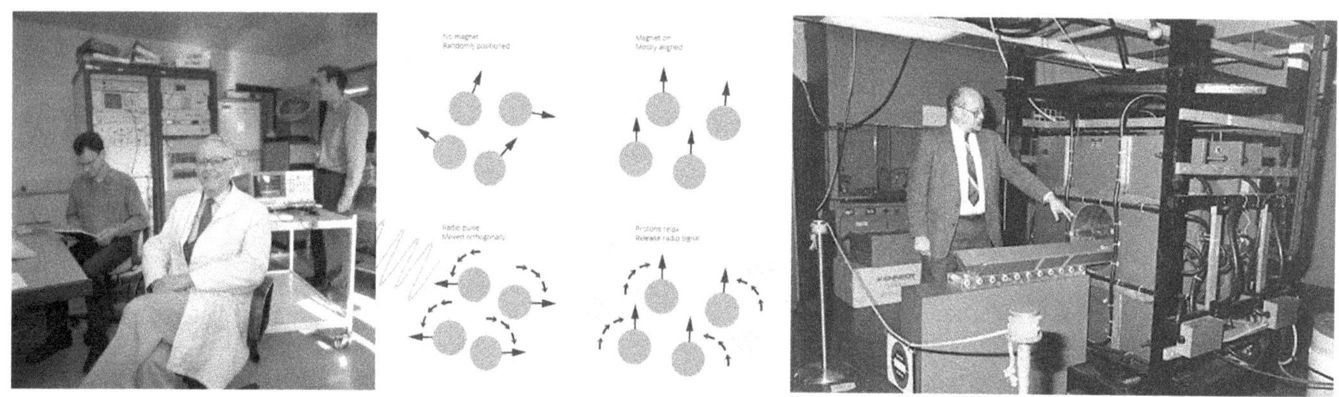

The scientists, who dared to scan the water molecules, of our body, (Which forms 60% of total body mass) into stunning medical Images. Rest is history, we are now blessed with this radiation free Imaging.

History

Paul Lauterbur was born on May 6, 1929, in Sidney, Ohio, USA. His journey into the world of MRI began in the 1970s when he discovered that magnetic gradients could be used to produce two-dimensional images of structures that could not be seen through other techniques. Working at Stony Brook University, Lauterbur conducted early experiments using NMR machines, often at night, to avoid disrupting the department's schedule. His seminal paper, initially rejected by Nature for its "fuzzy" images, eventually became a classic after he persuaded the editors to reconsider.

Sir Peter Mansfield was born on October 9, 1933, in Lambeth, London. After his education, he moved to the University of Nottingham, where he spent much of his career. Mansfield made significant advancements in MRI technology, including developing the technique for "slice selection" and fast imaging through echo-planar imaging, which made it possible to capture images much more quickly than before. His contributions were instrumental in translating MRI from a theoretical concept into a practical diagnostic tool.

Snippets

Paul Lauterbur's Pioneering Work: Lauterbur's innovative use of magnetic gradients to generate the first MRI images marked a paradigm shift in medical imaging, demonstrating MRI's potential by imaging a clam, green peppers, and distinguishing between two types of water.

Sir Peter Mansfield's Technical Innovations: Mansfield significantly advanced MRI technology by developing the "slice selection" technique and fast imaging protocols, including echo-planar imaging, which enabled rapid and precise MRI scans, revolutionizing diagnostic capabilities.

Collaboration and Persistence: Despite initial skepticism and technical challenges, the persistent efforts and collaboration between physicists, chemists, and engineers led to MRI's development into a vital diagnostic tool used worldwide.

Broad Applications: Today, MRI is indispensable across various medical fields, from neurology and oncology to orthopedics, thanks to the foundational work of Lauterbur and Mansfield, providing detailed views of the body's internal structures without ionizing radiation.

Early Researchers

Raymond Damadian. While not awarded the Nobel Prize alongside Lauterbur and Mansfield, Damadian's work was instrumental in the field. He was the first to propose the body's scanning using NMR and constructed the first MRI scanner, demonstrating its potential to distinguish between healthy and cancerous tissue based on differences in relaxation times.

Herman Y. Carr also made significant early contributions by producing the first one-dimensional MRI signal in 1952, a foundational step towards the development of MRI. Although his work did not immediately lead to the development of MRI as we know it today, Carr's experiments demonstrated the potential of magnetic resonance for creating images.

Erwin Hahn is known for discovering spin echoes, a phenomenon that underlies many MRI techniques. His work provided the theoretical basis for manipulating nuclear spins to generate signals that could be used to form images.

Richard Ernst further contributed to the development of MRI through his advancements in nuclear magnetic resonance spectroscopy, especially his work on Fourier Transform NMR, which significantly increased the sensitivity and resolution of NMR spectroscopy. Though Ernst's work is more directly associated with chemical analysis, the principles he developed are integral to the imaging techniques used in MRI.

Current Implications

Non-Invasive Diagnostics: MRI provides detailed images of the body's internal structures without the need for invasive procedures, reducing the risk to patients and allowing for safer diagnostic practices.

Comprehensive Medical Research: The ability of MRI to visualize soft tissues in great detail has opened new avenues for medical research, enabling the study of complex diseases, brain function, and the effects of various treatments at a level of detail previously unattainable.

Neuroscience and Neurology: MRI, particularly functional MRI (fMRI), has revolutionized neuroscience by allowing researchers and clinicians to observe brain activity in real-time, enhancing the understanding of brain function, development, and disorders.

Personalized Medicine: The detailed images produced by MRI enable personalized treatment plans for patients, particularly in oncology, where tumor size, location, and response to therapy can be monitored with precision.

Sports Medicine and Orthopedics: MRI's ability to clearly image soft tissue structures like ligaments, tendons, and cartilage has made it an invaluable tool in diagnosing sports injuries, contributing to more effective treatment and rehabilitation strategies.

Expansion into Other Fields: Beyond human medicine, MRI technology is increasingly used in veterinary medicine, materials science, and plant biology, showcasing its versatility and the broad potential for its application in various research fields.

Technological Advancements: The ongoing development of MRI technology, including faster imaging techniques and higher resolution capabilities, continues to expand its applications and improve patient care.

Impact and Products

Impact on Healthcare and Diagnosis

- Revolutionized Diagnostic Imaging: MRI has fundamentally changed how physicians diagnose and understand a wide range of conditions, from brain tumors to spinal injuries, without the risks associated with ionizing radiation.

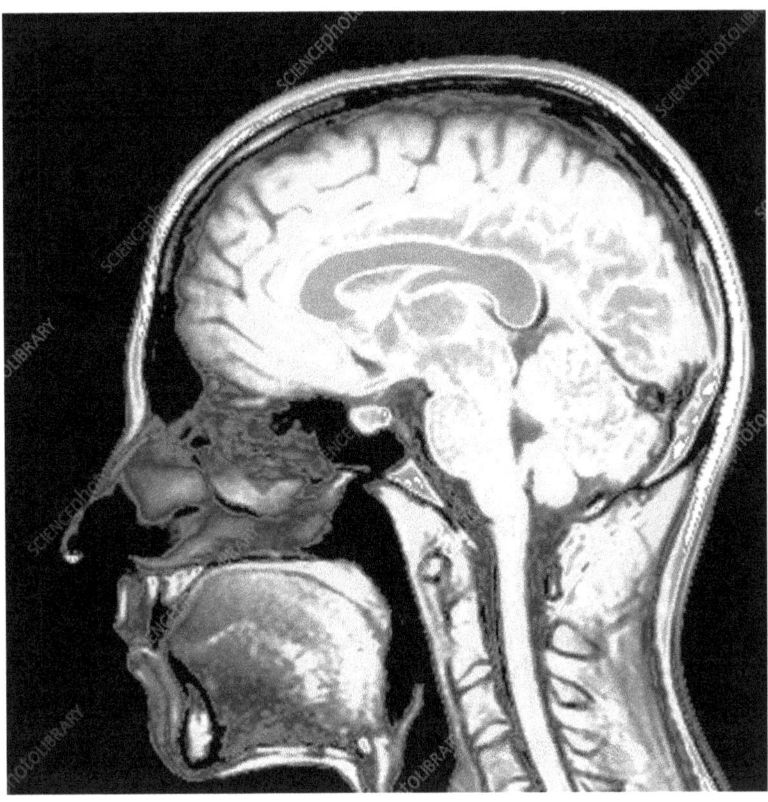

MRI techniques now evolved so much with functional and physiological Imaging

- Enhanced Patient Care: The ability to obtain clear, detailed images of soft tissues has improved the accuracy of diagnoses, the planning of surgeries, and the monitoring of treatment responses, leading to better patient outcomes.

Impact on Medical Research

- Advanced Neurological Research: MRI, especially functional MRI (fMRI), has been crucial in advancing our understanding of brain function, aiding in research on neurological diseases, cognitive neuroscience, and psychology.
- Contributed to Drug Development: By allowing detailed monitoring of how diseases progress and respond to treatments, MRI has become an indispensable tool in pharmaceutical research and the development of new therapies.

Technological Advancements and Products

- Development of Specialized MRI Techniques: Innovations such as diffusion tensor imaging (DTI), magnetic resonance angiography (MRA), and others have expanded the applications of MRI in medicine.
- Wide Range of MRI Machines: From high-field scanners offering exquisite detail to open and portable MRI systems designed for specific applications or patient comfort, the diversity of MRI technology has grown substantially.

Commercial and Economic Impact

- Growth of the MRI Industry: The MRI market has seen significant growth, with numerous companies manufacturing MRI machines and related technology, contributing to job creation and economic activity in the healthcare sector.
- Legal and Patent Landscape: The development of MRI technology has led to a complex landscape of patents and intellectual property rights, highlighting the commercial value and competitive nature of medical imaging technology.

Broader Applications Beyond Human Medicine

- Veterinary Medicine: MRI is used in veterinary practice to diagnose conditions in pets and livestock with the same level of detail as in humans.
- Industrial and Scientific Research: Non-medical applications of MRI, including material science, food industry, and plant biology, utilize MRI for its ability to provide detailed internal images without destructive testing.

The legacy of Lauterbur and Mansfield's MRI technology continues to grow, demonstrating the transformative power of their invention across multiple fields. The ongoing evolution of MRI technology promises to further expand its applications and impact, underscoring the enduring significance of their contribution to science and medicine.

RICHARD AXEL AND LINDA B. BUCK (2004)

The anatomical and molecular basis of the amazing sense of olfaction

In 2004, Richard Axel and Linda B. Buck were awarded the Nobel Prize in Medicine for their seminal discoveries on the olfactory system, elucidating how our sense of smell works through the identification of odorant receptors and the organization of the olfactory system.

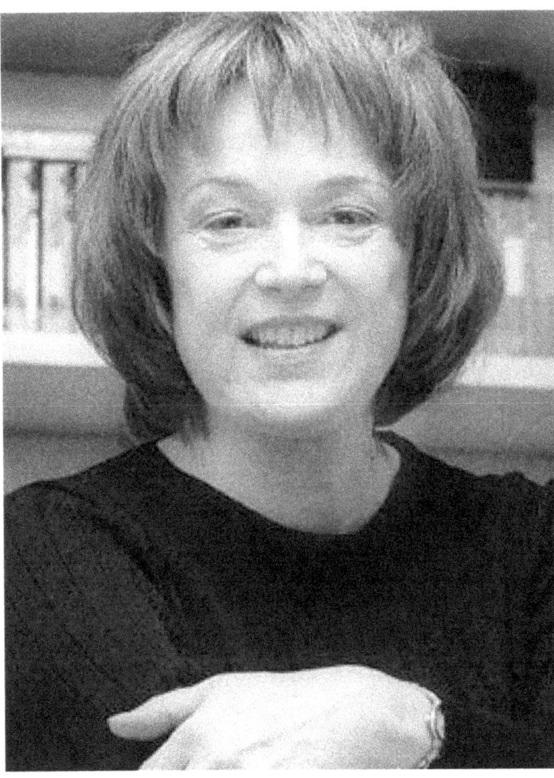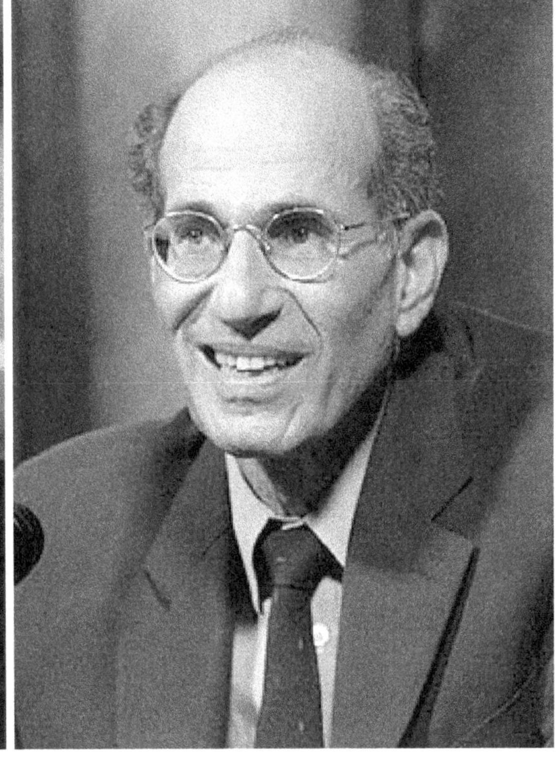

History

Richard Axel, born on July 2, 1946, in New York, USA, and Linda B. Buck, born on January 29, 1947, in Seattle, Washington, USA, embarked on research that would significantly advance our understanding of sensory perception. Axel's academic background includes an A.B. from Columbia University and an M.D. from Johns Hopkins University School of Medicine, leading to a distinguished career at Columbia University and the Howard Hughes Medical Institute. Buck pursued her B.S. in microbiology and psychology at the University of Washington, followed by a Ph.D. in immunology from the University of Texas Southwestern Medical Center, eventually collaborating with Axel at Columbia University.

Snippets

Their groundbreaking work revealed a complex system of about 1,000 genes coding for an equivalent number of olfactory receptors, demonstrating the molecular basis for odor detection and discrimination. This intricate system allows for the perception of a vast array of odors through the combination of signals from these receptors, sending electrical signals to the brain's olfactory bulb and translating them into distinct smells. Their research underscored the universality of olfactory mechanisms across different species, although humans have around 350 active olfactory receptors.

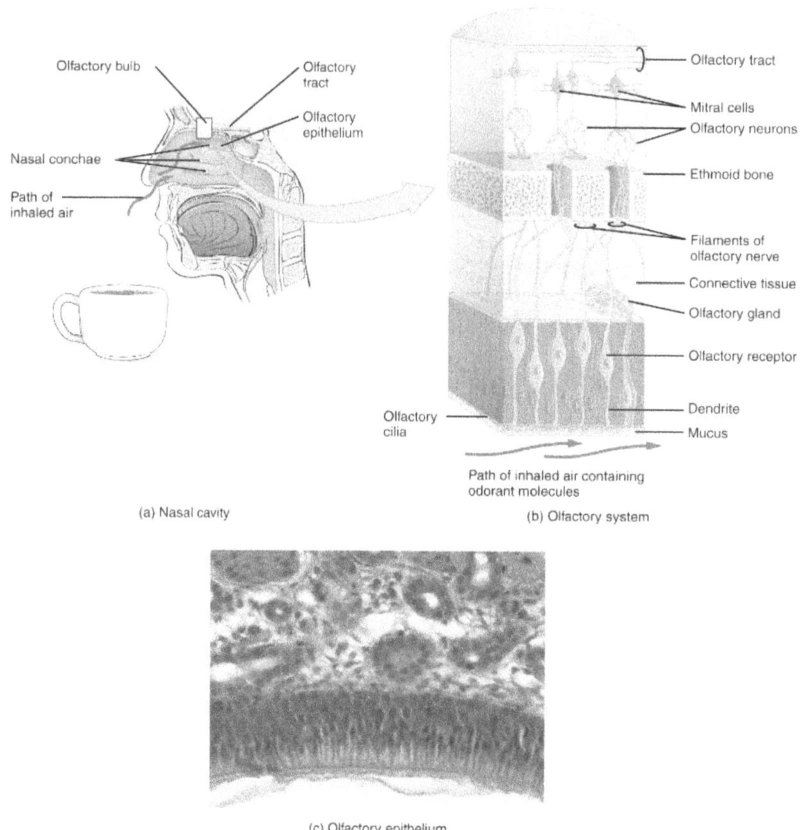

Current Implications

The elucidation of the olfactory receptor genes and the operational mechanisms of the olfactory system have profound implications for neuroscience, genetics, and molecular biology. Understanding how smells are detected and processed not only advances our knowledge of sensory systems but also opens pathways for researching neurobiological disorders and developing novel sensory prosthetics or therapies for smell and taste disorders.

Impact and Products

The contributions of Axel and Buck have had a lasting impact on the scientific community, influencing further research into sensory systems and genetic coding of sensory receptors. Their work has paved the way for future discoveries in how the brain processes complex sensory information, contributing to a broader comprehension of human perception and the neural basis of behavior.

BARRY MARSHALL AND J. ROBIN WARREN (2005)

Helicobacter Pylori : A new infective postulate in Peptic ulcer pathology

Barry Marshall and J. Robin Warren, both from Australia, were awarded the Nobel Prize in Medicine in 2005 for their discovery of the bacterium Helicobacter pylori and its role in causing gastritis and peptic ulcer disease. This groundbreaking work changed the understanding of stomach ulcers from being primarily caused by stress and lifestyle to an infectious disease model

History

Barry Marshall was born on September 30, 1951, in Kalgoorlie, Western Australia. He embarked on his medical career after obtaining a bachelor's degree from the University of Western Australia in 1974. Marshall's clinical interests and research led him to explore the underlying causes of chronic gastritis and peptic ulcers during his time at the Royal Perth Hospital.

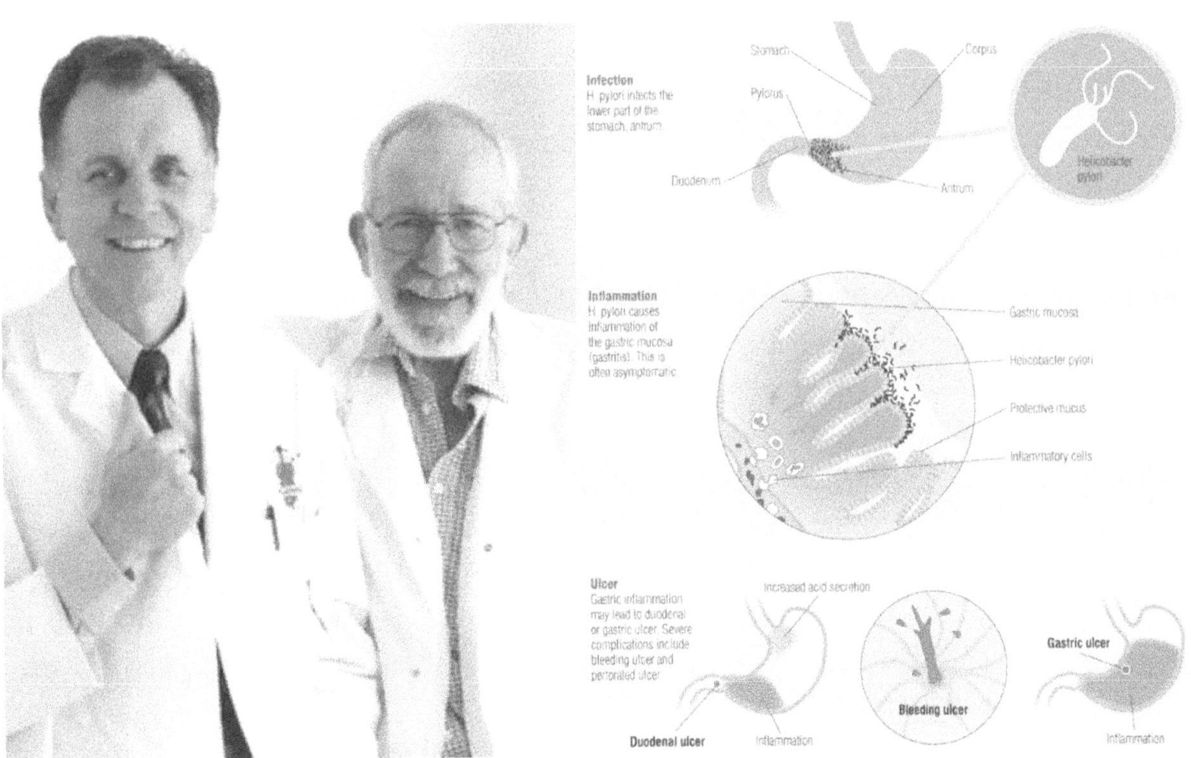

J. Robin Warren, born on June 11, 1937, in Adelaide, South Australia, was a pathologist with a keen interest in the stomach's lining and gastritis. His observations of small, curved bacteria in association with gastritis laid the groundwork for the collaboration with Marshall

In 1981, during Marshall's internal medicine fellowship at Royal Perth Hospital, the duo's paths converged. Warren's pathological insights combined with Marshall's clinical interest in gastritis to form a formidable research team. They hypothesized that the bacteria Warren observed, later named Helicobacter pylori, were directly linked to peptic ulcers and gastric cancer.

Facing skepticism from the scientific community, which largely dismissed the possibility that bacteria could survive in the stomach's acidic environment, Marshall and Warren persisted in their research. Their determination was epitomized in 1984 when Marshall famously ingested H. pylori to prove its role in causing gastritis, leading to a greater acceptance of their findings.

Snippets

Discovery of Helicobacter pylori: Barry Marshall and J. Robin Warren identified Helicobacter pylori in the early 1980s, linking it to gastritis and peptic ulcer disease, fundamentally changing the understanding of these conditions.

Challenging Medical Norms: Their hypothesis that a bacterial infection, not stress or lifestyle, causes stomach ulcers was initially met with skepticism. Marshall's self-experimentation, where he ingested H. pylori and developed gastritis, played a pivotal role in proving their theory.

Nobel Prize Recognition: In 2005, Marshall and Warren were awarded the Nobel Prize in Medicine for their groundbreaking work on H. pylori, confirming the bacterium's role in peptic ulcers and setting new standards for treatment.

Impact on Treatment: The identification of H. pylori led to the development of antibiotic treatments, drastically reducing the need for surgery in peptic ulcer disease and reshaping the management of gastric disorders.

Ongoing Research and Legacy: Marshall and Warren's discovery continues to influence the field of gastroenterology, with ongoing research into the broader implications of H. pylori infections, including their potential link to gastric cancer.

Early Researchers

André Dubois, who conducted significant research into gastrointestinal diseases and the microbiology of the stomach, contributing to the broader understanding that paved the way for the discovery of H. pylori. Another pioneer, Walter B. Cannon, known for his work on the physiological response to emotional stress, provided early insights into how the body's biological processes, including those in the stomach, are influenced by stress, a factor previously thought to be a primary cause of ulcers before Marshall and Warren's discovery.

The work of these individuals, among others, underscores the collaborative nature of scientific discovery. Their contributions, while perhaps not as widely recognized as those of Marshall and Warren, were essential in building the body of knowledge that allowed for the identification of H. pylori as a causative agent in peptic ulcer disease.

Current Implications

Shift in Treatment Paradigms: Prior to their discovery, peptic ulcers were primarily treated with medications to reduce stomach acid and surgical interventions. Now, the standard treatment includes antibiotics to eradicate H. pylori, effectively curing the underlying cause of the ulcers for many patients. This approach has drastically reduced the need for surgery related to peptic ulcers and improved treatment outcomes.

Prevention of Gastric Cancer: H. pylori infection is a known risk factor for the development of gastric cancer, one of the leading causes of cancer death worldwide. Early detection and treatment of H. pylori infection have become important strategies in preventing gastric cancer.

Impact on Public Health Policies: Understanding the role of H. pylori in gastrointestinal diseases has influenced public health strategies regarding the diagnosis and treatment of peptic ulcer disease. There is now a greater emphasis on testing for H. pylori in patients with gastric symptoms, leading to more targeted and effective treatment plans.

Research and Development: The discovery has spurred ongoing research into the relationship between chronic infections, inflammation, and cancer. It has opened new avenues for investigating other chronic conditions that may have a microbial component, expanding our understanding of human health and disease.

Diagnostic Developments: The need to detect H. pylori infection efficiently has led to the development of various diagnostic tests, including urea breath tests, stool antigen tests, and blood antibody tests. These non-invasive methods have made it easier to diagnose infections and monitor treatment success.

Global Health Considerations: With H. pylori infection rates being higher in developing countries, its identification as a causative agent in peptic ulcers and gastritis has important implications for global health initiatives, especially in regions with limited healthcare resources. Efforts to improve sanitation and reduce transmission are crucial in these settings.

Impact and Products

Development of Diagnostic Tools: The need to accurately diagnose H. pylori infection led to the creation of innovative diagnostic products, including the urea breath test, stool antigen tests, and serological assays. These tools have become standard in detecting H. pylori, facilitating early treatment and reducing the risk of severe gastrointestinal diseases.

Pharmaceutical Advances: The understanding of H. pylori's role in peptic ulcer disease revolutionized the development of targeted pharmaceutical treatments. Beyond the widespread use of antibiotics to eradicate the bacterium, this discovery has fueled the ongoing development of more effective, less side-effect-prone antibiotic regimens and adjunct therapies to enhance treatment outcomes and patient compliance.

Preventive Care Products: Knowledge of H. pylori's transmission and the conditions conducive to its proliferation has spurred the creation of products aimed at preventive care and hygiene, particularly in settings with higher risks of H. pylori infection. These range from water purification systems to personal hygiene products designed to reduce the spread of H. pylori.

Nutritional Supplements and Probiotics: The insight into how H. pylori affects the stomach lining and overall gastrointestinal health has encouraged the development and marketing of dietary supplements and probiotics aimed at supporting gut health. These products are designed to complement medical treatments for H. pylori infection and promote a healthy digestive system.

Technology and Research Platforms: The ongoing research into H. pylori and its mechanisms of infection and disease causation has led to the development of advanced research platforms and technologies. These include genomic sequencing of bacterial strains, in vitro models to study bacterial-host interactions, and in silico modeling to predict treatment outcomes. These technologies not only enhance our understanding of H. pylori but also contribute to the broader field of microbiology and infectious disease research.

Their work has not only transformed the approach to treating peptic ulcer disease but also contributed to the broader understanding of the role of microbes in human health and disease.

ANDREW Z. FIRE AND CRAIG C. MELLO (2006)

When Interference within RNA codes became an ultimate Innovation

Andrew Z. Fire and Craig C. Mello were awarded the Nobel Prize in Medicine in 2006 for their discovery of RNA interference (RNAi), a process where double-stranded RNA silences specific genes. This discovery has fundamentally changed our understanding of how genes are regulated and expressed.

History

Andrew Z. Fire, born on April 27, 1959, in Stanford, California, and Craig C. Mello, born on October 18, 1960, in New Haven, Connecticut, are the pioneering scientists behind the discovery of RNA interference (RNAi). Their collaboration, which culminated in this groundbreaking discovery, began in the realm of molecular biology, where they were intrigued by how genes are regulated and expressed within organisms.

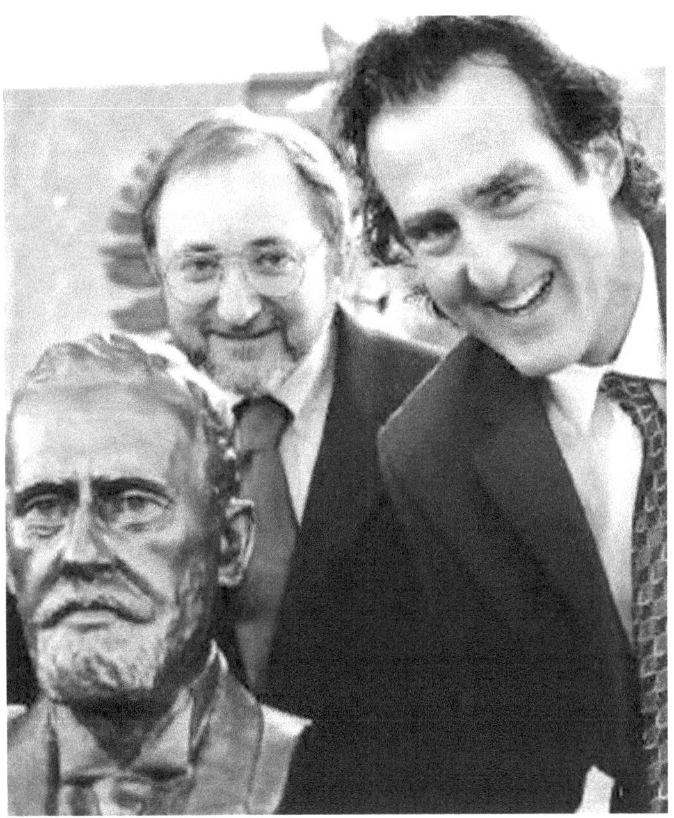

Their journey into the discovery of RNAi started in the late 1990s when they were working with the roundworm C. elegans. In 1998, they published a seminal paper that detailed their findings on

RNAi, revealing that double-stranded RNA (dsRNA) can silence specific genes within an organism. This process, where dsRNA leads to the targeted degradation of messenger RNA (mRNA), effectively prevents the mRNA from producing proteins and thus silences the gene.

This discovery was not just a significant scientific achievement but also a fundamental shift in understanding genetic regulation. It opened up new possibilities for genetic research and biotechnology, providing a powerful tool for scientists to explore gene function and regulation with unprecedented precision.

The collaboration between Fire and Mello, bridging their respective institutions – Stanford University School of Medicine for Fire and the University of Massachusetts Medical School for Mello – showcases the importance of cross-institutional partnerships in advancing scientific research. Their work has had a profound impact on the field of molecular biology, offering new avenues for exploring genetic diseases and developing novel therapeutic strategies.

Snippets

Discovery of RNAi: Andrew Z. Fire and Craig C. Mello's groundbreaking work revealed RNA interference (RNAi) as a natural process of gene silencing by double-stranded RNA.

Mechanism Unveiled: They demonstrated how RNAi could block messenger RNA, preventing specific genes from being expressed and thus silencing them. This process plays a crucial regulatory role in gene expression.

Significant Publication: Their findings were published in a seminal paper in 1998, highlighting RNAi's role in the roundworm C. elegans and opening up a new field of biological research.

Nobel Prize Awarded: For their discovery of RNA interference, Fire and Mello were awarded the Nobel Prize in Medicine in 2006, underscoring the significance of their work in understanding genetic regulation.

Applications in Research and Medicine: The discovery of RNAi has led to its use as a powerful tool in molecular biology for gene silencing, with applications in drug development, gene therapy, and the study of functional genomics.

Impact on Genetic Research: RNAi has revolutionized the way scientists study gene function and expression, offering a method to precisely control the flow of genetic information.

Early Researchers

Victor Ambros, whose discovery of the first microRNA in 1993 opened the door to understanding the intricate roles of small RNAs in gene regulation. Alongside him, Gary Ruvkun's work in identifying complementary genes that regulate development in C. elegans through small RNA molecules laid the groundwork for understanding the biological significance of RNAi. Their contributions, though not as widely recognized outside of scientific circles, were instrumental in setting the stage for Fire and Mello's discovery.

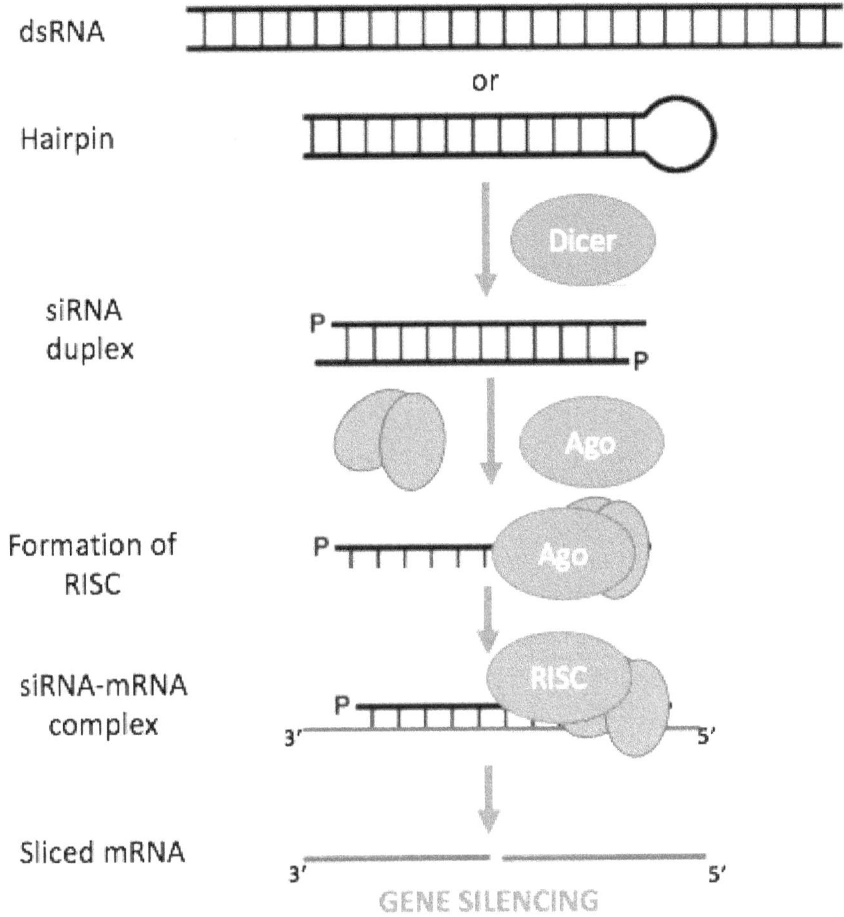

The mode of creation of small Interfering RNA

Another notable contributor is Thomas Tuschl, whose work on RNAi in mammalian cells further expanded the understanding of RNAi's potential, bridging the gap between basic science and therapeutic applications. His efforts in elucidating the mechanisms through which RNAi operates in different organisms highlighted the universal nature of this gene-silencing process.

These pioneers, among others, contributed layers of knowledge and innovation essential for the momentous discovery of RNAi. Their tireless exploration of genetic and RNA functions provided the essential building blocks upon which Fire and Mello could construct their groundbreaking work. In the grand narrative of scientific progress, it is important to remember these individuals whose curiosity, perseverance, and collaborative spirit helped unravel one of nature's most intricate biological processes.

Current Implications

Gene Function and Regulation: RNAi has become a fundamental tool in molecular biology and genetics for studying gene function. It allows researchers to "knock down" the expression of specific genes to understand their roles in biological processes and disease mechanisms.

Therapeutic Applications: The ability to silence genes implicated in diseases offers promising therapeutic potentials. RNAi-based therapies are being developed for various conditions, including viral infections, cancer, and genetic disorders. These therapies work by targeting and silencing harmful genes.

Drug Development: RNAi technology is also revolutionizing drug discovery and development. By silencing genes associated with disease, researchers can identify potential drug targets more efficiently and develop therapies that specifically target these genes.

Agriculture: In agriculture, RNAi is being used to develop crops that are resistant to pests and diseases, require fewer chemical inputs, and have improved nutritional profiles.

Functional Genomics: RNAi has facilitated the growth of functional genomics, enabling the large-scale analysis of gene functions and their contributions to various biological processes. This has implications for understanding complex diseases, improving crop yields, and even environmental conservation efforts.

Impact and Products

Therapeutic Products: The most direct impact has been in the development of RNAi-based drugs aimed at silencing the expression of disease-causing genes. This approach has led to the creation of new treatments for viral diseases, certain types of cancer, and genetic disorders. An example includes patisiran, approved for the treatment of hereditary transthyretin-mediated amyloidosis, a rare disease caused by the accumulation of misfolded protein.

Research Tools: RNAi has become an indispensable tool in genetic research, allowing scientists to study gene function by "turning off" specific genes in the laboratory. This has facilitated the development of kits and reagents for gene silencing, widely used in academic and pharmaceutical research to explore gene function, validate drug targets, and study disease mechanisms.

Agricultural Biotechnology: In agriculture, RNAi technology is being used to create genetically modified crops with improved traits, such as enhanced resistance to pests and diseases, improved nutritional content, and increased tolerance to abiotic stresses like drought and salinity. RNAi-based biopesticides, which target specific pests without harming other organisms, represent another innovative application in this field.

Veterinary Medicine: Similar to its applications in human medicine, RNAi is also being explored for treating diseases in animals. This includes the development of RNAi-based treatments for viral diseases in livestock, offering a new approach to managing animal health and preventing the spread of infectious diseases.

Diagnostics: Beyond therapeutics and agriculture, RNAi technology has potential applications in diagnostics. By detecting the presence or absence of specific RNA sequences, researchers can develop sensitive diagnostic tests for various diseases, including infectious diseases and cancers.

The foundational work of Fire and Mello has thus not only expanded our understanding of gene regulation but also opened up new avenues for innovation across multiple disciplines.

MARIO R. CAPECCHI, SIR MARTIN J. EVANS, AND OLIVER SMITHIES (2007)

The creation of "knock out mouse" provided unlimited research models of human disease in animals

In 2007, Mario R. Capecchi, Sir Martin J. Evans, and Oliver Smithies were awarded the Nobel Prize in Medicine for their groundbreaking work on gene targeting techniques using embryonic stem cells. This innovation has had a profound impact on biomedical research, particularly in the creation of animal models of human diseases, which are crucial for understanding disease mechanisms and testing new treatments.

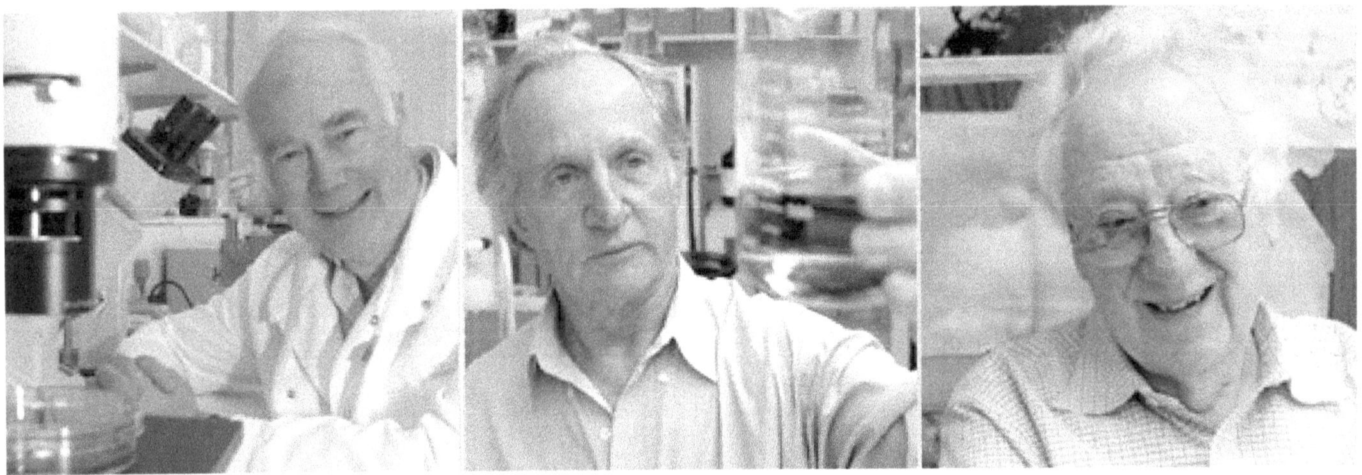

History

Mario R. Capecchi was born on October 6, 1937, in Verona, Italy, and faced a tumultuous childhood during World War II before moving to the United States, where he pursued a distinguished career in genetics. Sir Martin J. Evans, born on January 1, 1941, in Stroud, Gloucestershire, England, is celebrated for isolating and cultivating embryonic stem cells from mice, which laid the foundation for gene targeting. Oliver Smithies, born on June 23, 1925, in Halifax, England, and died on January 10, 2017, in Chapel Hill, North Carolina, USA, contributed significantly to this field by developing techniques to manipulate genes in mice, creating models for human diseases.

Snippets

Capecchi's research focused on developing methods to precisely alter genes within mice, a process that allows for the creation of "knockout mice" used to study genetic diseases. Evans's isolation of embryonic stem cells and his techniques for manipulating the mouse genome were pivotal in making targeted genetic modifications possible. Smithies's work, particularly his development of starch gel electrophoresis and his contributions to gene targeting, has been instrumental in understanding and treating genetic conditions.

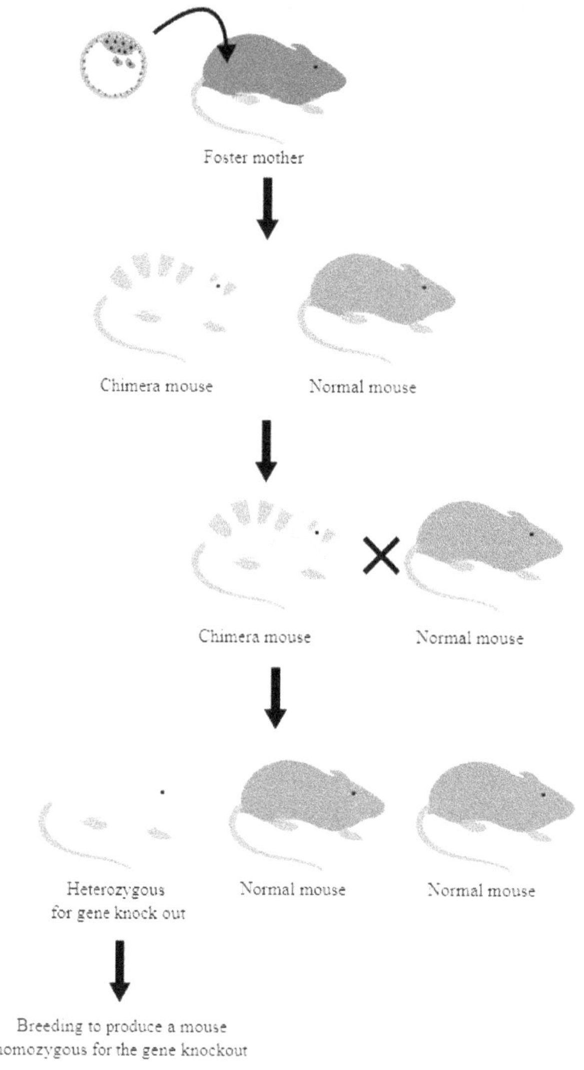

The scheme of creation of knock out mice

Current Implications

The collective work of these three scientists has revolutionized genetic research, enabling precise modifications of the genome in living organisms. This has opened up new avenues for the study of gene function, the understanding of disease processes at the genetic level, and the development of gene therapies for various conditions.

Impact and Products

The technique of gene targeting in mice, developed by Capecchi, Evans, and Smithies, is now a standard tool in molecular biology and genetic engineering. It has facilitated the creation of animal models for studying a wide range of human diseases, including cancer, heart disease, and neurological disorders, significantly advancing the field of medical research and offering new strategies for developing treatments and cures.

HARALD ZUR HAUSEN, FRANÇOISE BARRÉ-SINOUSSI, AND LUC MONTAGNIER (2008)

The studies on HIV and Papilloma virus and their link to cancer

In 2008, Harald zur Hausen, Françoise Barré-Sinoussi, and Luc Montagnier were collectively awarded the Nobel Prize in Medicine for their significant contributions to understanding and identifying viruses linked to cancer and AIDS, respectively.

History

Harald zur Hausen, born on March 11, 1936, in Gelsenkirchen, Germany, and passed away on May 28, 2023, in Heidelberg, Germany, was recognized for his discovery of the human papillomavirus (HPV) and its link to cervical cancer. His research facilitated the development of vaccines against HPV, contributing to cancer prevention efforts globally.

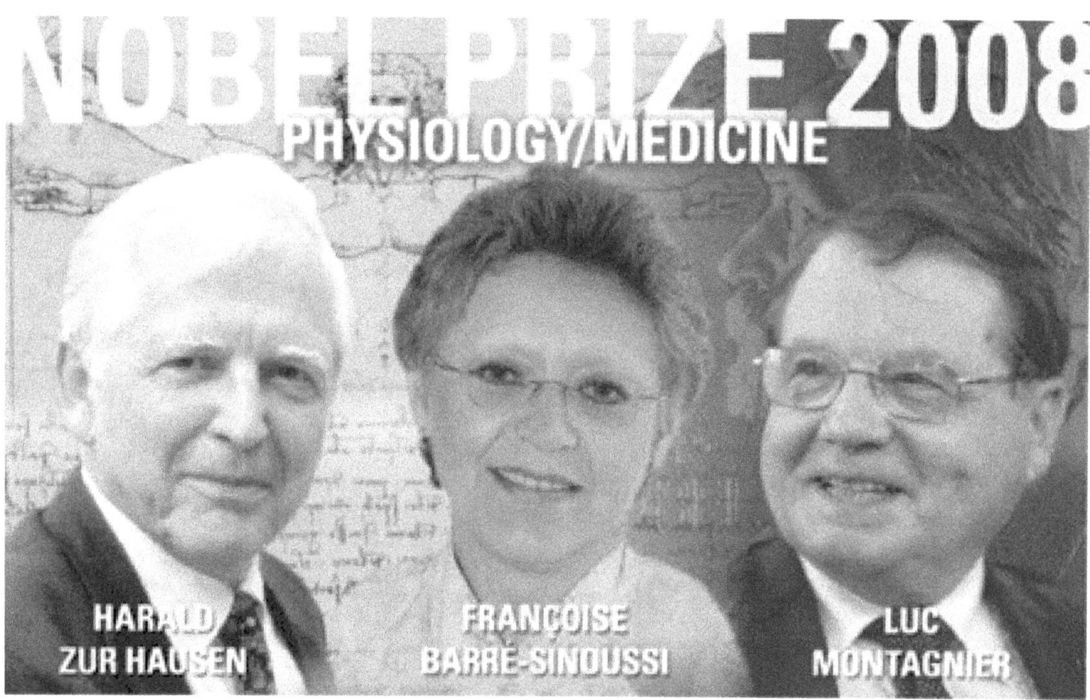

Françoise Barré-Sinoussi, born on July 30, 1947, in Paris, France, played a crucial role in identifying the human immunodeficiency virus (HIV) as the cause of acquired immunodeficiency syndrome (AIDS). Her career at the Pasteur Institute in Paris has been pivotal in AIDS research, from discovery through to seeking effective treatments.

Luc Montagnier, born in Chabris, France, and passed away on February 8, 2022, was integral to the early efforts to identify HIV. His work alongside Barré-Sinoussi marked a turning point in understanding and combating AIDS, leading to significant advancements in diagnosis, treatment, and prevention.

Snippets

Zur Hausen's groundbreaking work identified HPV as a primary cause of cervical cancer, challenging previous beliefs and leading to the development of preventive vaccines. Barré-Sinoussi and Montagnier's collaborative efforts in isolating and identifying HIV as the causative agent of AIDS laid the foundation for understanding this devastating disease and opened pathways for research on antiretroviral drugs.

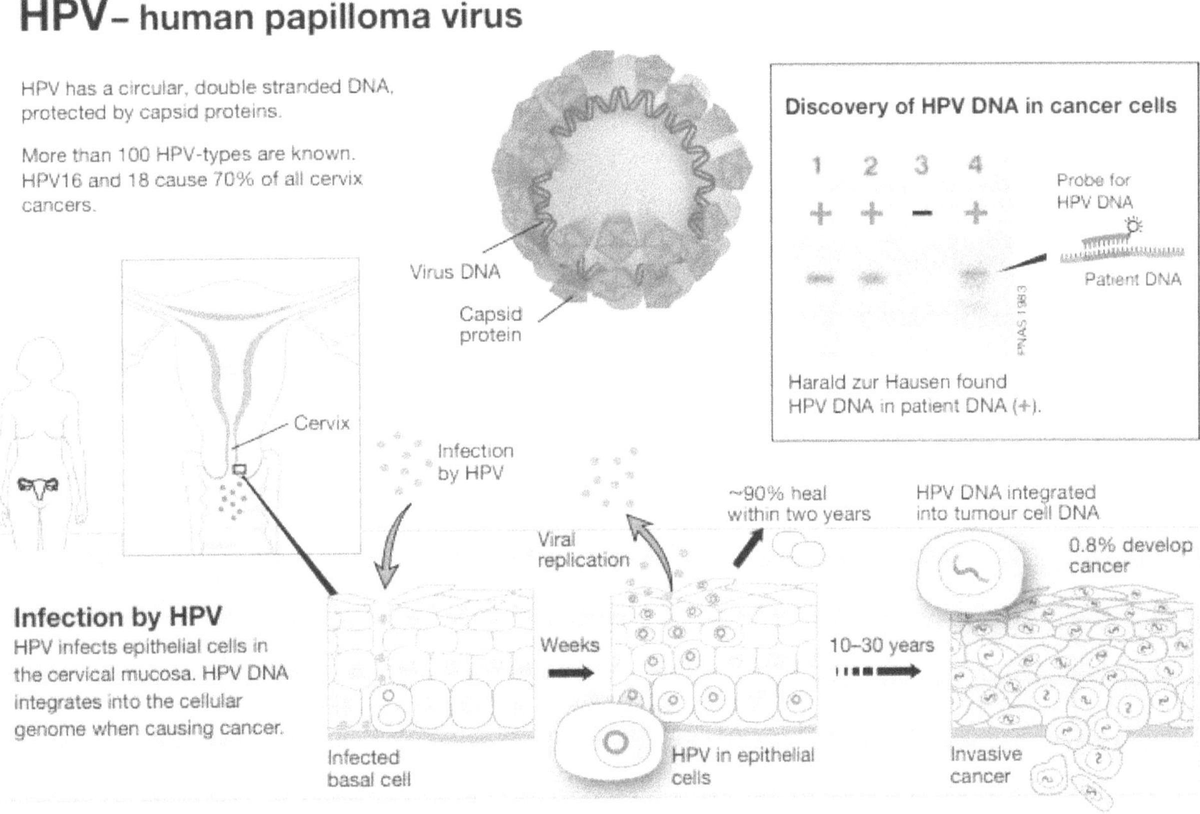

Current Implications

The discoveries by these laureates have had profound implications for public health, leading to the development of diagnostic tests, treatments, and vaccines that have saved or improved millions of lives worldwide. Their work has also emphasized the importance of scientific research in tackling global health challenges.

Impact and Products

The collective achievements of zur Hausen, Barré-Sinoussi, and Montagnier have significantly advanced medical science's ability to fight cancers caused by viruses and to manage and prevent HIV/

AIDS. Their contributions continue to inspire ongoing research and innovation in the fight against infectious diseases and cancer.

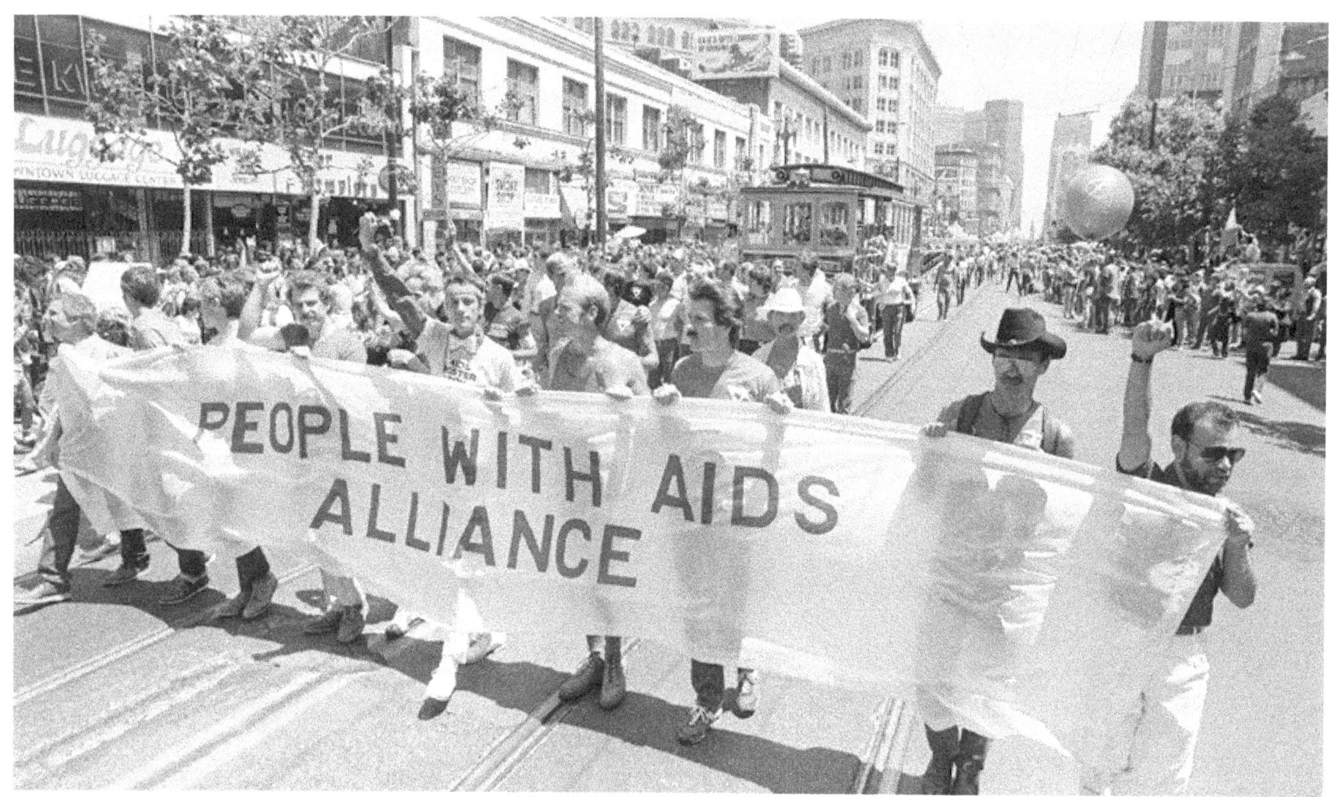

HIV infection had a tremendous impact on the globe with medical, social and economic challenge

ELIZABETH H. BLACKBURN, CAROL W. GREIDER, AND JACK W. *SZOSTAK (2009)*

The exposition of the hidden secrets about Telomeres in chromosome

Blackburn, Greider, and Szostak's pioneering research provided critical insights into chromosome protection mechanisms. Their discovery revealed that telomeres, repetitive DNA sequences at the ends of chromosomes, play a key role in preserving the genetic information during cell division

History

Elizabeth H. Blackburn was born on November 26, 1948, in Hobart, Tasmania, Australia. She embarked on a path that would lead her to major scientific discoveries, ultimately sharing the 2009 Nobel Prize in Medicine. Blackburn's early interest in biology and chemistry guided her educational journey, leading her to earn her Bachelor's and Master's degrees from the University of Melbourne, Australia, and her Ph.D. from the University of Cambridge, England, in 1975. Her postdoctoral work at Yale University further honed her research skills.

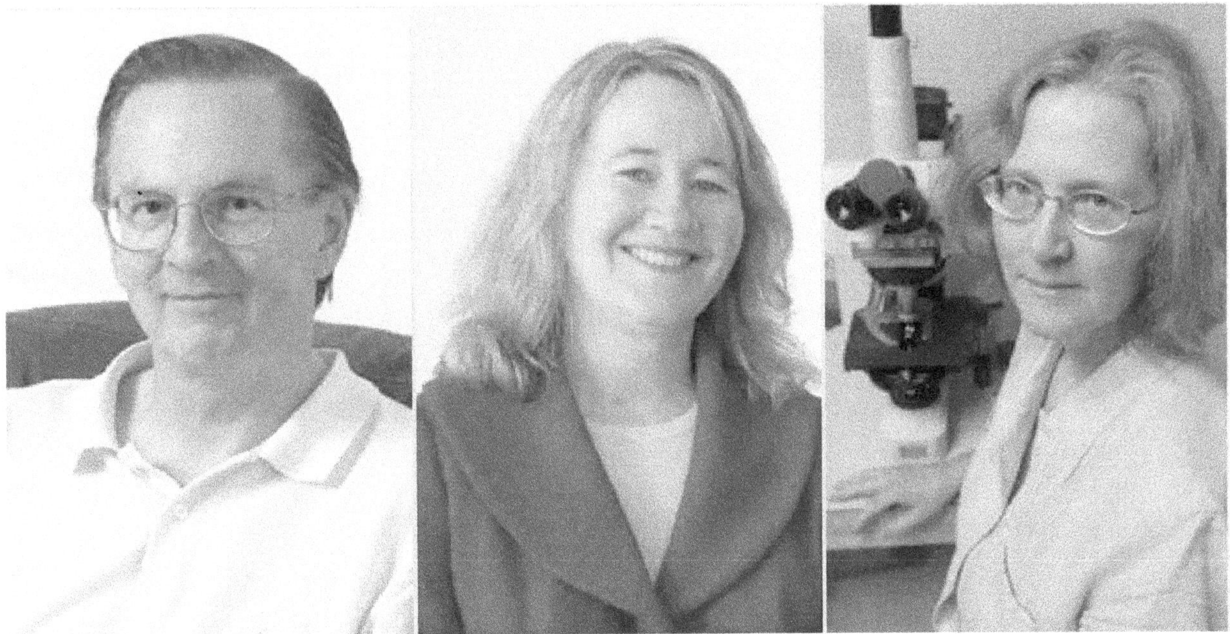

Carol W. Greider was born on April 15, 1961, in San Diego, California, USA. Inspired by the pioneering work of her mother and the scientific community around her, Greider pursued her passion for science. She received her Bachelor's degree in biology from the University of California, Santa Barbara, in

1983, and completed her Ph.D. at the University of California, Berkeley, in 1987, where she worked closely with Blackburn, making crucial advancements in the understanding of telomeres.

Jack W. Szostak was born on November 9, 1952, in London, United Kingdom, and moved to Canada during his childhood. His scientific journey began with undergraduate studies at McGill University, Montreal, where he developed an interest in molecular biology. Szostak furthered his education by obtaining a Ph.D. from Cornell University in 1977, which set the stage for his contributions to the field of genetics and chromosome biology.

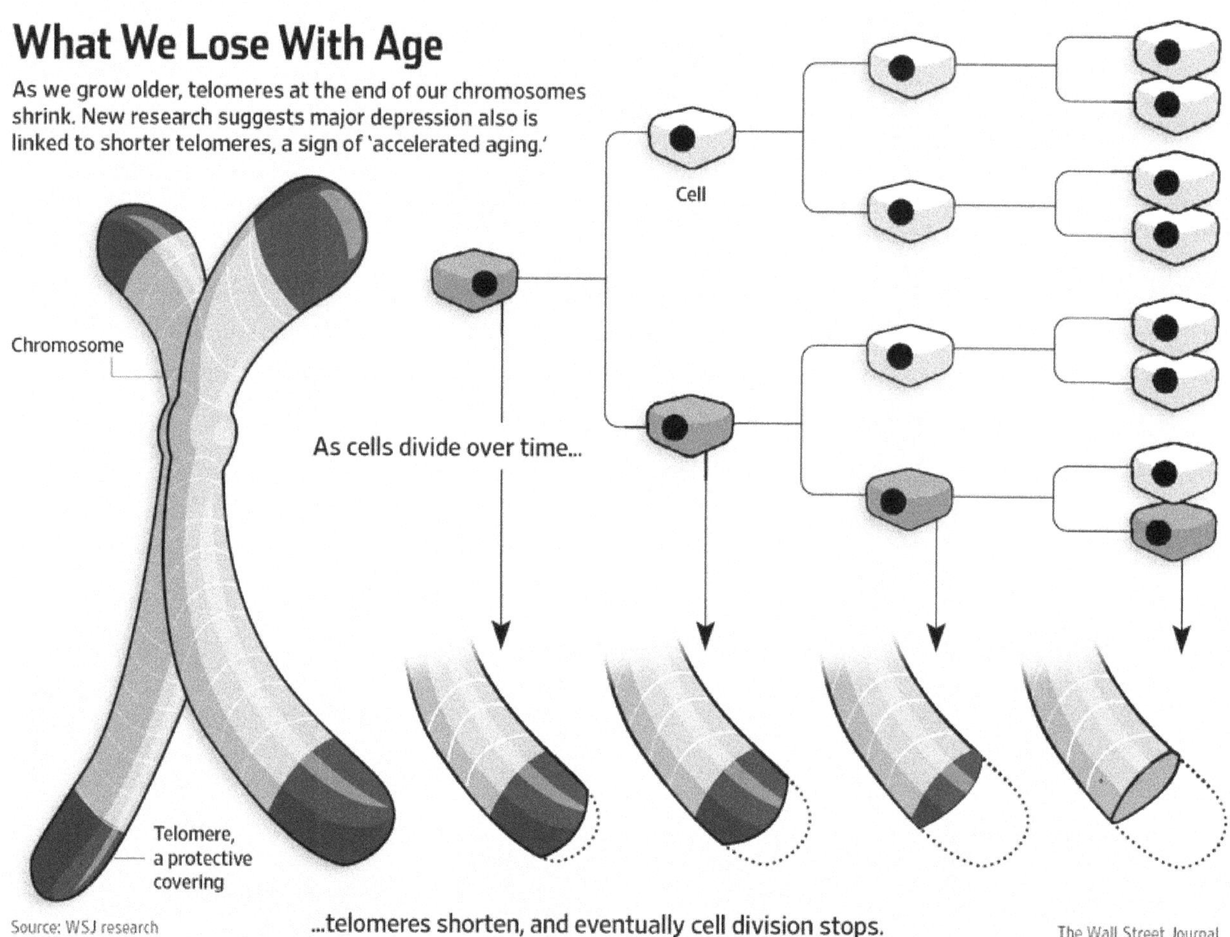

Snippets

Discovery of Telomeres and Telomerase: Their research unveiled the structure and function of telomeres, the protective caps at the ends of chromosomes, and telomerase, the enzyme responsible for maintaining telomere length.

Implications for Aging and Cancer: Their findings have crucial implications for understanding the mechanisms of aging and the development of cancer, particularly how cells can proliferate uncontrollably in cancer or become senescent as telomeres shorten with age.

Advances in Medicine: This discovery has led to new approaches in cancer treatment focusing on telomere and telomerase dynamics, as well as sparked research into anti-aging strategies and therapies.

Early Researchers

Hermann Muller, an American geneticist who, in the early 20th century, contributed to our understanding of the role of chromosomes in heredity. Although Muller's work was primarily focused on genetic mutations and their effects, his research helped build the genetic knowledge base that would later prove essential for understanding telomeres.

Another notable contributor is Barbara McClintock, whose discovery of "jumping genes" or transposable elements in corn highlighted the dynamic nature of the genome. While her work initially seemed distant from telomere research, the mechanisms of genetic regulation and chromosome protection she uncovered are closely related to the understanding of how telomeres function at the chromosomal ends.

Additionally, Leonard Hayflick's observation that human cells have a limited capacity to divide in culture, known as the "Hayflick limit," provided early evidence of cellular aging and hinted at the existence of biological mechanisms, like telomeres and telomerase, that control cell lifespan.

Current Implications

Understanding of Aging: Their discoveries have advanced our understanding of the biological mechanisms underlying aging. Telomere shortening is now recognized as a key factor in cellular aging, influencing how cells age and die.

Cancer Research and Treatment: The realization that cancer cells often reactivate telomerase to become "immortal" has prompted the development of anti-cancer strategies aimed at inhibiting telomerase. This approach holds promise for limiting the growth of tumors.

Stem Cell Research: Insights into telomere dynamics are crucial for stem cell research. Understanding how telomerase activity is regulated in stem cells could lead to methods to maintain stem cell potency, enhancing regenerative medicine's potential.

Development of Diagnostic Tools: Telomere length and telomerase activity are being explored as biomarkers for aging and disease, including cancer. This could lead to improved diagnostic tools and personalized treatment strategies.

Potential for Anti-aging Therapies: The prospect of manipulating telomerase to extend telomeres offers a tantalizing, albeit controversial, avenue for anti-aging therapies. While much research is needed, the idea of potentially delaying the aging process or treating age-related diseases by targeting telomeres and telomerase is an area of active investigation.

Impact and Products

Telomerase Inhibitors: In the field of cancer therapy, studies influenced by their work have resulted in the creation of telomerase inhibitors. These medications target and block the telomerase enzyme in cancer cells to restrict their capacity to sustain telomere length and continue reproducing endlessly.

Telomere Extension Treatments: Exploration into methods for artificially extending the length of telomeres in normal cells has been pursued as a potential anti-aging therapy. While still in the experimental phase, these treatments offer the promise of enhancing cell longevity and combating age-related diseases.

Diagnostic Tests for Telomere Length: The measurement of telomere length is being utilized as a diagnostic tool to assess biological aging and disease risk. Products that can accurately measure telomere length from blood samples are becoming available, offering insights into individual health status and predisposition to various diseases.

Personalized Medicine Approaches: Understanding the role of telomeres and telomerase in disease has opened avenues for personalized medicine. For instance, assessing telomerase activity levels in tumors can help tailor more effective, individualized treatment plans for cancer patients.

Research and Laboratory Tools: The study of telomeres and telomerase has led to the development of new laboratory tools and assays. These enable researchers to study telomere biology in greater detail, facilitating further discoveries in genetics, aging, and disease mechanisms.

The impact of Blackburn, Greider, and Szostak's research extends into pharmaceutical development, diagnostics, and the burgeoning field of regenerative medicine, illustrating the profound and lasting influence of their discoveries on science and health care.

ROBERT G. EDWARDS (2010)

The man who played the God's game and showed us babies can be grown in test tubes

Robert G. Edwards was awarded the Nobel Prize in Medicine in 2010 for his pioneering development of in vitro fertilization (IVF), a groundbreaking advancement in assisted reproductive technology.

History

Robert G. Edwards, born on September 27, 1925, in Batley, Yorkshire, embarked on a path that would revolutionize reproductive medicine. After serving in the British Army, Edwards pursued his passion for science, earning his undergraduate degree from Bangor University. His academic journey led him to the University of Edinburgh, where he was awarded a PhD in 1955 for his work under the supervision of R.A. Beatty and C.H. Waddington at the Institute of Animal Genetics and Embryology.

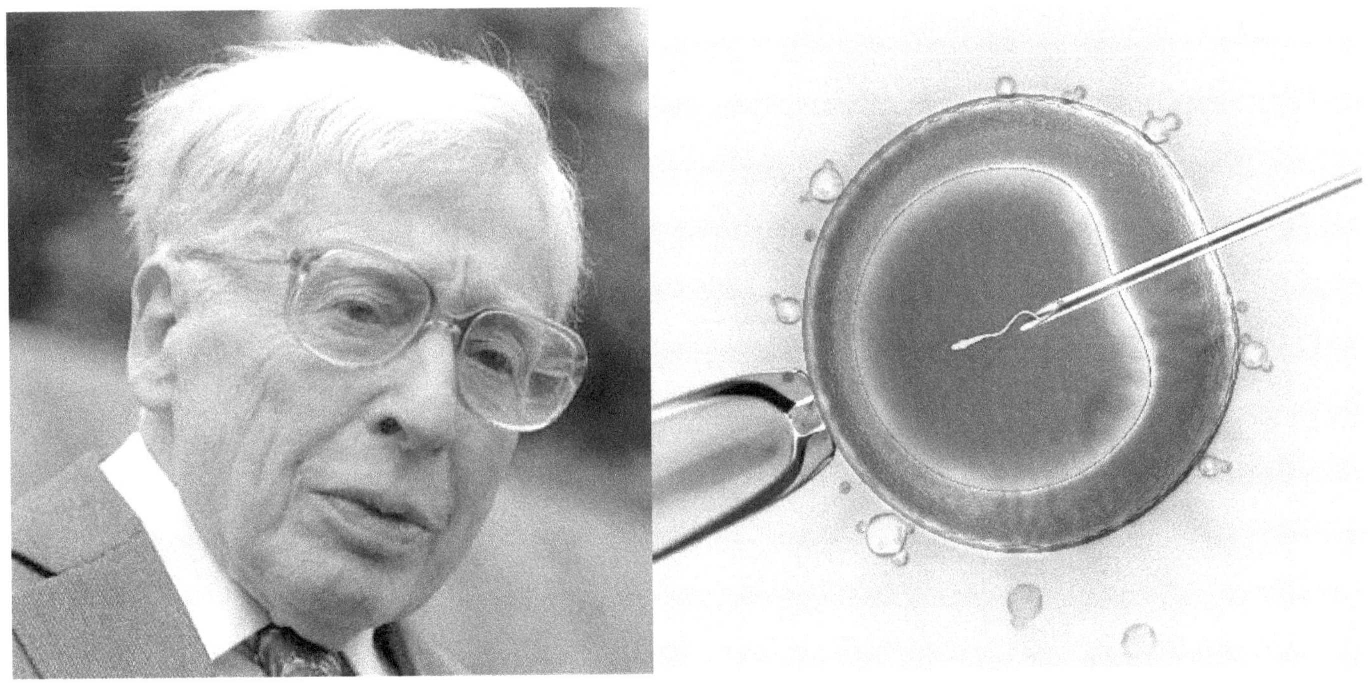

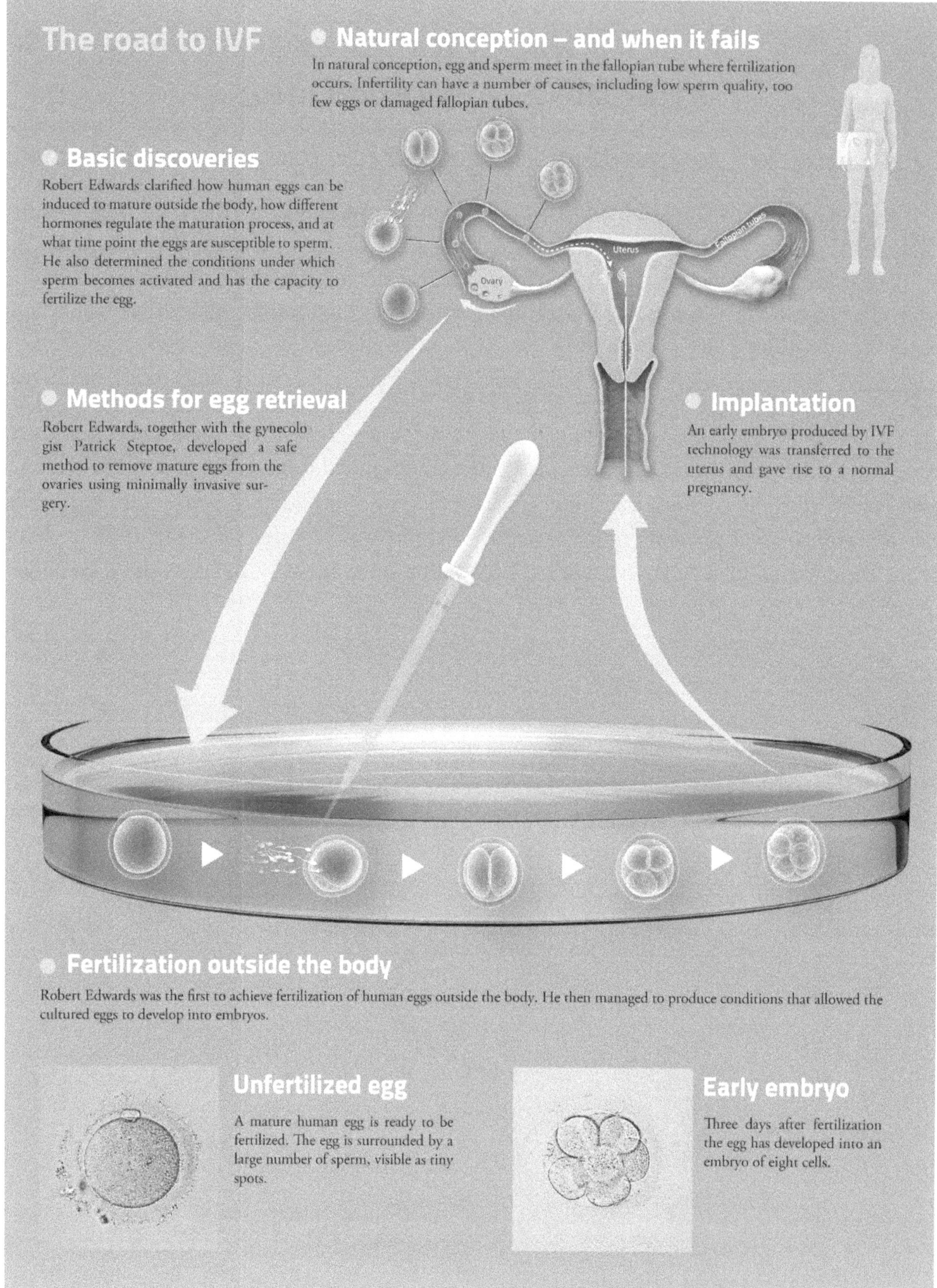

Courtesy Mattias Karlen at Nobel Committee 2012

His career, marked by a relentless pursuit of understanding human fertilization, took him across the globe, including a postdoctoral fellowship at the California Institute of Technology. Edwards's significant contributions began to take shape after he joined the University of Cambridge in 1963, where he shifted his focus towards the practical applications of his embryology research.

In the late 1960s, Edwards, along with gynaecological surgeon Patrick Steptoe, began to explore the possibilities of in vitro fertilization (IVF). This collaboration faced considerable skepticism and opposition from the broader medical and scientific communities, yet it was marked by pioneering spirit and innovation. By 1968, Edwards achieved fertilization of a human egg in the laboratory, setting the stage for a revolution in assisted reproductive technology.

The birth of Louise Brown on July 25, 1978, as the world's first baby conceived via IVF, marked the culmination of Edwards and Steptoe's efforts. This event not only made medical history but also sparked a global conversation on the ethical, social, and legal aspects of assisted reproduction.

Snippets

Pioneering IVF Research: Starting in the late 1960s, Edwards, alongside Patrick Steptoe, worked on fertilizing human eggs outside the body, leading to the birth of Louise Brown in 1978, the world's first "test-tube baby".

Establishment of Bourn Hall Clinic: Edwards and Steptoe founded the Bourn Hall Clinic, the world's first IVF clinic, to continue their work and train new specialists in reproductive medicine.

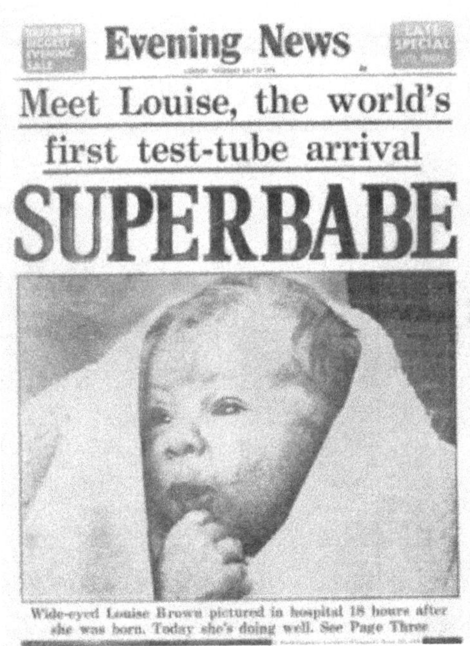

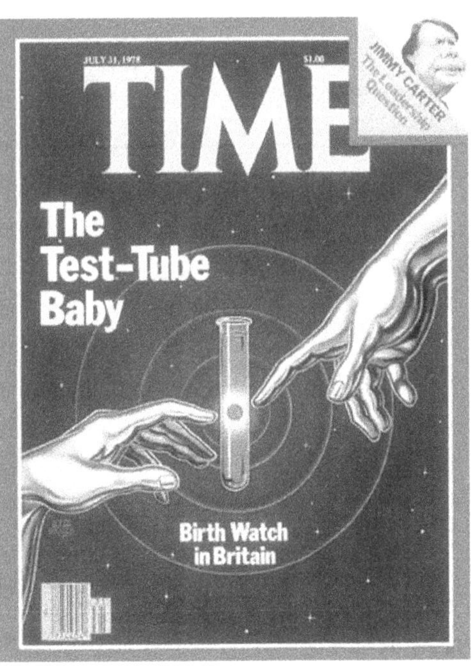

Impact on Reproductive Medicine: IVF has become a widespread therapy worldwide, with millions of babies born using this technology. The method has seen significant improvements over the years, enhancing treatment success rates.

Recognition and Controversy: Edwards's work received global recognition and numerous awards, though it also sparked ethical, social, and legal debates about assisted reproductive technologies.

Early Researchers

Walter Heape, a British physiologist who, in the late 19th and early 20th centuries, conducted the first successful embryo transplantation in rabbits, demonstrating the possibility of manipulating embryos outside the maternal body. This experiment laid the groundwork for the future of reproductive technologies, including IVF.

Another significant contributor was Gregory Pincus, an American biologist whose research in the mid-20th century focused on mammalian eggs and hormone-induced ovulation. Pincus's work on in vitro fertilization of rabbit ova provided essential insights into the mechanisms of fertilization and early embryo development.

Min Chueh Chang, working in the United States during the mid-20th century, made pivotal discoveries in sperm capacitation and fertilization, further advancing the understanding of the reproductive process necessary for the development of IVF.

These scientists, among others, contributed to the body of knowledge that enabled Edwards and his colleagues to achieve the first successful IVF pregnancy. Their work, though not as widely recognized, was instrumental in overcoming the scientific and technical challenges that had previously made assisted reproduction seem like an impossible dream.

Current Implications

Widespread Treatment for Infertility: IVF has become a cornerstone treatment for various forms of infertility, enabling millions of individuals and couples worldwide to conceive children they otherwise might not have been able to have. The technology has evolved to improve success rates and reduce risks, making it more accessible to a broader population.

Advancements in Genetic Screening: The use of IVF has facilitated the growth of preimplantation genetic diagnosis (PGD) and screening (PGS), allowing for the genetic testing of embryos. This has significant implications for preventing hereditary diseases and understanding genetic disorders, offering families the chance to reduce the risk of passing on genetic conditions.

Ethical, Social, and Legal Debates: IVF and related technologies have sparked ongoing ethical discussions concerning the implications of assisted reproductive technologies, including concerns about "designer babies," the rights of donors and surrogates, and the regulation of fertility clinics. These discussions have led to varied regulations and guidelines across different countries.

Research and Development: The techniques developed through IVF research have also propelled advancements in related fields, including stem cell research and regenerative medicine. The ability to manipulate and study embryos in the lab has opened new avenues for understanding human development and disease.

Impact on Family Dynamics: IVF has expanded the concept of family for many, offering options for single parents, same-sex couples, and older parents to conceive. This shift has contributed to ongoing conversations about the nature of parenthood and family in the 21st century.

Impact and Products

Expansion of Assisted Reproductive Technologies (ART): Following the success of IVF, there has been a proliferation of related reproductive technologies, including Intracytoplasmic Sperm Injection (ICSI) for severe male infertility, egg and embryo freezing for fertility preservation, and surrogacy options for those who cannot carry a pregnancy.

Development of Fertility Drugs: The IVF process is closely tied to the use of fertility drugs that stimulate the ovaries to produce multiple eggs. The development and refinement of these drugs have been directly influenced by the needs of IVF procedures, leading to more effective and safer treatments for patients undergoing fertility treatments.

Cryopreservation Techniques: The need to preserve embryos and gametes for future IVF cycles has driven advancements in cryopreservation techniques. This includes the vitrification process, which has significantly improved the survival rate of thawed embryos and eggs, enhancing the overall success rate of ART cycles.

Genetic Testing Services: IVF has facilitated the growth of genetic testing services, such as Preimplantation Genetic Testing (PGT), allowing for the detection of genetic abnormalities before embryo transfer. This has not only improved the success rates of IVF by selecting the healthiest embryos but also reduced the risk of genetic diseases being passed on to the next generation.

Fertility Tracking and Management Apps: The desire to conceive has spurred the development of numerous fertility tracking apps and devices that help individuals and couples track ovulation and fertility windows, optimizing the chances of natural conception or timing for IVF treatments.

Specialized IVF Equipment: The IVF field has seen the introduction of specialized laboratory equipment designed to mimic the conditions of the human body as closely as possible, such as advanced incubators that maintain the ideal environment for embryo development and microscopes for intricate procedures like ICSI.

The introduction of IVF by Edwards has not only provided hope to millions of individuals and couples facing infertility but also sparked continuous innovation in reproductive technologies and treatments. These advancements reflect the dynamic nature of the field and its ongoing commitment to improving outcomes for patients seeking to build their families.

BRUCE A. BEUTLER, JULES A. HOFFMANN, AND RALPH M. STEINMAN (2011)

Invention of dendritic cells and the Immune surveillance system

In 2011, Bruce A. Beutler, Jules A. Hoffmann, and Ralph M. Steinman were collectively awarded the Nobel Prize in Medicine for their significant contributions to our understanding of the immune system. Their discoveries have been pivotal in revealing how the body's innate and adaptive immunity responses are activated.

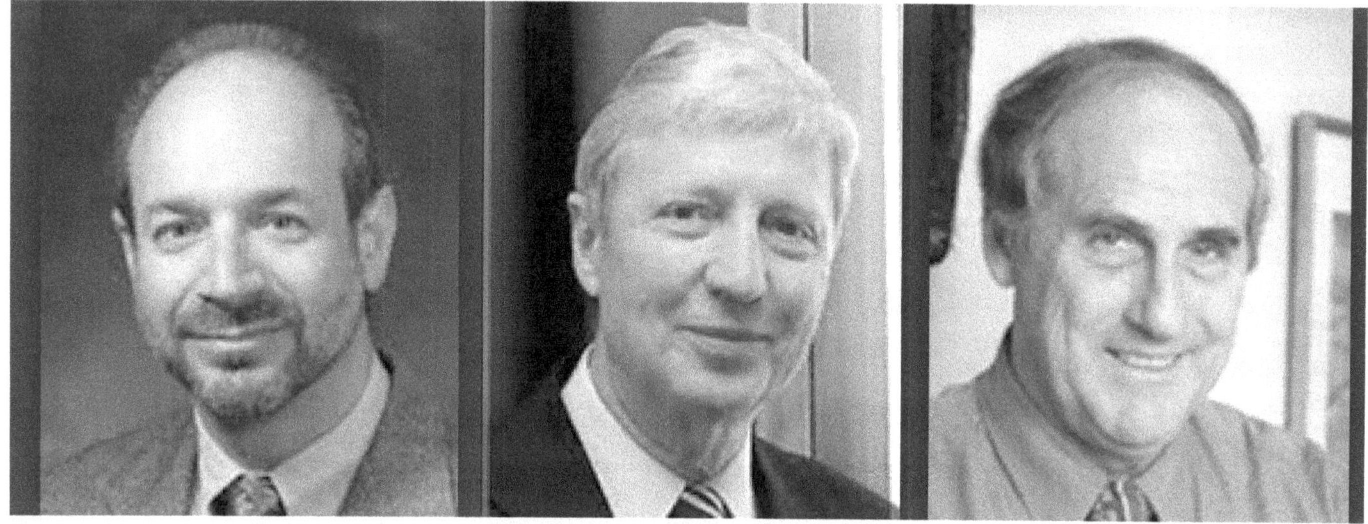

History

Bruce A. Beutler, born on December 29, 1957, in Chicago, Illinois, USA, played a key role in identifying receptor proteins that can recognize bacteria and other pathogens, thus activating the innate immune system. Jules Hoffmann, born on August 2, 1941, in Echternach, Luxembourg, contributed to this field by discovering the Toll gene in fruit flies, a critical component of the innate immune response. Ralph M. Steinman, born on January 14, 1943, in Montreal, Canada, and passed away just days before the announcement of the Nobel Prize, was honored for his discovery of dendritic cells, which bridge innate and adaptive immunity by presenting antigens to T cells.

Snippets

The work of Beutler and Hoffmann unveiled mechanisms of the innate immune system, the body's first line of defense against infection, by showing how specific receptor proteins recognize and combat pathogens. Steinman's discovery of dendritic cells has been crucial for understanding how the immune system is alerted to the presence of pathogens and how it remembers and responds more efficiently to future encounters with the same pathogens.

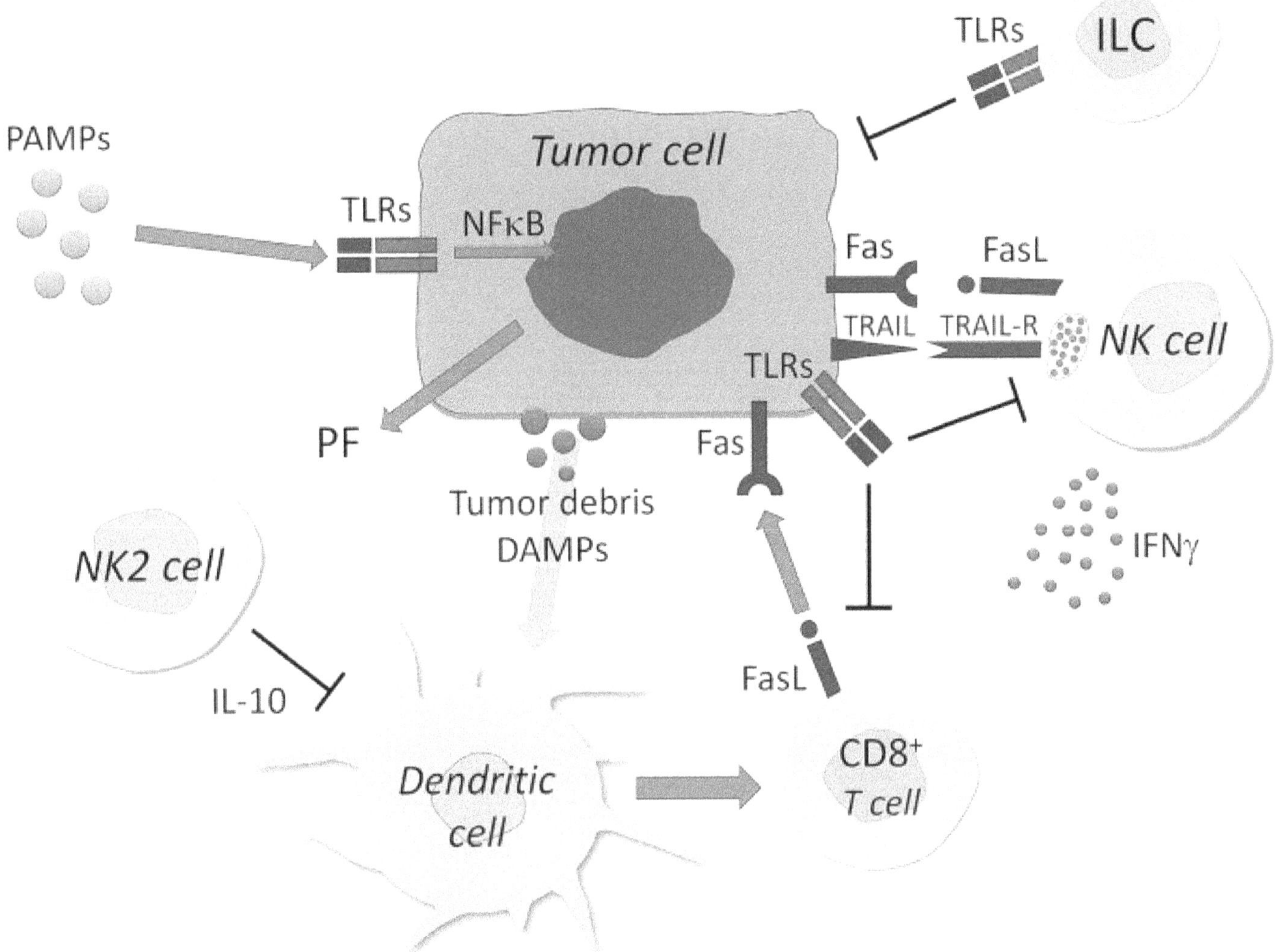

PF — proinflammatory factors
ILC — innate lymphoid cell

Current Implications

These discoveries have profoundly impacted medical research and treatment strategies, especially in developing vaccines and understanding autoimmune diseases, allergies, and cancer. By elucidating the pathways that activate the immune system, their work has opened new avenues for therapeutic interventions targeting immune responses.

Impact and Products

The collective contributions of Beutler, Hoffmann, and Steinman have advanced the field of immunology, providing insights into the complex mechanisms of the immune system and paving the way for innovative treatments for a wide range of diseases. Their groundbreaking research continues to inspire ongoing studies aimed at unlocking the full potential of immunotherapy and vaccine development, offering hope for new ways to fight infectious diseases and cancer.

SIR JOHN B. GURDON AND SHINYA YAMANAKA (2012)

Technique to create pluripotent stem cells and resetting the clock of life

In 2012, Sir John B. Gurdon and Shinya Yamanaka were awarded the Nobel Prize in Medicine for their groundbreaking discovery that mature cells can be reprogrammed to become pluripotent, fundamentally changing our understanding of cell development and potential.

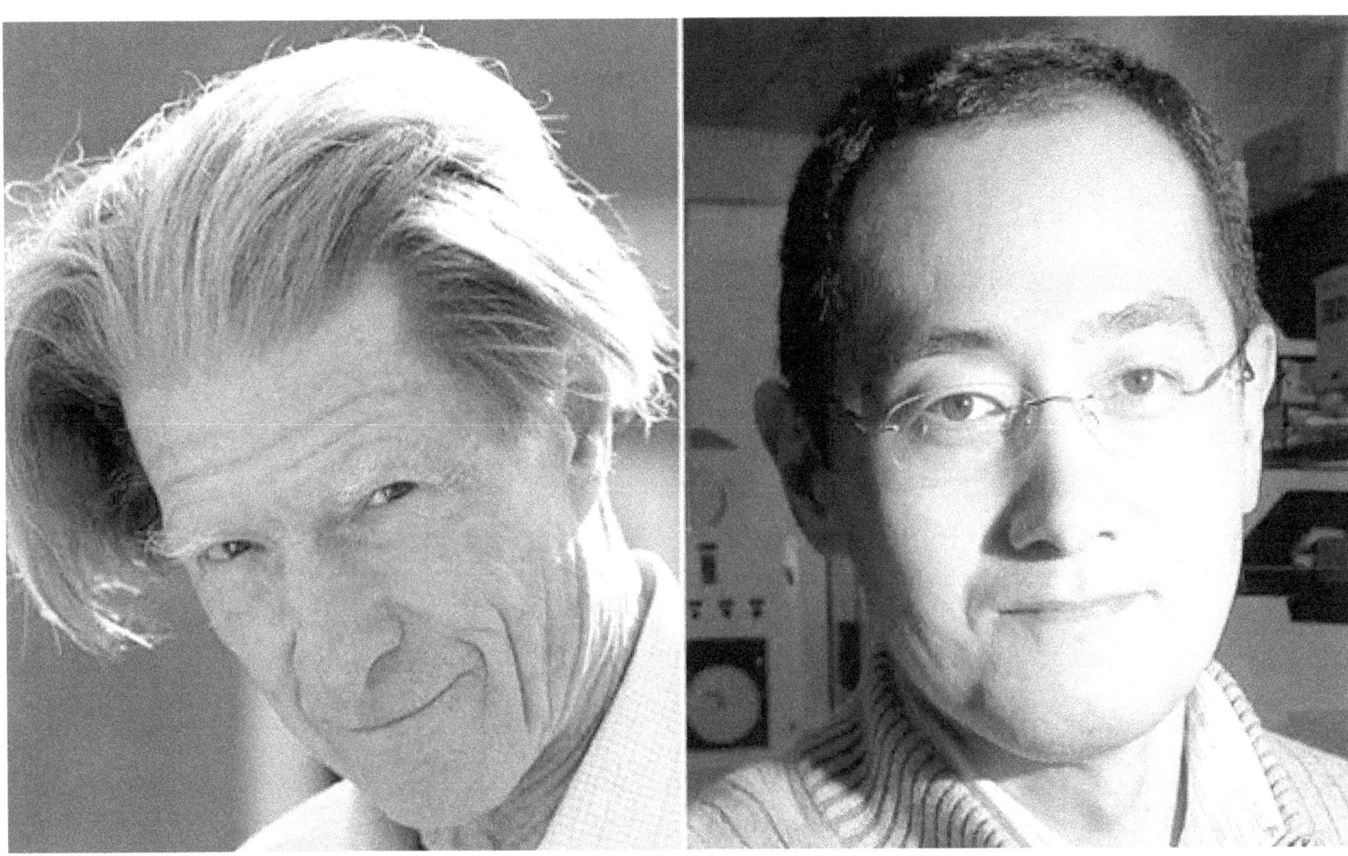

History

Sir John B. Gurdon, born on October 2, 1933, in Dippenhall, United Kingdom, pioneered research that challenged the irreversible nature of cell specialization. Despite early academic challenges, Gurdon's passion for science led him to significant discoveries in cellular biology, specifically in nuclear transplantation and cloning. Shinya Yamanaka, born on September 4, 1962, in Osaka, Japan, extended Gurdon's findings by identifying factors that could reprogram adult cells to a pluripotent state, effectively turning back the cellular clock.

Snippets

Gurdon's landmark experiment in 1962 involved transplanting the nucleus from a mature cell into an egg cell devoid of its nucleus, leading to the development of a fully formed frog. This experiment demonstrated that the cell's nucleus retained all the information needed to develop into any cell type. Yamanaka, building on this concept, identified a set of four genes that, when introduced into adult skin cells, could reprogram these cells to an embryonic-like state, termed induced pluripotent stem cells (iPSCs).

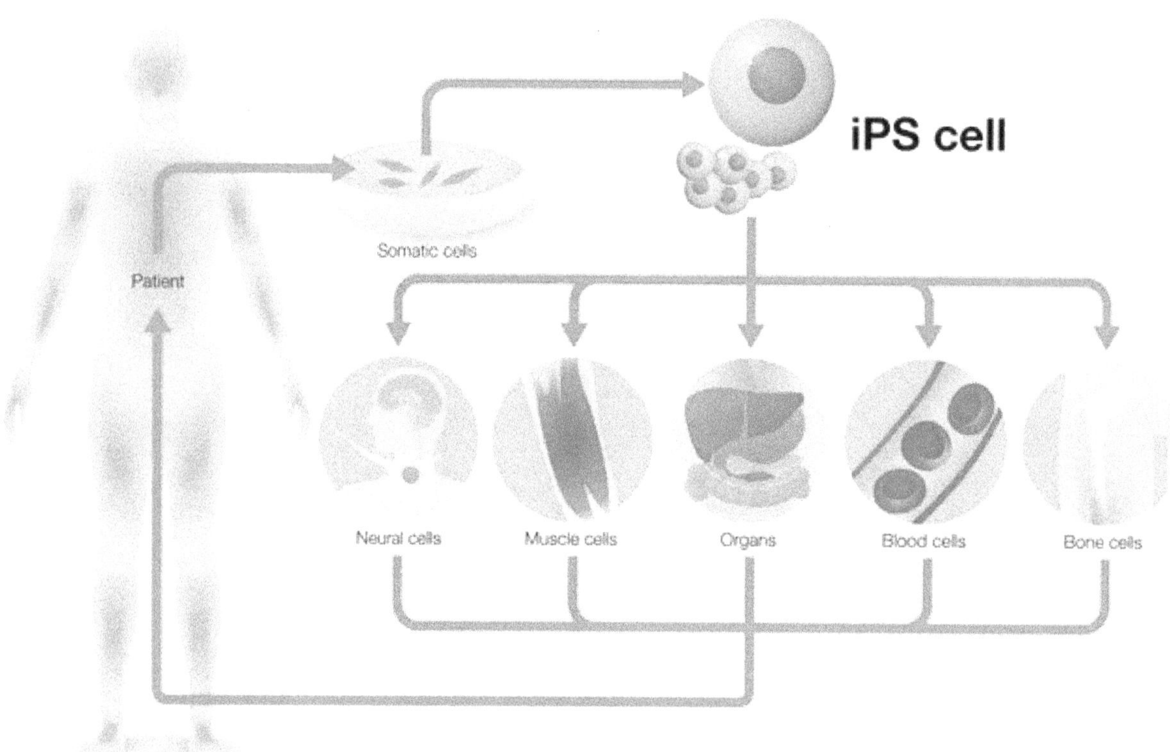

Current Implications

The discoveries by Gurdon and Yamanaka have revolutionized biomedical research, opening new avenues for regenerative medicine, drug discovery, and our understanding of diseases. iPSC technology has the potential to generate patient-specific cell types for therapy, model diseases in a dish, and test pharmacological treatments, reducing the reliance on animal models and offering new insights into disease mechanisms.

Impact and Products

The work of Gurdon and Yamanaka has not only provided profound insights into cellular biology and the potential for cell-based therapies but also underscored the plasticity of the cellular state. Their research has laid the groundwork for future innovations in treating degenerative diseases, personalized medicine, and tissue regeneration, highlighting the transformative power of understanding and manipulating cellular fate.

JAMES E. ROTHMAN, RANDY W. SCHEKMAN, AND THOMAS C. SÜDHOF (2013)

Cellular science at its best, scientists who found the Intra – cytoplasmic traffic regulators

In 2013, James E. Rothman, Randy W. Schekman, and Thomas C. Südhof were awarded the Nobel Prize in Medicine for their discoveries concerning the regulation of vesicle traffic, a critical transport system in our cells. Their research provides insight into how cells transport molecules.

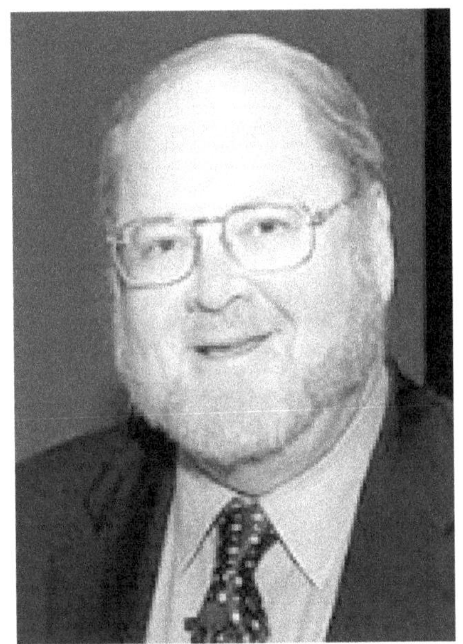

James E. Rothman

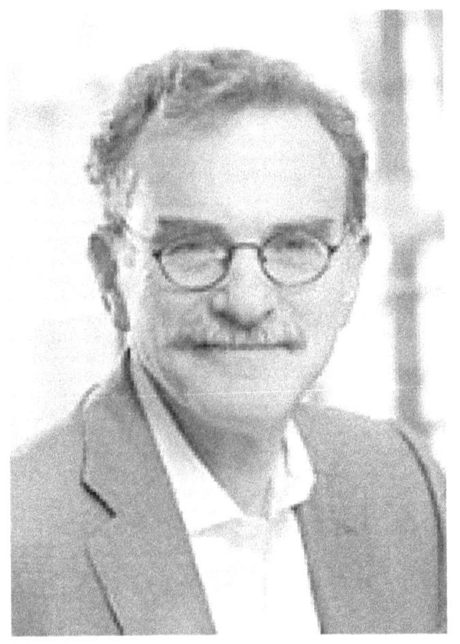

Randy W. Schekman

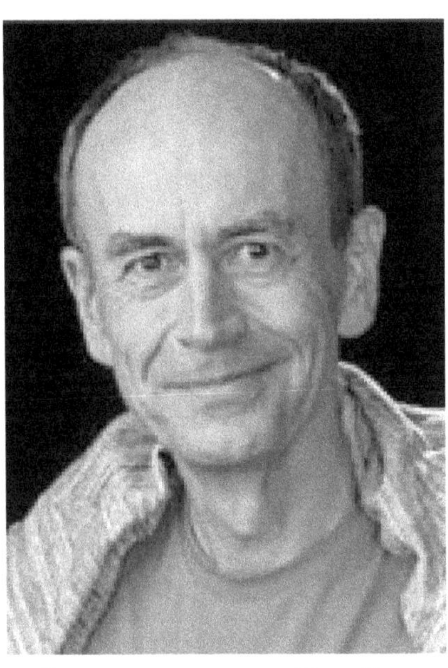

Thomas C. Südhof

History

James E. Rothman was born on November 3, 1950, in Haverhill, Massachusetts, USA. He conducted significant research at several prestigious institutions, including Yale University, where he was affiliated at the time of the award. Randy W. Schekman, born on December 30, 1948, in Saint Paul, Minnesota, USA, carried out his Nobel-recognized work at the University of California, Berkeley. Thomas C. Südhof, born on December 22, 1955, in Göttingen, Germany, contributed to this field while at Stanford University.

Snippets

Rothman's work revealed the process by which vesicles fuse with their target compartments within the cell, ensuring that molecules are delivered to the right location. Schekman discovered a set of genes that are required for vesicle traffic in yeast, providing insights into the components necessary for vesicular transport. Südhof's research focused on how vesicles release neurotransmitters in the brain, a crucial step in the communication between neurons.

Current Implications

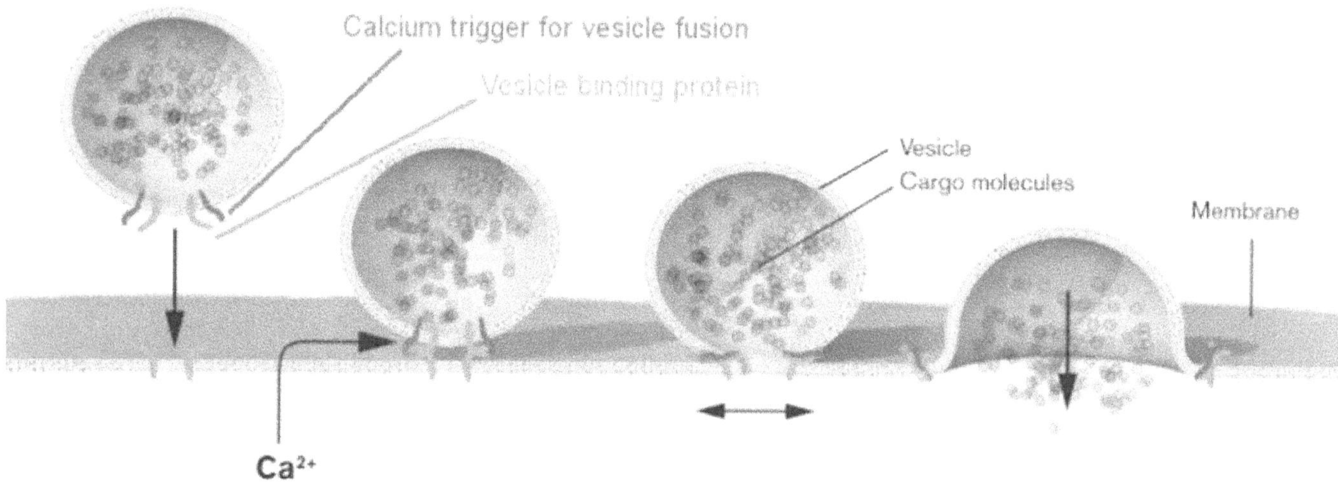

Their combined discoveries have significantly advanced our understanding of cellular organization and the mechanics behind molecular transport within and between cells. This knowledge is vital for comprehending various diseases, including neurological and metabolic disorders, where vesicle traffic is affected.

Impact and Products

The work of Rothman, Schekman, and Südhof has laid the foundation for exploring new treatments for diseases related to vesicle transport and secretion. Their achievements have opened new research avenues in cell biology and medicine, highlighting the importance of basic scientific research in uncovering the mechanisms of life at the cellular level.

JOHN O'KEEFE, MAY-BRITT MOSER, AND EDVARD I. MOSER (2014)

This trio's dramatic discovery of cortical grid cells that is the core of human Geo-positioning and balance system

In 2014, John O'Keefe, May-Britt Moser, and Edvard I. Moser were awarded the Nobel Prize in Medicine for their discoveries of cells that constitute a positioning system in the brain, often referred to as the brain's "inner GPS." Their pioneering work has significantly enhanced our understanding of spatial memory and navigation.

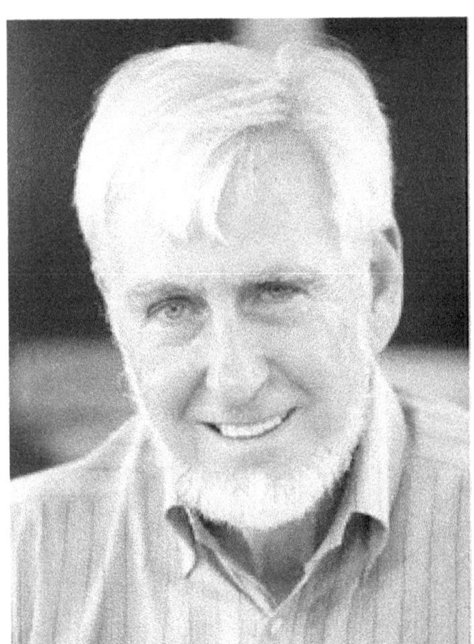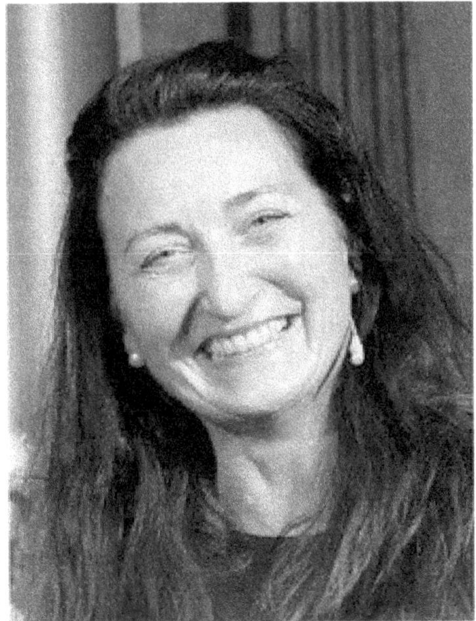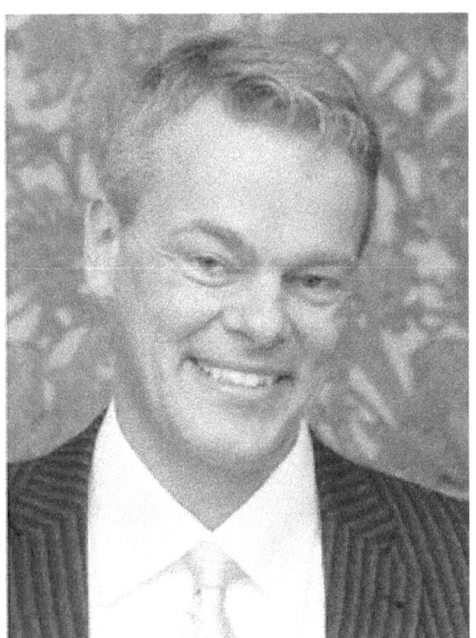

History

John O'Keefe, born on November 18, 1939, in New York, NY, USA, conducted foundational research at University College London, where he discovered "place cells" in the hippocampus that become activated when an animal is in a specific location. May-Britt Moser and Edvard I. Moser, both from Norway, discovered "grid cells" in the entorhinal cortex that create a coordinate system for precise positioning and pathfinding. These discoveries are pivotal for understanding how the brain processes spatial information and guides navigation.

Snippets

The work of O'Keefe in the 1970s opened the field by identifying cells in the hippocampus that were activated in specific spatial locations. Building on this, the Mosers, in 2005, identified a different type of cell that generates a hexagonal grid of spatial coordinates. These cells work together to form the brain's navigation system, allowing organisms to understand their location and navigate their environment.

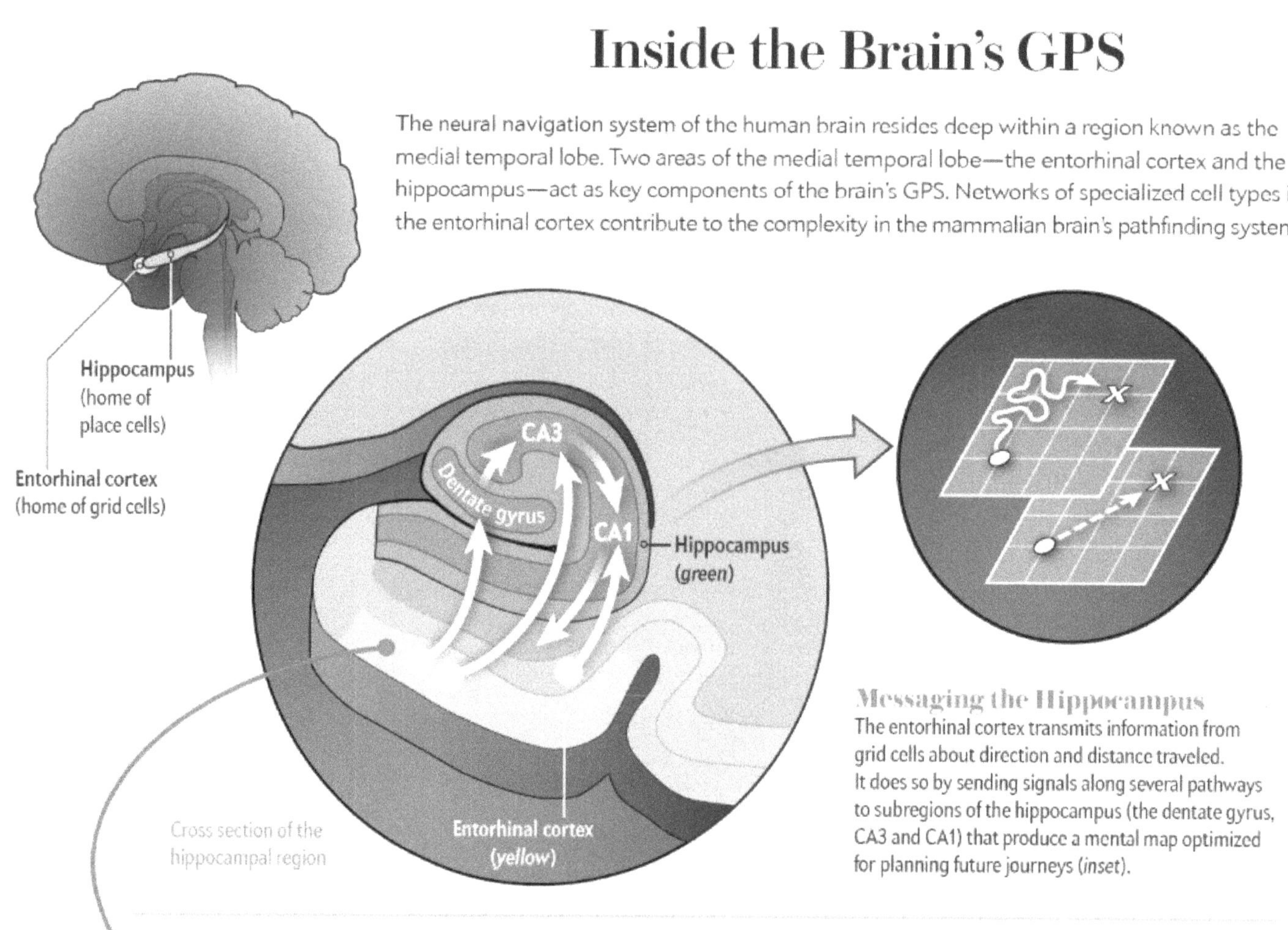

Image Credit: Jen Christiansen

Current Implications

The implications of their research are vast, influencing neuroscience, psychology, and even technology development for navigation tools. Understanding the neural basis of spatial memory and navigation aids in the study of Alzheimer's disease and other neurological conditions where navigation and memory are impaired.

Impact and Products

The collective contributions of O'Keefe and the Mosers have significantly advanced our understanding of cognitive processes and laid the groundwork for future research in brain function and memory. Their discoveries have potential applications in developing treatments for diseases involving memory loss and spatial disorientation.

WILLIAM C. CAMPBELL, SATOSHI ŌMURA, AND YOUYOU TU (2015)

Discovery of Ivermectin and Artemisinin, in our fight against filariasis and malaria

The 2015 Nobel Prize in Medicine was awarded to William C. Campbell, Satoshi Ōmura, and Youyou Tu for their groundbreaking discoveries in the treatment of parasitic diseases, fundamentally changing the approach to combating these global health challenges.

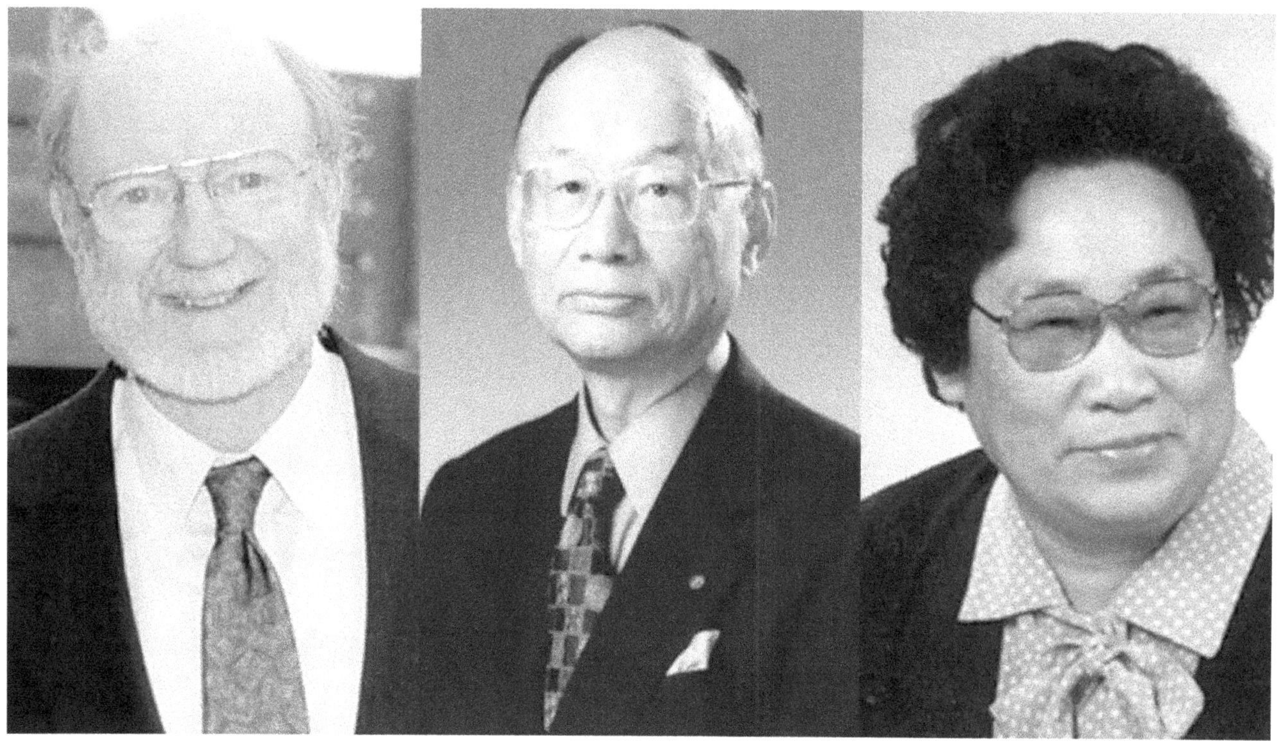

NEW NOBELS William C. Campbell (left), Satoshi Ōmura (center) and Youyou Tu (right) received the Nobel Prize in medicine or physiology for identifying drugs that fight parasites.

History

William C. Campbell was born in 1930 in Ramelton, Ireland. His career, notably in the United States, focused on parasitology and led to the discovery of Ivermectin, which was further developed into Ivermectin, a drug instrumental in treating river blindness and lymphatic filariasis.

Satoshi Ōmura, born in 1935 in the Yamanashi Prefecture of Japan, is a microbiologist and biochemist. His work on isolating natural products led to the discovery of Ivermectin. Ōmura's contributions to extracting and identifying unique compounds from soil bacteria were crucial in developing new pharmaceuticals.

Youyou Tu was born in 1930 in Ningbo, Zhejiang, China. She is renowned for her discovery of artemisinin, a drug that has dramatically reduced mortality rates from malaria. Tu's work was significantly inspired by ancient Chinese herbal texts, leading her to identify and extract the active component from Artemisia annua (sweet wormwood).

Snippets

Discovery of Ivermectin: Campbell and Ōmura's work led to the discovery of Ivermectin, revolutionizing treatment for river blindness and lymphatic filariasis, diseases affecting millions globally.

Artemisinin Against Malaria: Youyou Tu's research into traditional Chinese medicine culminated in the discovery of Artemisinin, significantly reducing mortality rates from malaria and transforming global health policies.

Global Impact: Their collective discoveries have provided effective treatments for debilitating parasitic diseases, saving countless lives and contributing to the ongoing fight against global health threats.

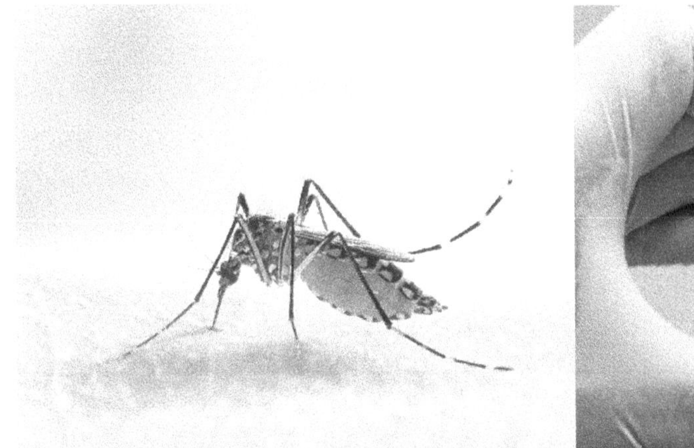
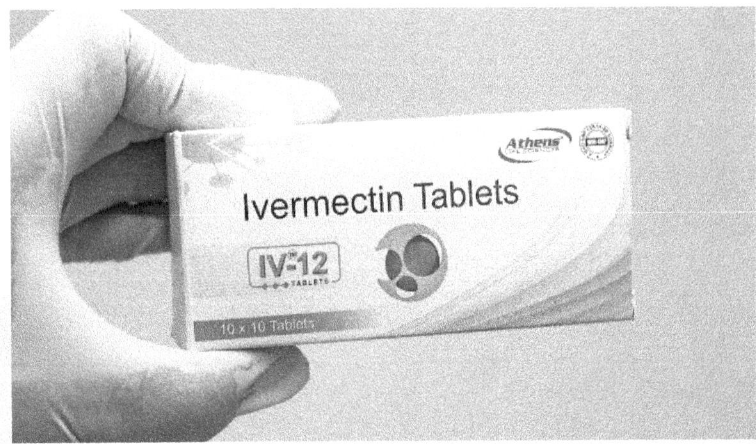

Early Researchers

Researchers in the early 20th century began laying the groundwork for understanding parasitic life cycles and their interaction with human hosts, contributing to the foundational knowledge necessary for later breakthroughs in therapy development. Scientists such as Paul Müller, who discovered the insecticidal properties of DDT, played a significant role in combating malaria-carrying mosquitoes, indirectly influencing future strategies for disease control.

In the world of traditional medicine, the efforts of early practitioners and herbalists, who documented and tested the medicinal qualities of plants, have been priceless. Their shared wisdom, handed down through generations, offered vital understandings for Youyou Tu's Artemisinin research.

Furthermore, the early pioneers in the field of antibiotic discovery, such as Alexander Fleming, Selman Waksman, and Gerhard Domagk, set the stage for the exploration of natural products as sources of new medicines. Their successes inspired subsequent generations of scientists, including Ōmura, to search for novel compounds in nature that could be harnessed to fight infections.

Current Implications

Revolutionizing Treatment for Parasitic Diseases: The discovery of Ivermectin from the research of Campbell and Ōmura has been instrumental in controlling river blindness and lymphatic filariasis, significantly reducing their prevalence. This has had a monumental impact on public health in affected regions, improving the quality of life for millions.

Malaria Therapy Advancements: Youyou Tu's discovery of Artemisinin has transformed the treatment of malaria, a disease that continues to claim hundreds of thousands of lives annually. Artemisinin-based combination therapies (ACTs) are now the standard treatment for malaria, contributing to a substantial decrease in malaria mortality rates globally.

Influencing Global Health Policies: The success of these therapies has influenced global health policies, with organizations like the World Health Organization (WHO) adopting guidelines that incorporate these treatments. This has led to coordinated international efforts to distribute these life-saving drugs to the communities most in need.

Stimulating Further Research: Their achievements have encouraged further research into parasitic diseases, leading to better understanding, prevention, and treatment strategies. The work has also underscored the importance of exploring natural products and traditional medicine as potential sources for new drugs.

Ethical, Social, and Economic Considerations: The widespread use of these treatments has raised important questions regarding drug resistance, access to medication, and the ethical considerations of drug development and distribution. These discussions continue to shape the landscape of global health initiatives and pharmaceutical research.

Impact and Products

Ivermectin Production and Distribution: Following the discovery of its efficacy against parasitic diseases, Ivermectin has been produced and distributed on a global scale, becoming a cornerstone in the treatment of river blindness and lymphatic filariasis. Pharmaceutical companies have developed formulations of Ivermectin that are now used worldwide, significantly reducing the incidence of these diseases in endemic regions.

Artemisinin-Based Therapeutics: The extraction and synthesis of Artemisinin inspired the pharmaceutical industry to produce a range of Artemisinin-based combination therapies (ACTs), which are now the standard treatment for malaria recommended by health authorities worldwide. These drugs have been pivotal in reducing the mortality rates of malaria, particularly in Sub-Saharan Africa and Southeast Asia.

Research Tools for Drug Discovery: The research methodologies developed by Ōmura and Campbell in isolating and identifying Ivermectin have influenced the pharmaceutical industry's approach to drug discovery, particularly in the screening of natural products for medicinal properties. Similarly, Tu's approach to extracting Artemisinin from sweet wormwood has underscored the value of traditional knowledge in guiding modern pharmaceutical research.

Global Health Initiatives: The success of these treatments has led to the formation of global health initiatives focused on distributing these life-saving medications. Programs funded by international organizations, governments, and NGOs have been essential in providing these drugs to populations at risk, highlighting the importance of international cooperation in global health.

Advancements in Parasitology and Pharmacology: Beyond their immediate therapeutic applications, the discoveries have spurred advancements in the fields of parasitology and pharmacology, leading to a deeper understanding of the mechanisms of parasitic diseases and the development of new therapeutic targets.

The impact of their work is reflected not only in the lives saved and improved through these treatments but also in the ongoing innovation in medical research and public health initiatives aimed at eradicating parasitic diseases.

YOSHINORI OHSUMI (2016)

Autophagy, the purposeful self-digestion of misbehaving cells, which is different from apoptosis

Yoshinori Ohsumi was awarded the 2016 Nobel Prize in Medicine for his discoveries of mechanisms for autophagy. His pioneering work elucidated how cells recycle their content, a fundamental process in cellular maintenance and health.

History

Yoshinori Ohsumi, born on February 9, 1945, in Fukuoka, Japan, has carved a significant path in cell biology, particularly through his groundbreaking work on autophagy. His academic journey began with his education at the University of Tokyo, where he obtained both his bachelor's degree in 1967 and his Ph.D. in 1974. Following his doctoral studies, Ohsumi expanded his research horizons internationally as a postdoctoral fellow at Rockefeller University in New York City.

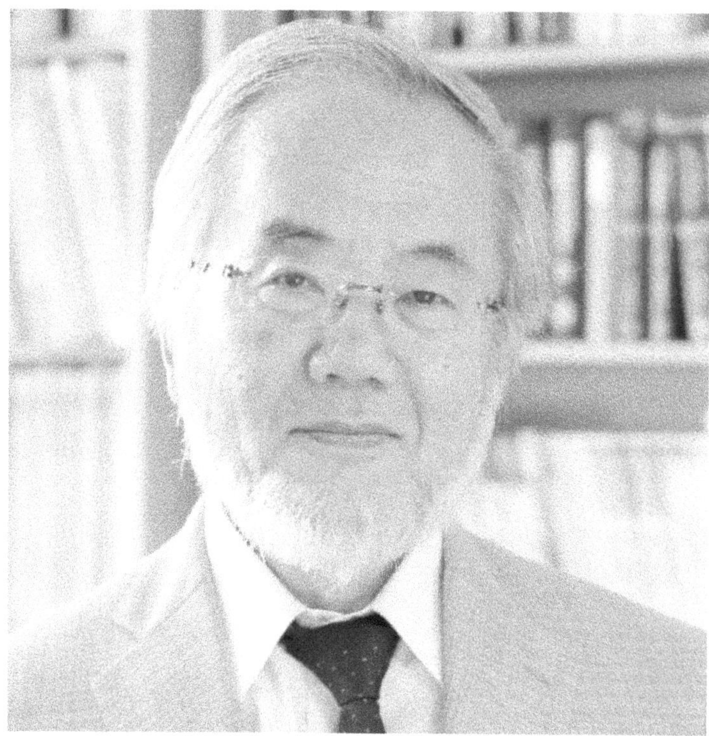

Upon returning to Japan in 1977, Ohsumi joined the University of Tokyo as a research associate. His dedication and pioneering research in the field of cellular biology propelled him through the

"""

ranks, leading to a position as a professor at the National Institute for Basic Biology in Okazaki City by 1996. Ohsumi's academic journey did not stop there. He also held a professorship at the Graduate University for Advanced Studies in Hayama from 2004 to 2009. Even after his official retirement in 2014, Ohsumi continued to contribute to the scientific community as a Professor at the Institute of Innovative Research at the Tokyo Institute of Technology, where he leads the Cell Biology Research Unit.

Ohsumi's foray into the world of autophagy began in earnest in 1988, focusing on yeast vacuole physiology. His fascination with cellular degradation processes, known as autophagy, or "self-eating," had been described and studied extensively in animal cells. Ohsumi's innovative research in the 1990s, particularly through mutational screening of yeast cells, identified essential genes enabling cells to undergo autophagy, laying the groundwork for understanding this critical biological process.

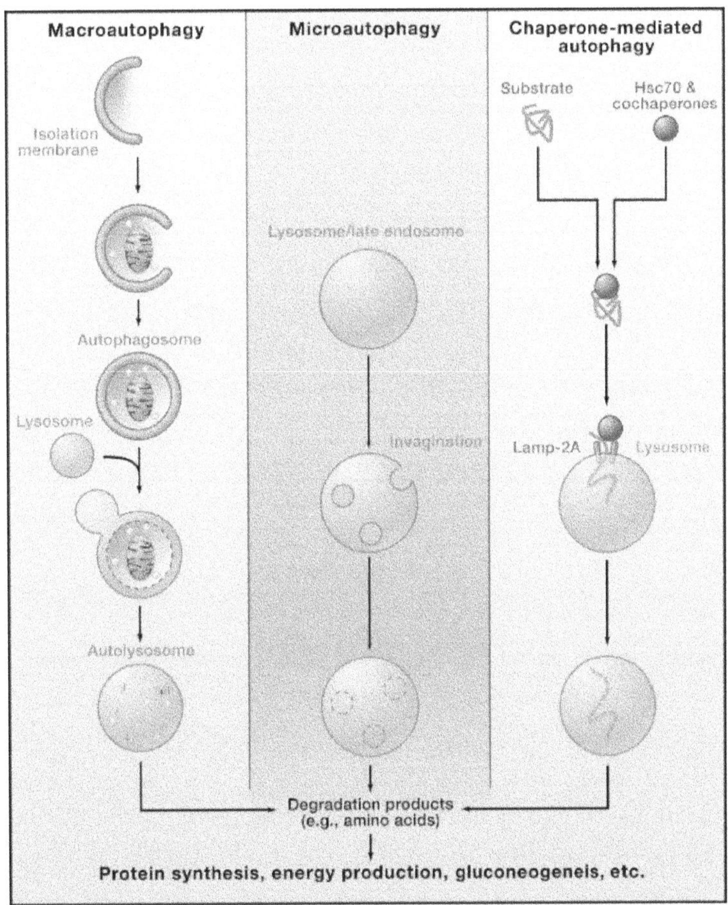

The principle of autophagy

Snippets

Yoshinori Ohsumi's Autophagy Discovery: Ohsumi's pivotal discovery in the late 1980s and 1990s unraveled the genetic underpinnings of autophagy in yeast, revealing the cellular process where cells break down and recycle their own components.

Foundational Work: Beginning his autophagy research at the University of Tokyo, Ohsumi identified the genes essential for autophagy through mutational screening, laying the groundwork for understanding this crucial biological mechanism.

Global Impact on Medicine and Biology: Ohsumi's discoveries have profound implications for understanding diseases linked to autophagy dysfunction, including cancer and neurodegenerative disorders, opening new avenues for therapeutic interventions.

Continued Legacy: Even after retirement, Ohsumi remains active in research as head of the Cell Biology Research Unit at the Tokyo Institute of Technology, continuing to contribute to the field of cell biology and autophagy research.

Early Researchers

Christian de Duve, who coined the term "autophagy" in 1963, is among the notable figures whose work laid the groundwork for understanding the cell's internal recycling process. De Duve's identification of lysosomes and peroxisomes illuminated the intricate pathways of cellular degradation and recycling, providing a conceptual framework that would later support Ohsumi's autophagy research. George Palade, another luminary, contributed profoundly to our knowledge of cell organelles and their functions, earning him a Nobel Prize for his work on the endoplasmic reticulum and the discovery of ribosomes. These cellular structures are now known to play crucial roles in the autophagic process, illustrating the interconnectedness of cellular components and functions.

Albert Claude, alongside de Duve and Palade, is credited with pioneering the use of electron microscopy for biological studies, which has become an essential tool in autophagy research. Their combined efforts in elucidating cell structure and function have been pivotal in the development of cell biology as a discipline.

Current Implications

Medical Research and Disease Treatment: Ohsumi's work has opened up new pathways in the study of diseases where autophagy plays a crucial role. Conditions such as cancer, neurodegenerative disorders like Alzheimer's and Parkinson's disease, and infectious diseases are now studied with a lens that considers autophagy's role in disease progression and potential treatment strategies.

Drug Development: The understanding of autophagy mechanisms is guiding the development of new therapeutic drugs aimed at manipulating the autophagy pathway. By targeting the autophagy process, researchers hope to develop treatments that can either enhance or inhibit autophagy to treat diseases.

Aging and Longevity: Autophagy is also linked to aging and lifespan extension. Research suggests that enhancing autophagy can help clear damaged cells, potentially slowing down the aging process and increasing lifespan, which has implications for studies in gerontology and developing anti-aging interventions.

Nutritional Science: The process of autophagy is influenced by nutrition and fasting. This connection has spurred research into how dietary interventions can modulate autophagy, leading to potential dietary guidelines and interventions for health maintenance and disease prevention.

Genetic Studies: Ohsumi's identification of the genes involved in autophagy has fueled genetic research aimed at understanding how variations in these genes affect human health and susceptibility to diseases. This area of research holds promise for personalized medicine, where treatments might be tailored based on an individual's genetic makeup regarding autophagy-related genes.

Cellular Stress Response: Autophagy plays a critical role in the cellular response to stress, including oxidative stress, starvation, and infection. Understanding how cells use autophagy to survive under adverse conditions is vital for developing strategies to protect cells in various diseases and conditions.

Impact and Products

Impact on Scientific Research and Healthcare

- **Enhanced Understanding of Disease Mechanisms:** Ohsumi's discoveries have deepened our understanding of the cellular mechanisms underlying numerous diseases, including cancer, neurodegenerative diseases, and infections. This enhanced understanding is crucial for developing targeted therapies.
- **Foundational Research in Autophagy:** The identification and characterization of autophagy-related genes have become a cornerstone of cellular biology, influencing countless research projects and studies aimed at unraveling the complexities of cellular processes.
- **Basis for Novel Therapeutic Targets:** The autophagy pathway, thanks to Ohsumi's work, is now recognized as a potential therapeutic target for various conditions. Modulating autophagy holds promise for treating diseases where either too much or too little autophagy is part of the pathology.

Development of Products and Therapies

- **Autophagy-Modulating Pharmaceuticals:** The insights gained from Ohsumi's research have spurred the development of drugs designed to modulate autophagy. These include potential treatments for conditions where autophagy's role is critical, offering a new avenue for therapeutic intervention.
- **Diagnostic Tools:** Understanding autophagy has led to the development of new diagnostic markers and tools for diseases associated with autophagy dysfunction. Detecting alterations in autophagy-related pathways can aid in the early diagnosis of certain conditions, improving patient outcomes.
- **Nutritional Interventions:** The link between autophagy and nutrition has inspired the creation of dietary supplements and regimens aimed at enhancing autophagy for health benefits. These

interventions are based on the premise that activating autophagy through certain dietary practices can contribute to better health and potentially extend lifespan.

The ongoing exploration of autophagy-related pathways and mechanisms continues to uncover new potentials for improving human health and understanding the fundamental processes of life.

JEFFREY C. HALL, MICHAEL ROSBASH, AND MICHAEL W. YOUNG (2017)

The phenomenal discovery of period genes and Internal body clock

Jeffrey C. Hall, Michael Rosbash, and Michael W. Young were awarded the 2017 Nobel Prize in Medicine for their discoveries of molecular mechanisms controlling the circadian rhythm, the internal biological clock that regulates the daily physiological cycles of living organisms.

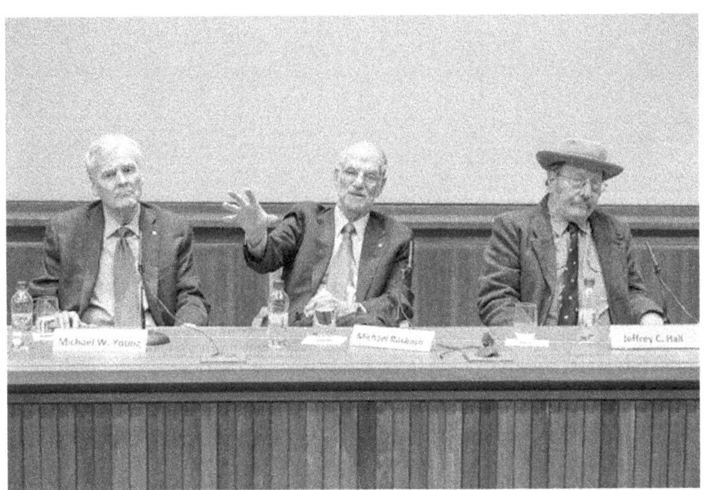

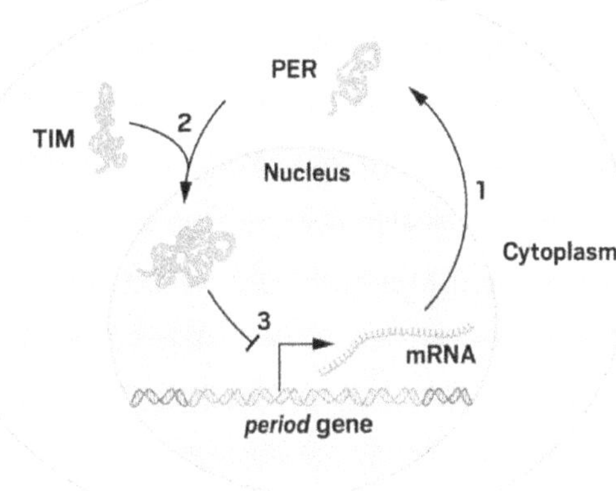

History

Jeffrey C. Hall was born on May 3, 1945, in New York, USA. He embarked on his journey into genetics and chronobiology after obtaining his Ph.D. in Genetics from the University of Washington. Hall's career includes significant periods at Brandeis University and the University of Maine, where his research focused on the neurological mechanisms of the fruit fly, Drosophila melanogaster, a model organism that played a crucial role in their circadian rhythm studies.

Michael Rosbash, born in 1944 in Kansas City, Missouri, USA, pursued his education in biophysics, earning a Ph.D. from the Massachusetts Institute of Technology. Rosbash joined Brandeis University, where his collaboration with Hall began. Their work concentrated on isolating the period gene in Drosophila, which was critical in understanding the molecular makeup of the circadian clock.

Michael W. Young, born on March 28, 1949, in Miami, USA, completed his doctoral studies at the University of Texas at Austin, focusing on genetics. Young's research at Rockefeller University furthered the understanding of the circadian rhythm through the discovery of additional genes in

Drosophila that regulate the clock, including timeless and doubletime, elucidating the cycle of the circadian rhythm.

Snippets

Discovery of the Period Gene: Hall, Rosbash, and Young's foundational work in isolating the period gene in Drosophila melanogaster marked a turning point in understanding the genetic basis of circadian rhythms, demonstrating how mutations in this gene disrupted the fruit fly's biological clock.

Elucidation of the Molecular Mechanism: Their research revealed that the period gene's protein product accumulates during the night and is degraded during the day, elucidating the molecular mechanism that underpins the circadian rhythm and explaining how this cycle is maintained in organisms.

Identification of Additional Clock Genes: Furthering their groundbreaking work, Michael W. Young discovered additional genes, such as timeless and doubletime, that play critical roles in regulating the circadian clock, offering a more comprehensive view of the circadian rhythm's genetic control.

Impact on Health and Medicine: Their discoveries have profound implications for understanding human health, shedding light on how disruptions in circadian rhythms can influence sleep patterns, behavior, metabolic disorders, and susceptibility to various diseases.

Early Researchers

Colin Pittendrigh, often referred to as the father of chronobiology, who in the mid-20th century, laid the groundwork for understanding biological rhythms. His work on the fruit fly Drosophila melanogaster and other organisms helped establish the principles of circadian rhythms and their adaptiveness in natural environments. Pittendrigh's concept of the "circadian oscillator" was instrumental in framing subsequent research in the field, including the work of Hall, Rosbash, and Young.

Another significant figure is Jürgen Aschoff, a German biologist who, alongside Pittendrigh, contributed to the foundational theories of circadian rhythms, including the Aschoff's Rule, which describes how circadian rhythms change under continuous light conditions. Aschoff's extensive research on human circadian rhythms in the absence of external cues provided critical insights into the endogenous nature of the biological clock.

Franz Halberg is credited with coining the term "circadian" and is known for his extensive research on biological rhythms, particularly in human physiology. His work emphasized the ubiquity and importance of circadian rhythms in health and disease, laying the groundwork for understanding the temporal structure of biological systems.

Erwin Bünning, a German biologist, made significant contributions to the field of plant physiology and chronobiology. His experiments in the early 20th century on the circadian rhythms of plants highlighted the endogenous nature of these rhythms, suggesting that similar mechanisms might exist in animals and humans.

Current Implications

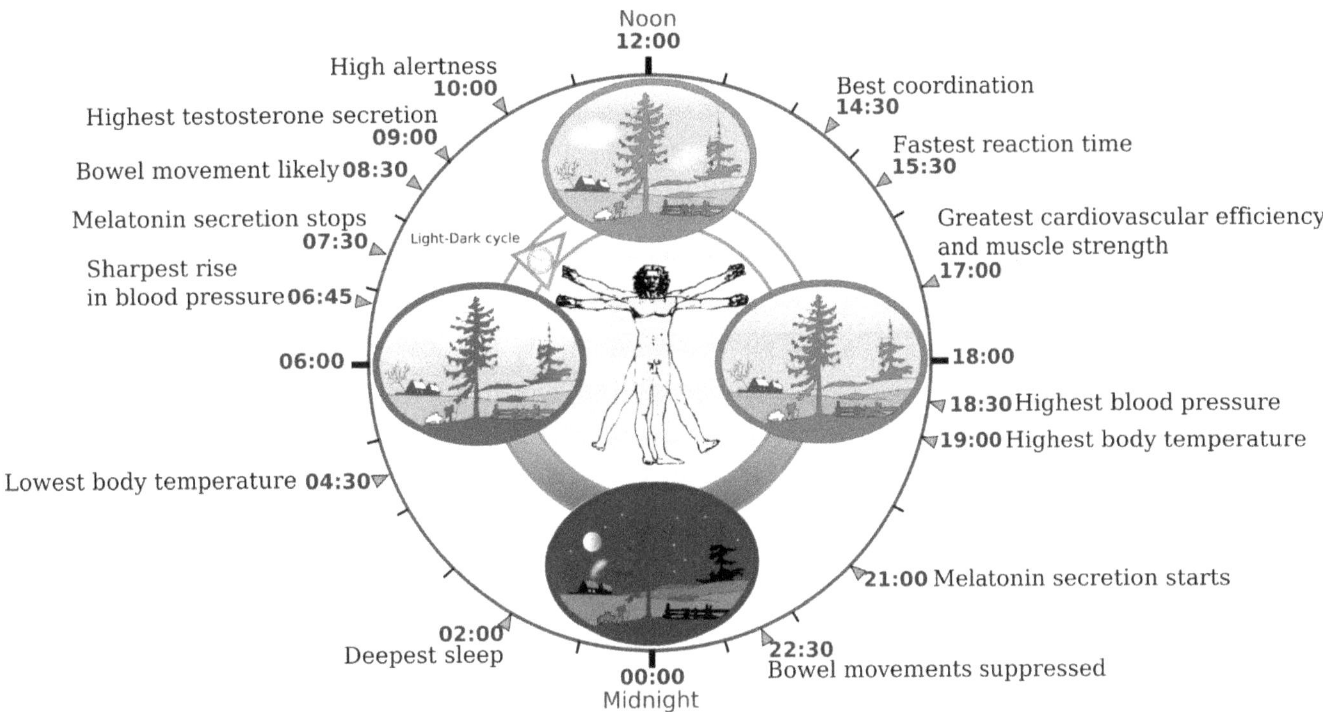

Sleep Disorders: The identification of genes controlling the circadian rhythm has directly impacted the understanding and treatment of sleep disorders. Insights into the genetic basis of sleep regulation are guiding the development of new therapeutic approaches for conditions like insomnia, delayed sleep phase disorder, and others.

Mental Health: There is a growing recognition of the link between circadian rhythm disruptions and mental health issues, including depression, bipolar disorder, and anxiety. Understanding the molecular mechanisms of circadian rhythms is aiding in the exploration of novel treatment strategies that align with the body's natural biological clock.

Chronopharmacology: The field of chronopharmacology, which studies the effects of drug timing on therapeutic outcomes, has been significantly influenced by circadian biology. Timing medication in harmony with the body's circadian rhythms can enhance drug efficacy and minimize side effects, offering a personalized approach to treatment.

Cancer Treatment: Circadian rhythm research is influencing cancer treatment protocols. Certain chemotherapies may be more effective when administered at specific times of the day, potentially reducing toxicity and improving outcomes based on the timing of cell cycle and DNA repair processes.

Metabolic Disorders: The links between circadian rhythms, metabolism, and obesity are subjects of intense study. Disruptions in circadian rhythms have been associated with increased risk for metabolic syndromes, diabetes, and obesity, highlighting the importance of synchronizing eating patterns and activity levels with the body's internal clock.

Jet Lag and Shift Work: Understanding the molecular basis of circadian rhythms offers potential solutions for mitigating the effects of jet lag and the health risks associated with shift work. Strategies to quickly re-synchronize the body's internal clock can improve the quality of life for frequent travelers and shift workers.

Impact and Products

Advancements in Sleep Medicine

- Personalized Medicine for Sleep Disorders: Insights into the circadian rhythm have enabled more personalized approaches to diagnosing and treating sleep disorders, such as insomnia and sleep phase disorder, improving treatment efficacy and patient outcomes.
- Chronotherapy: The application of timing in treatment administration, known as chronotherapy, has been enhanced by understanding circadian rhythms. This approach optimizes the effectiveness of various medications by aligning them with the body's biological clock.

Development of Health and Wellness Products

- Wearable Technology: Wearables and apps that monitor sleep patterns and provide recommendations to improve sleep quality have been developed, leveraging the science behind circadian rhythms. These technologies help users align their activities with their natural sleep-wake cycles.
- Light Therapy Devices: Based on the understanding that light exposure influences circadian rhythms, light therapy devices have been designed to treat seasonal affective disorder (SAD) and adjust the body's clock, particularly useful for shift workers and those experiencing jet lag.

Implications for Workplace and Education

- Workplace Design: Knowledge of circadian rhythms has influenced workplace design, encouraging the incorporation of natural light and the adjustment of work schedules to match employees' biological clocks, thereby enhancing productivity and well-being.
- School Start Times: Research on adolescent circadian rhythms has advocated for later school start times to align with teenagers' natural sleep patterns, supporting better academic performance and mental health.

Therapeutic Interventions for Diseases

- Cancer Treatment: The circadian rhythm's role in cell cycle regulation has informed the timing of chemotherapy treatments, aiming to maximize efficacy while minimizing side effects.
- Metabolic and Cardiovascular Health: Understanding the circadian regulation of metabolism has led to novel strategies in managing metabolic syndrome and cardiovascular diseases, emphasizing the timing of food intake and physical activity.

Their work inspires innovations in healthcare, technology, and lifestyle products, showcasing the potential of chronobiological principles to enhance human health and wellbeing.

JAMES P. ALLISON AND TASUKU HONJO (2018)

Truly a breaking news : Releasing the inappropriate breaks and unlocking the Immune system

In 2018, James P. Allison and Tasuku Honjo were jointly awarded the Nobel Prize in Medicine for their revolutionary discovery of cancer therapy by inhibition of negative immune regulation. This pivotal research has established a new pillar in cancer treatment, known as immunotherapy, which leverages the body's immune system to combat cancer cells more effectively.

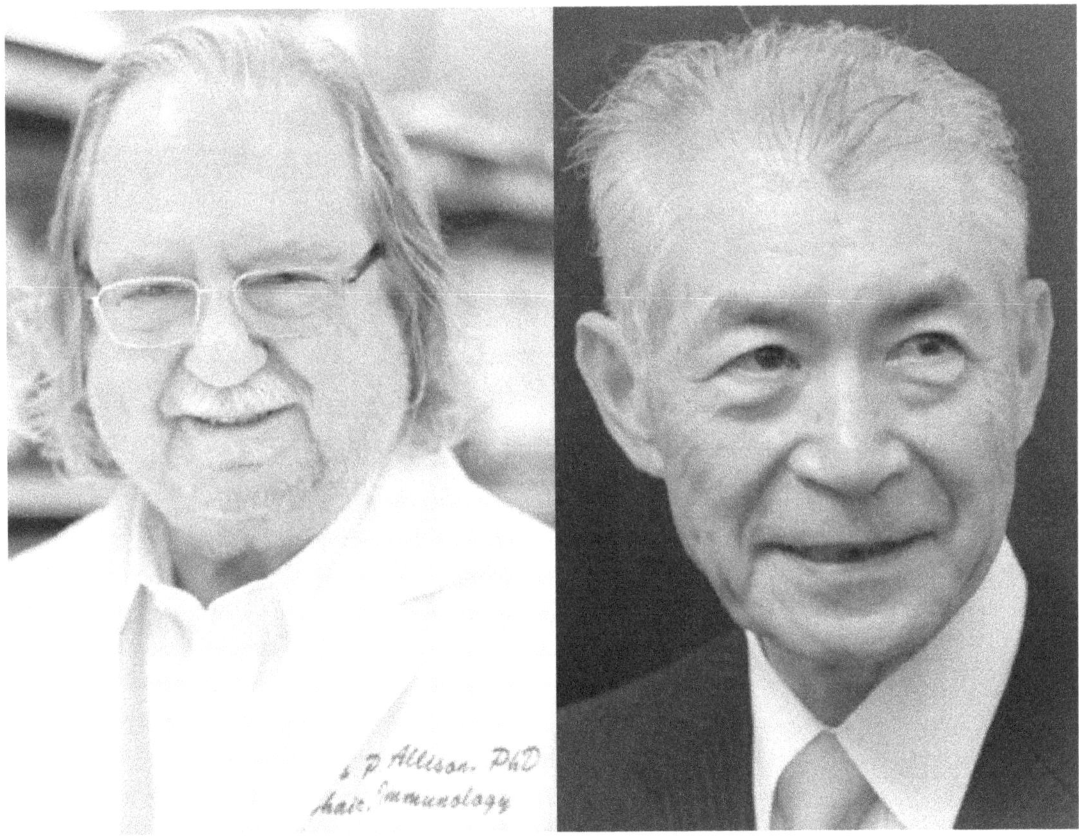

History

James P. Allison, born on August 7, 1948, in Alice, Texas, USA, has had a distinguished career in immunology, contributing significantly to the understanding of the immune system's role in cancer. His educational journey culminated in a Ph.D. from the University of Texas in Austin in 1973, after which he held positions at several prestigious institutions, including the University of Texas MD Anderson Cancer Center and the Parker Institute for Cancer Immunotherapy.

Tasuku Honjo, born on January 27, 1942, in Kyoto, Japan, has been a professor at Kyoto University since 1984. His education in medicine and subsequent Ph.D. from Kyoto University laid the groundwork for his extensive research in immunology, particularly his discovery of the protein PD-1, which acts as a brake on the immune system.

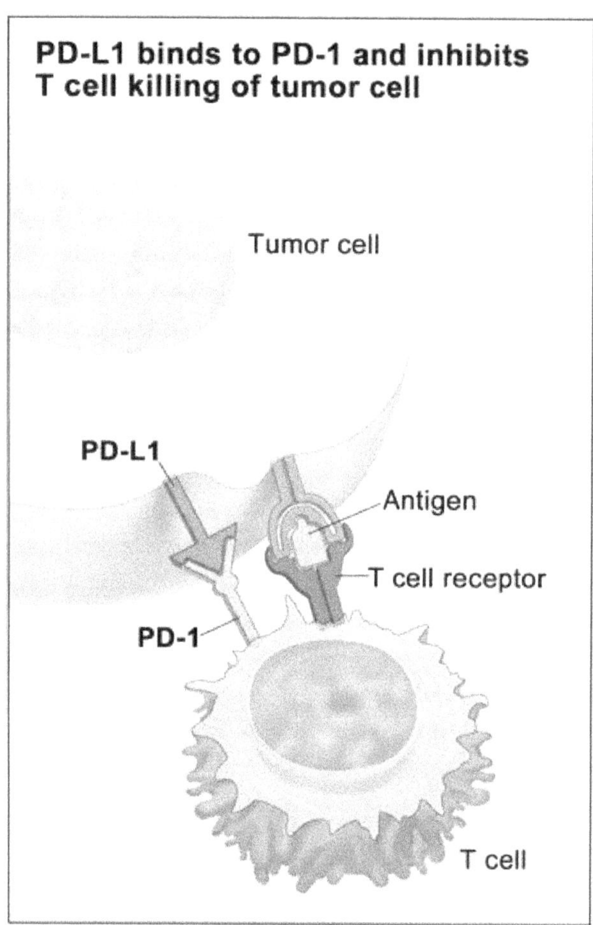

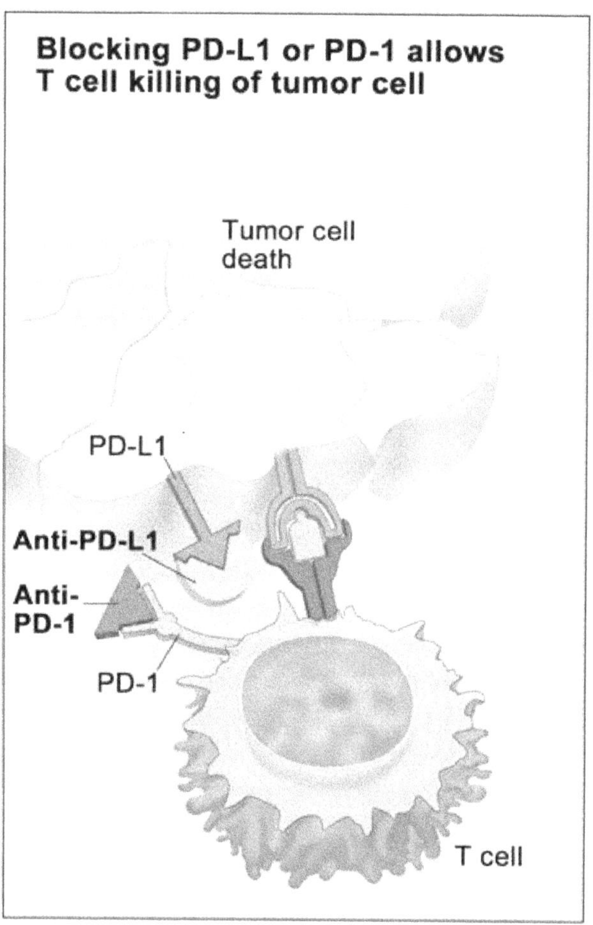

Snippets

Allison's research in the mid-1990s focused on a protein known as CTLA-4 that functions as a brake on the immune system. He developed the concept of blocking this brake to allow the immune system to attack tumors, leading to the development of new cancer treatments.

Honjo discovered PD-1, another protein that inhibits the immune system, and elucidated its role in regulating the immune response. This discovery paved the way for developing therapies that enhance the immune system's ability to fight cancer by targeting PD-1.

Current Implications

The work of Allison and Honjo has transformed cancer treatment, offering new hope to patients with previously untreatable forms of cancer. Immunotherapy has become a key component of cancer treatment alongside surgery, chemotherapy, and radiation therapy.

Impact and Products

The discoveries made by Allison and Honjo have led to the development of immunotherapeutic drugs that significantly improve survival rates for cancer patients. Their research continues to inspire ongoing studies aimed at understanding and harnessing the immune system to combat various diseases.

WILLIAM G. KAELIN JR., SIR PETER J. RATCLIFFE, GREG SEMENZA L (2019)

Sensing the rhythm of life : Pivotal research in cellular sensing mechanisms of oxygen

In 2019, their groundbreaking contributions to our understanding of how cells sense and adapt to oxygen availability were honored with the Nobel Prize in Medicine, highlighting the global impact of their discoveries on medical science

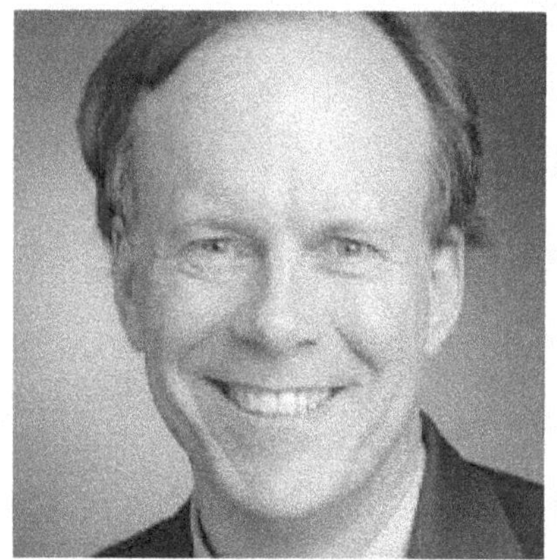

William G. Kaelin, Jr.
Dana-Farber Cancer Institute,
Harvard Medical School

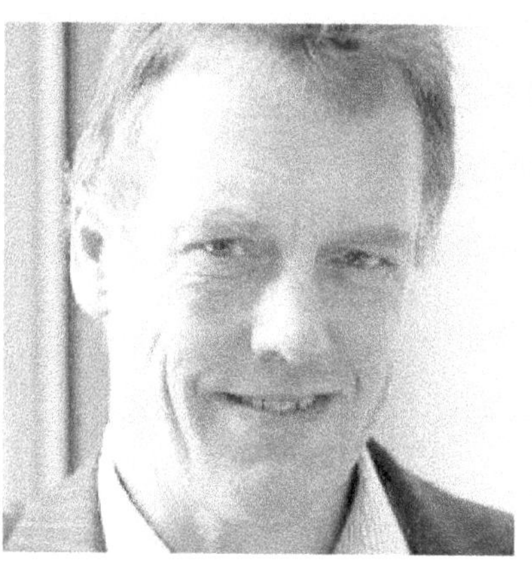

Peter J. Ratcliffe
University of Oxford, Francis
Crick Institute

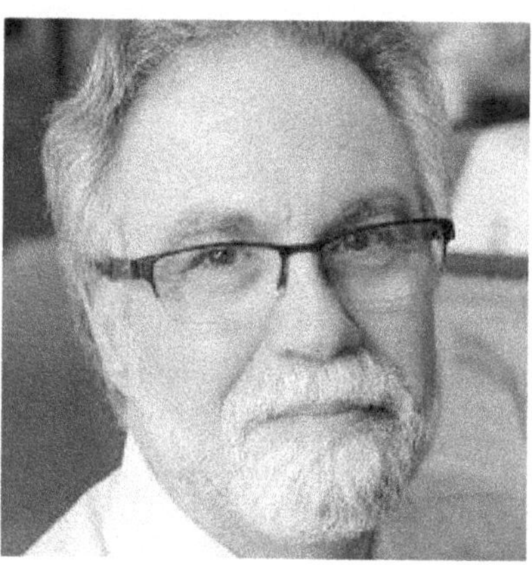

Gregg L. Semenza
Johns Hopkins University
School of Medicine

History

William G. Kaelin Jr., born in New York City in 1957, initially showcased a strong affinity for mathematics and science during his academic pursuits. Despite an early disinterest in biology due to its descriptive nature, a pivotal summer program at Florida Atlantic University ignited his passion for applying quantitative skills to biological questions. This experience, coupled with his undergraduate studies in mathematics and chemistry at Duke University and medical training at Johns Hopkins Hospital and Dana-Farber Cancer Institute, set the stage for his contributions to understanding how cells sense and adapt to oxygen levels.

Sir Peter J. Ratcliffe navigated his early medical education at St. Bartholomew's Hospital in London with a keen interest in the diagnostic process and a broad engagement with various medical specialties. Despite early uncertainty about his career path, an inclination towards practical and solvable scientific questions guided him toward nephrology and ultimately, the study of cellular oxygen sensing. His clinical training and subsequent research were characterized by a determination to uncover the mechanisms by which cells detect and respond to oxygen, a quest that led him from London to Oxford and into groundbreaking research.

Gregg L. Semenza, like his colleagues, was drawn to the mysteries of cellular function and regulation. His work focused on the genetic and molecular basis of oxygen sensing in cells, contributing to the trio's collective discovery of the mechanisms that allow cells to adapt to varying oxygen levels. This discovery has vast implications for medical science, particularly in understanding diseases where oxygen availability is a critical factor.

Snippets

Discovery of Oxygen Sensing Mechanisms: Kaelin, Ratcliffe, and Semenza discovered the molecular machinery that cells use to sense and adapt to changing oxygen levels, a fundamental process for cellular survival.

Genetic Contributions: They identified specific genes that are essential for the cellular response to hypoxia (low oxygen conditions), which play crucial roles in physiological and pathological processes.

Implications for Disease: Their work has significantly advanced our understanding of diseases where oxygen availability is crucial, such as cancer, where tumor growth is influenced by oxygen levels, and anemia, characterized by inadequate oxygen transport.

Therapeutic Developments: The identification of oxygen-sensing pathways has opened new avenues for developing treatments targeting these mechanisms, offering potential new therapies for anemia and cancer.

Early Researchers

Otto Warburg, whose early 20th-century work on cellular respiration highlighted the importance of oxygen in the metabolism of tumor cells, sparking interest in the relationship between oxygen and cellular processes. Warburg's observations opened up new questions about how cells adapt to changes in oxygen levels, which would later be crucial in understanding cancer's development and progression.

Another noteworthy pioneer is Christian Bohr, known for the Bohr effect, describing how blood's oxygen-binding affinity is inversely related to acidity and carbon dioxide concentration. This fundamental discovery about hemoglobin's behavior under different oxygen conditions laid important groundwork for studying cellular oxygen sensing mechanisms.

Linus Pauling further contributed to this area by elucidating the molecular structure of hemoglobin and how its oxygen-binding capacity changes, which was pivotal in understanding oxygen transport at the molecular level, setting the stage for later discoveries about oxygen sensing within cells.

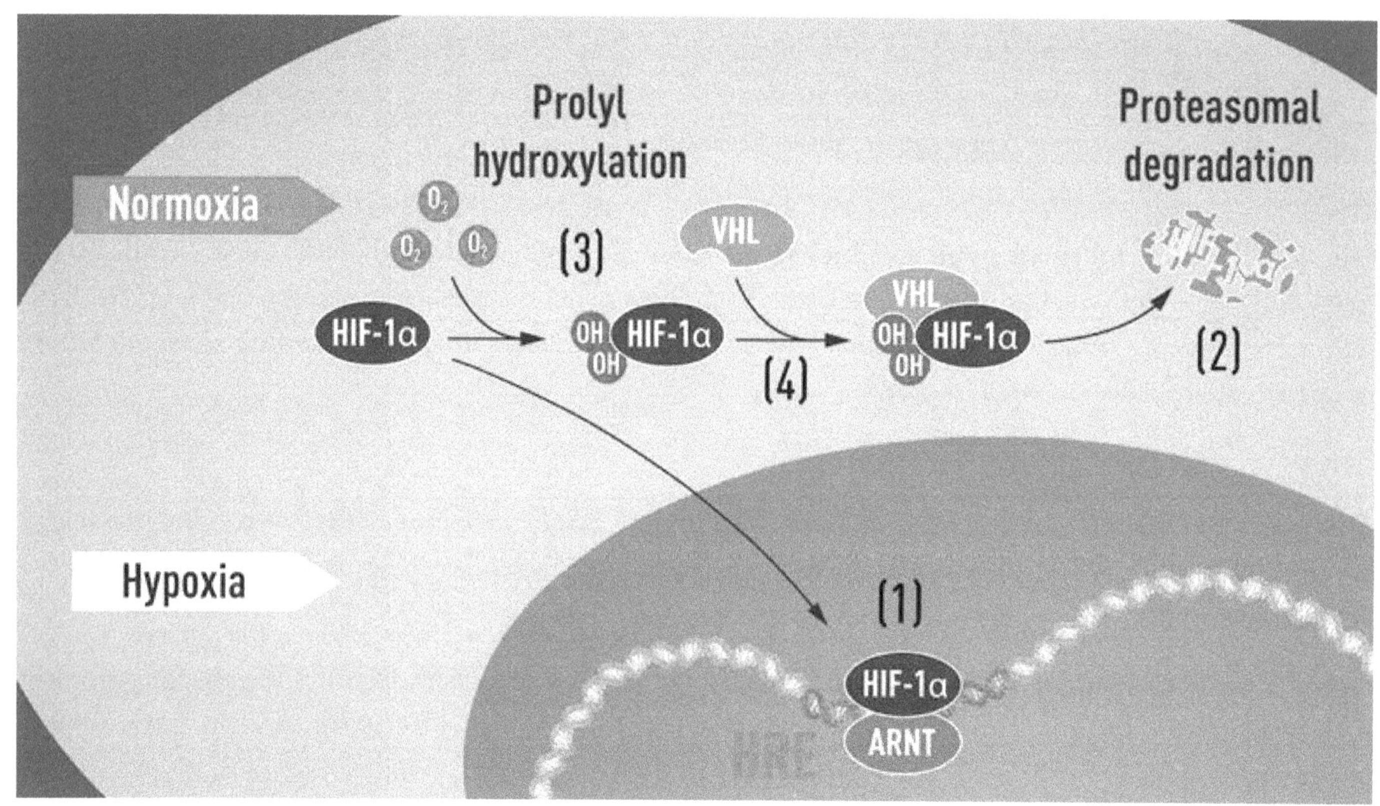

Source: © The Nobel Committee for Physiology or Medicine. Illustrator: Mattias Karlén

Current Implications

Cancer Research and Treatment: Understanding the mechanisms of oxygen sensing has opened new avenues in cancer research, particularly in targeting the hypoxic environments of tumors. Tumors often grow rapidly and outstrip their blood supply, leading to low oxygen levels. The Nobel Prize-winning work has helped in developing therapies aimed at manipulating the oxygen-sensing pathways to combat tumor growth and resistance to treatments.

Anemia and Cardiovascular Diseases: Insights into cellular responses to low oxygen levels have led to better understanding and treatments of diseases like anemia, where the body doesn't have enough red blood cells to carry adequate oxygen to its tissues. This research has also informed approaches to managing ischemic conditions, such as stroke and heart attacks, where oxygen supply to tissues is compromised.

Chronic Kidney Disease: Given the kidneys' role in erythropoietin production—a hormone that stimulates red blood cell production in response to oxygen levels—the work by Kaelin, Ratcliffe, and Semenza has implications for understanding and treating chronic kidney disease and its complications.

Development of Drugs: The molecular pathways involved in oxygen sensing are targets for new drugs that could potentially treat a range of conditions more effectively, from chronic anemia to cancers that thrive in low-oxygen environments.

Athletic and Physical Performance: This research has also impacted the field of sports science and medicine, particularly in understanding how oxygen availability affects muscle metabolism, endurance, and recovery. It has implications for training regimens and for the treatment of injuries in athletes.

Understanding Metabolic Disorders: The role of oxygen in metabolic processes means that the Nobel laureates' discoveries have implications for understanding and treating metabolic disorders, including diabetes and obesity.

Implications for Aging: Research into how cells detect and respond to oxygen also touches on the aging process, as oxygen metabolism and cellular stress responses linked to autophagy and longevity are influenced by oxygen levels.

Impact and Products

Healthcare and Therapeutic Advances

- **New Therapeutic Targets:** The elucidation of oxygen-sensing pathways has identified novel targets for drug development, particularly for diseases where oxygen availability is a key factor, such as chronic wounds or ischemic conditions.
- **Advancements in Anemia Treatment:** The understanding of how cells respond to low oxygen levels has directly influenced the development of more effective treatments for anemia, including drugs that stimulate erythropoiesis by mimicking hypoxic conditions.

Biotechnology and Drug Development

- **Drug Formulations for Cancer:** Knowledge about oxygen-sensing mechanisms has been instrumental in designing drugs that target the hypoxic tumor microenvironment, aiming to inhibit tumor growth and overcome resistance to chemotherapy.
- **Erythropoiesis-Stimulating Agents:** The biotech industry has leveraged insights into erythropoietin regulation under hypoxic conditions to develop erythropoiesis-stimulating agents, improving quality of life for patients with kidney disease and cancer.

Diagnostic Tools

- **Oxygen Monitoring Technologies:** Innovations in monitoring tissue oxygenation, inspired by the cellular mechanisms identified by Kaelin, Ratcliffe, and Semenza, have led to the development of advanced diagnostic tools, enhancing patient care in critical and chronic conditions.

Environmental and Industrial Applications

- **Cultivation and Bioreactor Design:** Understanding how cells adapt to oxygen availability has informed the optimization of cell culture conditions and bioreactor designs for more efficient production of biopharmaceuticals and tissue engineering.

Research and Scientific Tools

Genetic and Cellular Models: The creation of genetic and cellular models to study hypoxia-inducible factors (HIFs) and their pathways has become a vital resource for researchers exploring a wide array of biological and medical questions.

Their contributions continue to inspire a broad range of advancements aimed at improving human health and understanding the fundamental processes of life.

HARVEY J. ALTER, MICHAEL HOUGHTON, AND CHARLES M. RICE (2020)

The three warriors in virology, who could zero in on Hepatitis C structure

The trio was awarded the Nobel Prize in 2020 for their discovery of the Hepatitis C virus. This groundbreaking work has significantly contributed to the fight against liver disease worldwide.

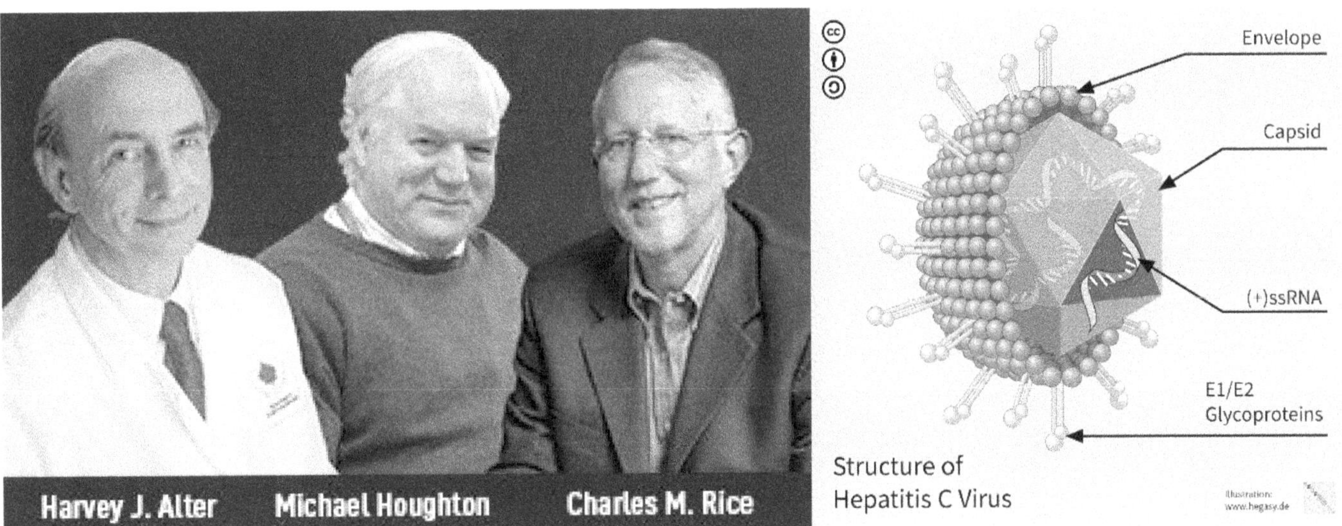

History

Harvey J. Alter

Harvey J. Alter was born on September 12, 1935, in New York, NY, USA. He is an American medical researcher renowned for his work in the discovery of the Hepatitis C virus. Alter's career is distinguished by his dedication to understanding and preventing blood-borne infectious diseases. At the time of the Nobel Prize award, he was affiliated with the National Institutes of Health in Bethesda, MD, USA. His pioneering studies in the 1970s, focusing on the occurrence of hepatitis in patients who had received blood transfusions, led to the groundbreaking discovery that a previously unknown virus, which was neither Hepatitis A nor B, was causing the disease.

Michael Houghton

Michael Houghton, born in 1949 in the United Kingdom, moved to Canada where he continued his research. His work has been instrumental in the virology field, particularly in the identification of the Hepatitis C virus. Houghton's affiliation at the time of receiving the Nobel Prize was with the

University of Alberta in Edmonton, Canada. In 1989, Houghton and his colleagues managed to isolate the genome of the Hepatitis C virus, an RNA virus belonging to the Flavivirus family, marking a pivotal moment in the scientific community's ability to diagnose and treat this disease.

Charles M. Rice

Charles M. Rice was born on August 25, 1952, in Sacramento, CA, USA. A virologist whose work has significantly advanced our understanding of hepatitis, Rice was affiliated with Rockefeller University in New York, NY, USA, when awarded the Nobel Prize. His contributions to the field include demonstrating that a specific region of the Hepatitis C virus's genome was crucial for its ability to cause the disease, thus providing the evidence needed to affirm that this virus alone was responsible for Hepatitis C. His research in 1997 was critical in paving the way for the development of effective treatments.

Snippets

Discovery of the Hepatitis C Virus: Alter, Houghton, and Rice's combined efforts led to the identification of the Hepatitis C virus, a groundbreaking achievement in the field of virology that has had profound implications for global health.

Filling a Crucial Gap in Infectious Disease: Before their work, the medical community was aware of Hepatitis A and B, but cases of chronic hepatitis remained unexplained. Their discovery of Hepatitis C filled this critical gap, identifying the cause of these unexplained cases.

Pioneering Blood Screening: Their discovery was pivotal in the development of blood screening tests for Hepatitis C, drastically reducing the risk of transmission through blood transfusions and improving the safety of blood banks worldwide.

Foundation for Antiviral Therapy: The identification of the Hepatitis C virus was crucial in the development of targeted antiviral therapies, significantly improving outcomes for patients with Hepatitis C and offering hope for a cure.

Global Health Impact: Hepatitis C affects millions of individuals globally, leading to liver diseases such as cirrhosis and liver cancer. The work of Alter, Houghton, and Rice has been instrumental in combating this virus, saving countless lives.

Early Researchers

Dr. Baruch Blumberg, who won the Nobel Prize in Medicine in 1976 for his discovery of the Hepatitis B virus, and for developing the diagnostic test and vaccine against it. Blumberg's work not only paved the way for blood screening methods but also highlighted the significant impact viral hepatitis had on global health, setting the stage for future hepatitis research.

Dr. Daniel Bradley, a virologist with the Centers for Disease Control and Prevention (CDC), made seminal contributions to understanding hepatitis caused by blood transfusion, known as non-A, non-B hepatitis, which would later be identified as Hepatitis C. Bradley's work in the 1970s and 1980s on the transmission and characterization of this mysterious agent laid critical groundwork for the eventual isolation of the Hepatitis C virus.

Another key contributor was Dr. Ralf F. Pettersson, a Swedish scientist who made significant advancements in molecular biology techniques that were crucial for the identification and genetic analysis of viruses, including what would become known as Hepatitis C.

Dr. Alfred Prince, a virologist, significantly contributed to the early understanding of hepatitis viruses and was among the first to hypothesize the existence of a hepatitis virus other than A or B, further motivating the search for what would be identified as Hepatitis C.

Current Implications

Improved Diagnostic Tests: The identification of the Hepatitis C virus has enabled the development of precise diagnostic tests, allowing for early detection and monitoring of the virus in patients.

Enhanced Blood Supply Safety: The discovery has dramatically improved the safety of blood transfusions by facilitating the development of effective screening tests for Hepatitis C in blood banks, significantly reducing the risk of transmission.

Development of Targeted Therapies: The understanding of the Hepatitis C virus at the molecular level has been crucial in the development of antiviral drugs specifically targeting the virus, leading to highly effective treatments that can cure Hepatitis C in most cases.

Vaccine Research: Although a vaccine for Hepatitis C is not yet available, the foundational work of Alter, Houghton, and Rice continues to inform ongoing research efforts aimed at developing a preventive vaccine.

Global Health Policies: The discovery has influenced public health policies worldwide, with increased emphasis on screening, prevention, and treatment of Hepatitis C. It has also highlighted the need for global strategies to combat viral hepatitis as a public health concern.

Educational Impact: The comprehensive understanding of Hepatitis C has become a crucial component of medical education, informing new generations of healthcare professionals about the diagnosis, management, and prevention of this virus.

Future Research Directions: The groundwork laid by their discovery opens up new research avenues, including the study of viral replication mechanisms, host-virus interactions, and the long-term impact of Hepatitis C on liver health.

Impact and Products

Advanced Blood Screening Tests: The creation of sensitive blood screening tests for Hepatitis C has been one of the most direct outcomes, greatly enhancing the safety of blood transfusions and organ transplants worldwide.

Antiviral Drugs: A range of direct-acting antiviral (DAA) drugs has been developed, transforming Hepatitis C from a potentially fatal disease to a curable condition within weeks. These drugs specifically target viral proteins to inhibit the replication of the virus.

Diagnostic Kits: Rapid and reliable diagnostic kits for Hepatitis C have been developed, enabling healthcare providers to perform quick testing and early diagnosis, crucial for effective treatment outcomes.

Genetic Sequencing Technologies: The research into Hepatitis C has spurred advancements in genetic sequencing technologies, allowing for detailed viral genome analysis which is vital for both research purposes and personalized medicine approaches.

Liver Health Monitoring Tools: The understanding of Hepatitis C's impact on liver health has led to the innovation of non-invasive liver health monitoring tools. These tools help in assessing liver fibrosis and cirrhosis without the need for a biopsy, improving patient care and monitoring.

These products and developments underscore the wide-ranging impact of discovering the Hepatitis C virus, highlighting how a single scientific breakthrough can lead to numerous advancements across different areas of healthcare and public health.

DAVID JULIUS AND ARDEM PATAPOUTIAN (2021)

Molecular reconstruction of Ion channels that sense touch and temperature

In 2021, David Julius and Ardem Patapoutian were jointly awarded the Nobel Prize in Medicine for their discoveries concerning the receptors for temperature and touch. This work has significantly advanced our understanding of how sensory inputs are detected and processed by the nervous system.

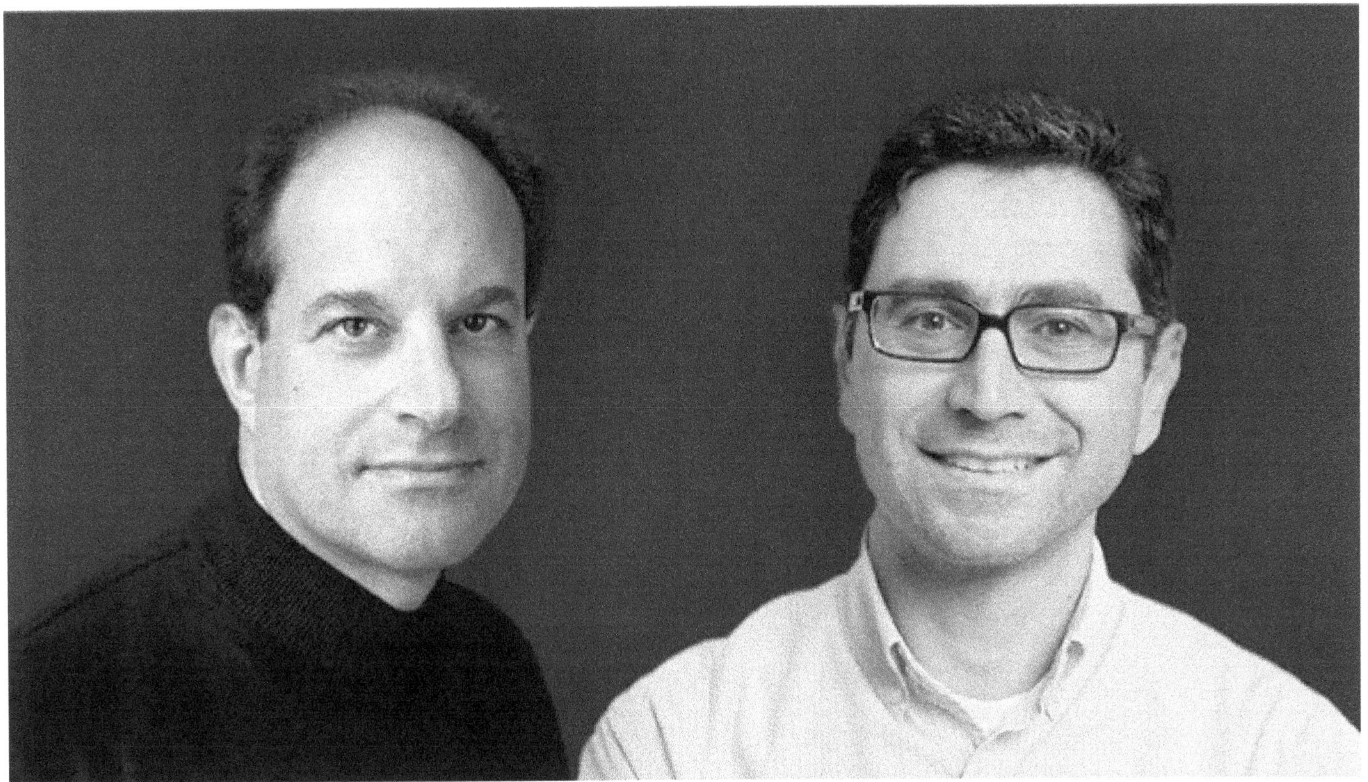

History

David Julius was born on November 4, 1955, in New York, NY, USA, and has conducted much of his research at the University of California, San Francisco. Ardem Patapoutian, born on October 2, 1967, in Beirut, Lebanon, has been a key figure at Scripps Research in La Jolla, CA, USA. Both scientists have contributed to the field of sensory perception through their innovative research.

Snippets

Julius utilized capsaicin, the spicy component of chili peppers, to identify a receptor in nerve cells that responds to heat, marking a breakthrough in understanding how temperature sensations are converted into electrical signals in the nervous system. Patapoutian discovered a novel class of ion channels activated by mechanical forces, uncovering the molecular basis of pressure and touch sensations. Together, their work has illuminated the mechanisms through which our bodies perceive and respond to the external environment.

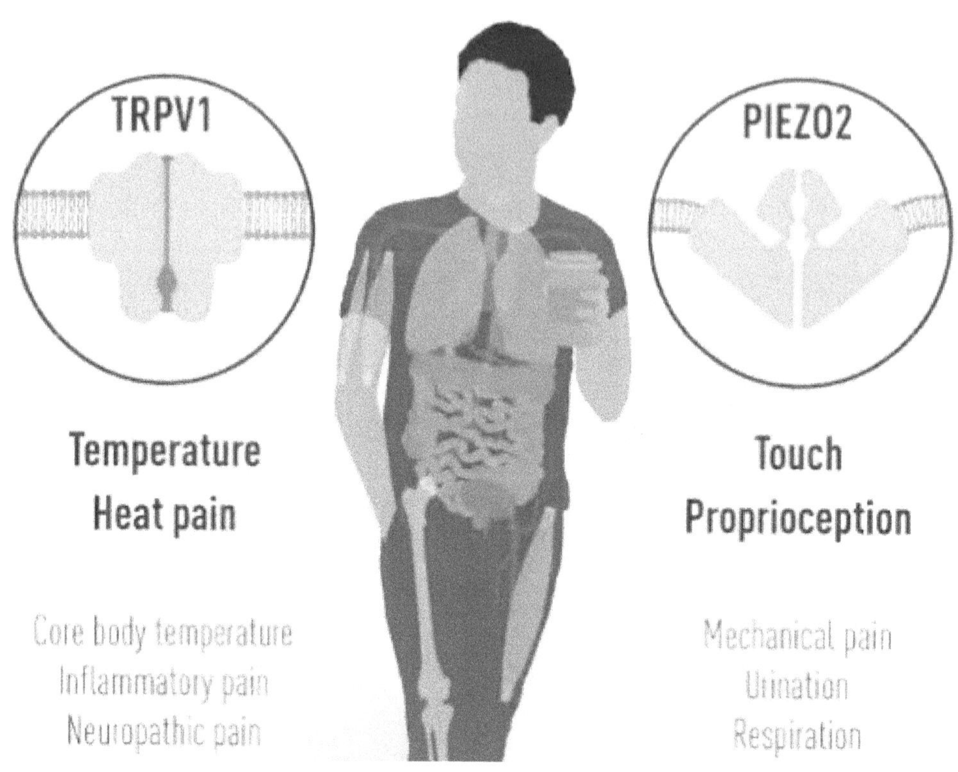

Discoveries by the winners of Nobel Prize 2021 in Medicine have explained how heat, cold and touch can initiate signals in our nervous system.

Current Implications

The discoveries made by Julius and Patapoutian have broad implications, not only enhancing our grasp of sensory perception but also paving the way for research into pain management, proprioception, and other aspects of neurobiology. Their work offers potential pathways for developing new treatments for chronic pain conditions and other sensory disorders.

Impact and Products

The contributions of Julius and Patapoutian to the understanding of sensory systems have had a profound impact on neuroscience, leading to a deeper appreciation of the complexity of sensory processing. Their work continues to inspire further research into the molecular underpinnings of sensation and the development of therapies to address sensory-related conditions.

SVANTE PÄÄBO (2022)

A passionate pioneer in paleo-genomics

Svante Pääbo was awarded the Nobel Prize in 2022 for his revolutionary discoveries regarding the genomes of extinct hominins and their impact on human evolution, establishing the field of paleo-genomics.

History

Born in Stockholm in 1955, Pääbo's scientific quest was influenced by a profound curiosity about human origins and what distinguishes us from our extinct relatives. His path took him to the Max Planck Institute for Evolutionary Anthropology in Leipzig, Germany, where he dedicated over three decades to unraveling the genetic secrets of Neanderthals and other extinct hominins.

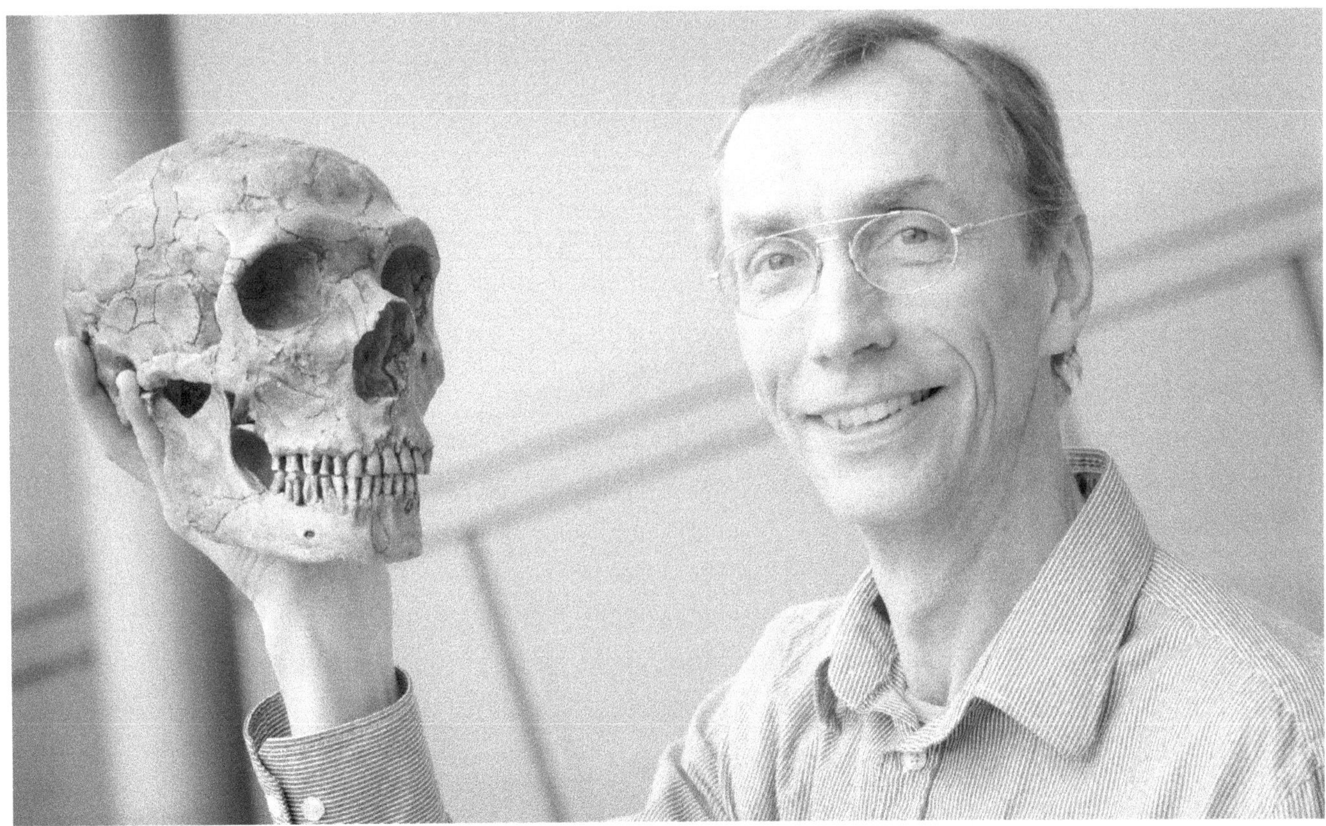

Pääbo's work was pioneering in that it bridged the gap between archaeology, paleontology, and genetics, fields that had previously operated largely in parallel with one another. Before Pääbo's innovations, our understanding of human evolution was primarily based on the study of fossils and artifacts. These relics provided invaluable insights into the physical appearance and environments of our ancestors but offered limited information on the genetic evolution that underpins what makes Homo sapiens unique.

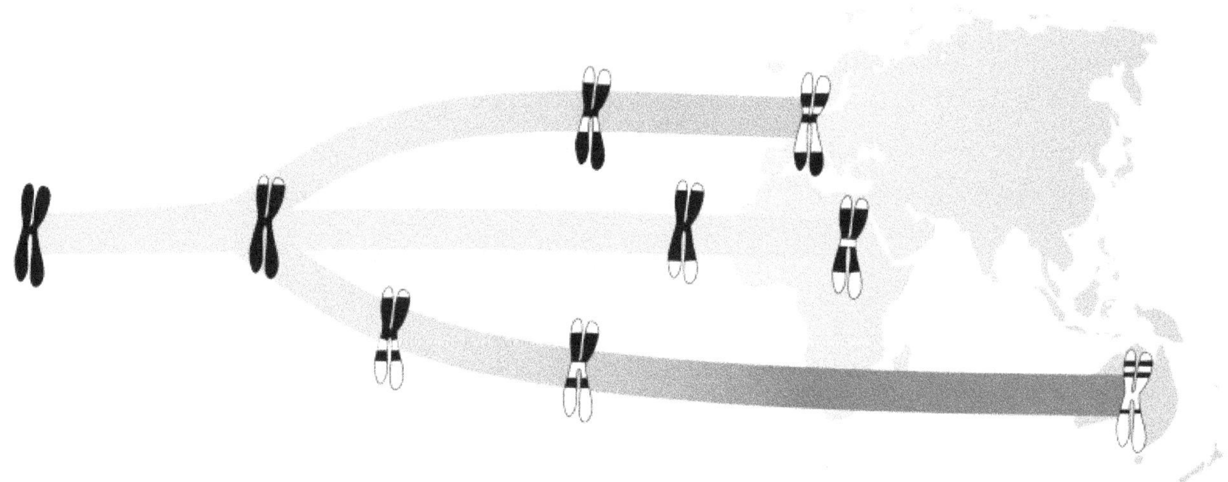

Transcontinental tracking of genes

The turning point came with Pääbo's revolutionary technique to extract and analyze DNA from ancient bones, a concept that faced skepticism due to the fragile nature of DNA, which degrades over time, and the risk of contamination from modern genetic material. Yet, Pääbo's persistence and innovative methods led to the successful sequencing of the Neanderthal genome, a feat that was once considered impossible. This achievement not only proved that extracting ancient DNA was feasible but also opened the door to comparative genomics between modern humans and our closest extinct relatives.

Pääbo didn't stop with Neanderthals. His discovery of Denisovans from a single finger bone expanded the known family tree of hominins, introducing a previously unknown group that contributed genetically to modern humans. This work underscored the complex web of interbreeding and migration that characterizes human history, challenging the simplistic view of a linear progression from ancient to modern humans.

Snippets

Pioneered Paleogenomics: Pääbo's work laid the foundation for the field of paleogenomics, using groundbreaking techniques to extract and sequence DNA from ancient bones, a task previously thought Impossible.

Sequenced the Neanderthal Genome: Achieving the first successful sequencing of the Neanderthal genome, Pääbo provided unprecedented insights into the genetic makeup of our closest extinct relatives.

Discovered the Denisovans: Through the analysis of a single finger bone, Pääbo identified a previously unknown group of ancient humans, the Denisovans, expanding our understanding of human ancestry.

Revealed Interbreeding Among Hominins: His research showed that early humans interbred with Neanderthals and Denisovans, with genetic legacies from these extinct hominins still present in modern human DNA.

Impacted Modern Human Physiology and Disease: The genetic contributions from Neanderthals and Denisovans have been linked to various aspects of modern human physiology and disease susceptibilities, highlighting the ongoing influence of our ancient relatives.

Advanced Ancient DNA Research Techniques: Pääbo's methods for extracting and analyzing ancient DNA have revolutionized the field, enabling other scientists to explore genetic materials from the past and uncover more about human history and evolution.

Early Researchers

Allan Wilson, a molecular biologist whose innovative use of mitochondrial DNA to trace human evolutionary history laid the groundwork for later studies on ancient DNA. Wilson's work in the 1970s and 1980s on the "Mitochondrial Eve" hypothesis proposed that all modern humans have a common ancestor, a concept that sparked considerable debate and further research into human origins.

Another key figure is Bryan Sykes, who, along with his team at the University of Oxford, provided early evidence for the retrieval of ancient DNA from human remains. Sykes's work in the late 1980s and early 1990s on the genetic analysis of the Cheddar Man, a Late Upper Paleolithic human from England, demonstrated the feasibility of extracting and studying ancient human DNA, setting the stage for future discoveries.

Rebecca Cann and Mark Stoneking, collaborators with Wilson, also deserve mention for their role in the early application of mitochondrial DNA to trace human lineages and migrations. Their research contributed significantly to the understanding of human evolution and migration patterns out of Africa.

The pioneering work in the field of ancient DNA is not limited to humans. Thomas H. Morgan and Svante Pääbo himself conducted some of the earliest studies extracting DNA from Egyptian mummies and extinct animals, exploring the limits of DNA preservation and extraction techniques that would later be applied to Neanderthal and Denisovan genomes.

Current Implications

Advancements in Genetic Research: Pääbo's techniques for extracting ancient DNA have revolutionized the field, enabling the study of genetic material from extinct species and providing a direct look into the past. This has broadened our understanding of genetic evolution and diversity.

Insights into Human Evolution: By comparing the genomes of modern humans with those of Neanderthals and Denisovans, researchers have gained invaluable insights into human evolution, migration patterns, and how our species has adapted over time.

Understanding of Modern Human Health: The discovery that modern humans carry DNA from extinct hominins has implications for our understanding of contemporary human health, including our susceptibility to certain diseases and conditions.

Cultural and Historical Recontextualization: Pääbo's discoveries have reconfigured our understanding of human history, challenging previous notions about the distinctiveness of Homo sapiens and providing a more nuanced view of our relationship with other hominins.

Ethical and Philosophical Questions: The ability to extract and analyze ancient DNA raises ethical and philosophical questions about identity, privacy, and our responsibilities toward our ancestors and their remains.

Influence on Anthropology and Archaeology: The field of paleogenomics has bridged the gap between genetics and archaeology, allowing for a multidisciplinary approach to studying ancient human societies and their environments.

Impact and Products

Public Exhibitions and Museums: Museums around the world have updated their exhibitions to include the latest findings on Neanderthals, Denisovans, and their connection to modern humans, often featuring replicas of ancient artifacts and interactive displays based on Pääbo's work.

Documentaries and Media Content: Numerous documentaries and media content exploring human history have been produced, drawing on the revelations about our ancient relatives made possible by Pääbo's research, making complex scientific discoveries accessible to a wider audience.

Genetic Testing Services: Commercial genetic testing services now often include information on an individual's Neanderthal ancestry, offering insights into genetic heritage and health predispositions linked to ancient human DNA.

Research Software and Databases: The development of specialized software and databases for analyzing ancient DNA sequences has been a direct outcome of the need to handle and interpret the complex data generated by studies of ancient genomes.

Collaborative International Research Projects: Pääbo's work has spurred international collaborations aimed at mapping the genetic history of human populations worldwide, combining efforts from genetics, archaeology, and anthropology to deepen our understanding of human diversity and evolution.

Through his contributions, we have gained not just a deeper understanding of our genetic past but also valuable tools and frameworks for exploring the complexities of human history and evolution.

KATALIN KARIKÓ AND DREW WEISSMAN (2023)

Modern messengers, whose mRNA vaccine fought the Covid pandemic with varied success

Katalin Karikó and Drew Weissman were awarded the Nobel Prize in 2023 for their pioneering discoveries concerning nucleoside base modifications in mRNA, which were crucial for the development of effective mRNA vaccines against COVID-19. Their work overcame significant challenges related to the stability and delivery of mRNA, leading to a new era in vaccine technology.

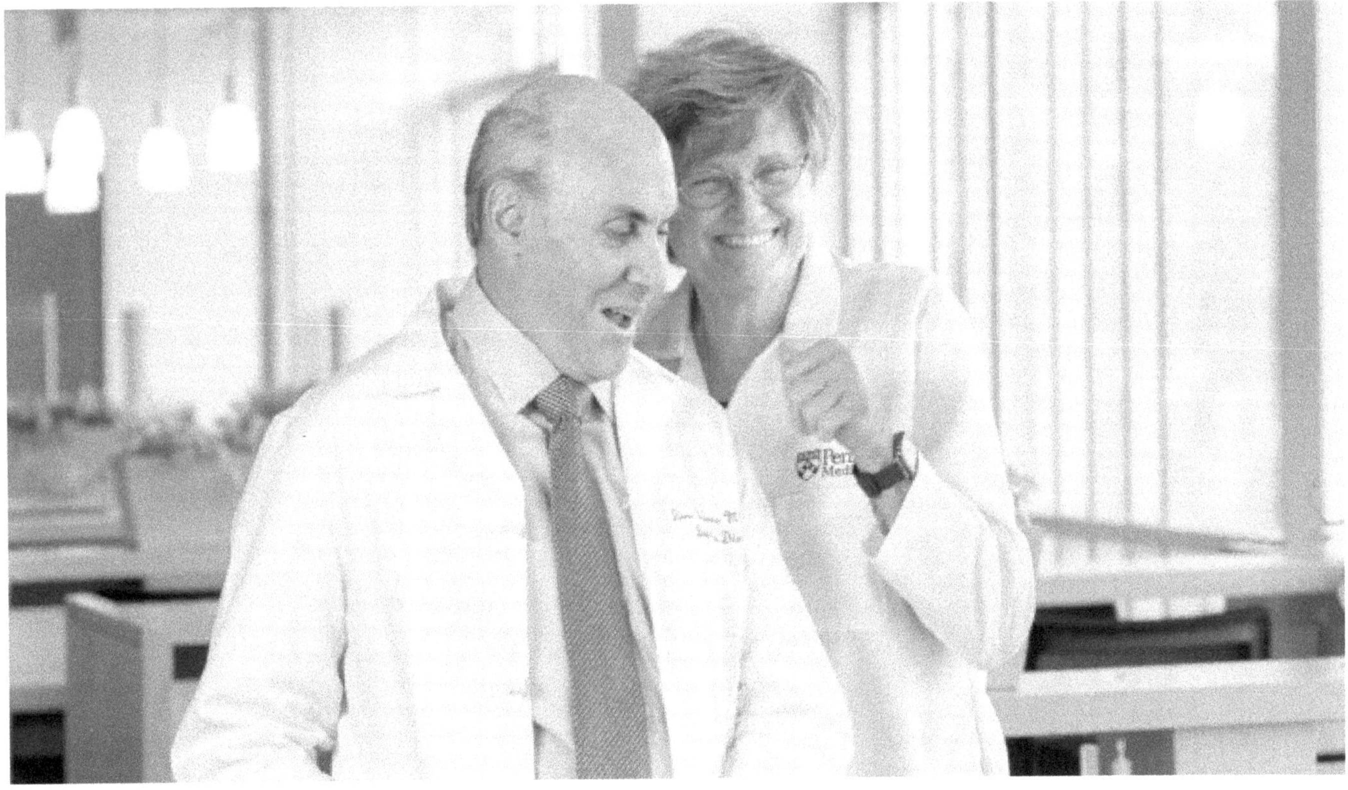

History

Katalin Karikó was born on January 17, 1955, in Szolnok, Hungary. She embarked on her scientific journey fueled by a steadfast belief in the therapeutic potential of messenger RNA (mRNA), a path that would ultimately revolutionize vaccine development and therapeutic interventions. Despite facing early skepticism and funding challenges, Karikó's dedication to her vision laid the groundwork for the use of mRNA in medicine. Her affiliation at the time of the Nobel Prize award included Szeged University in Hungary and the University of Pennsylvania in the United States. Karikó's work, particularly from the early 1990s onwards, played a pivotal role in overcoming the significant scientific hurdles associated with mRNA, including its instability and innate immunogenicity.

Drew Weissman, born on May 13, 1959, in the United States, brought an immunological perspective to the partnership with Karikó. His research focused on understanding the intricacies of the immune system, particularly dendritic cells' role in immune responses. Weissman's work at the University of Pennsylvania, where he crossed paths with Karikó, was instrumental in identifying the mechanism by which mRNA could be used effectively as a therapeutic tool without triggering harmful inflammatory responses. Their collaborative efforts led to the discovery of modified nucleosides in mRNA, a breakthrough that paved the way for the development of mRNA vaccines, including those against COVID-19.

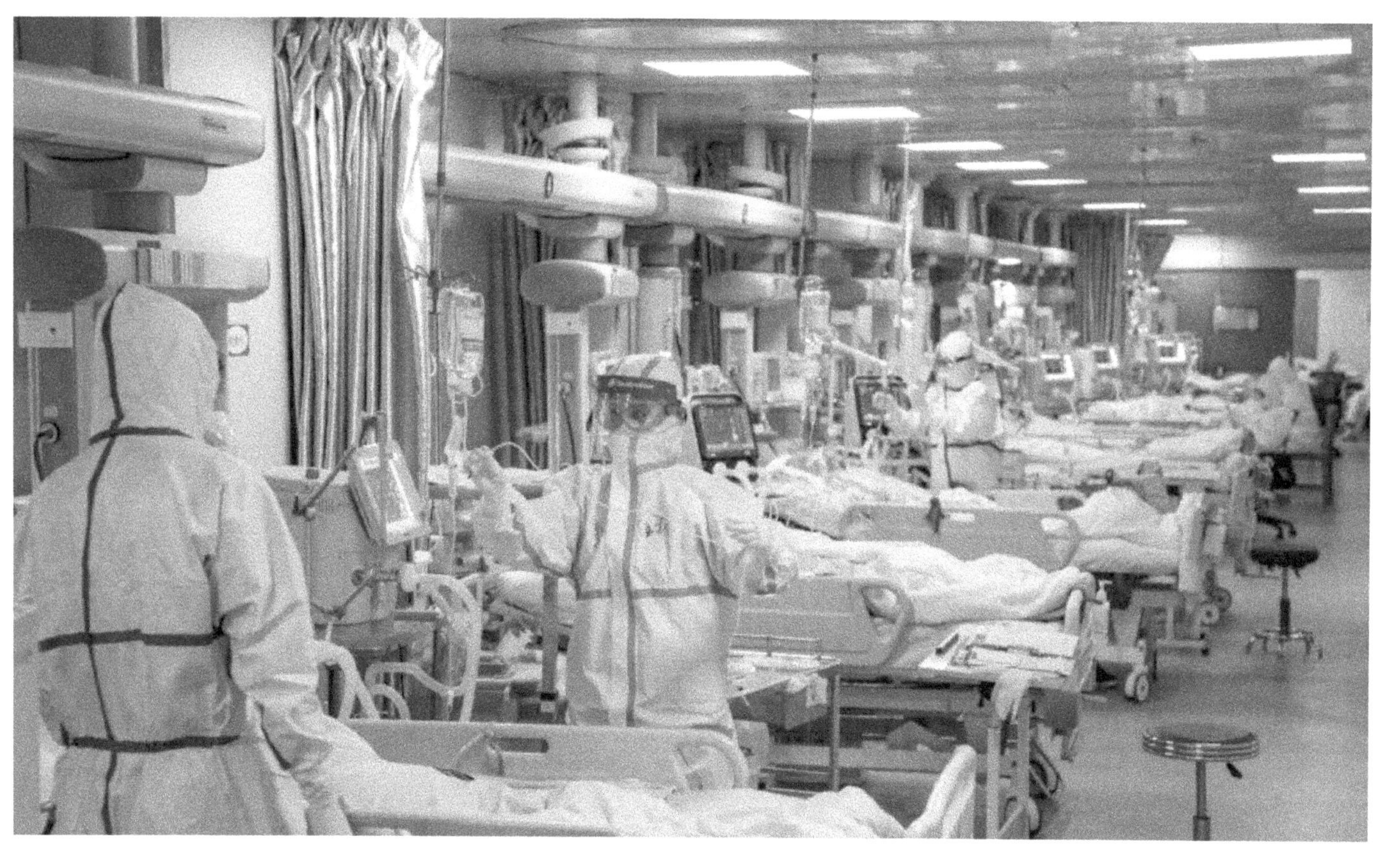

Hope we have learnt some important lessons of truth from this Neo-pandemic

Snippets

Overcoming mRNA Challenges: Karikó and Weissman's work addressed the challenge of mRNA's inherent instability and its tendency to trigger immune responses, which were significant obstacles in its therapeutic use.

Modified Nucleosides: Their pivotal discovery that incorporating modified nucleosides into mRNA could prevent unwanted immune reactions was a game-changer, enabling the safe use of mRNA as a therapeutic tool.

Foundations for mRNA Vaccines: This breakthrough laid the groundwork for the development of mRNA vaccines, most notably against COVID-19, showcasing the potential for rapid vaccine development in response to emerging infectious diseases.

Inspiring Future Research: Their success has opened new avenues for using mRNA technology, not only in vaccines but also in potential therapies for cancer and other diseases, highlighting the versatility and promise of mRNA-based treatments.

Early Researchers

Paul Zamecnik, who, along with Mahlon Hoagland and Mary Stephenson, discovered transfer RNA (tRNA) in the late 1950s, unraveling a crucial component of protein synthesis. This discovery was pivotal, as it unveiled the process by which mRNA carries genetic instructions from DNA to the cell's protein-making machinery, setting the stage for future explorations into mRNA's role in biology and medicine.

Another significant figure was Sydney Brenner, who, with his colleagues, laid the groundwork for understanding mRNA's function in protein synthesis during the early 1960s. Brenner's work was instrumental in elucidating the nature of mRNA and its critical role in translating genetic information into proteins, a foundational concept that underpins the mRNA vaccine technology.

Ralph Steinman's discovery of dendritic cells in 1973 provided invaluable insights into the immune system's intricacies. Understanding dendritic cells' role in initiating and regulating immune responses was crucial for the later development of mRNA vaccines, which rely on these cells to present antigens and elicit protective immunity.

The development of lipid nanoparticles, critical for delivering mRNA into cells without degradation, also owes much to earlier pioneers like Pieter Cullis and his team, who explored the use of lipid bilayers to encapsulate and protect nucleic acids in the 1970s and 1980s. This technology was crucial in overcoming one of the significant challenges Karikó and Weissman faced: the delivery of mRNA to cells without invoking an immune response that would destroy it.

Current Implications

Revolution in Vaccine Development: The success of mRNA vaccines against COVID-19 has revolutionized the field of vaccine development, demonstrating the potential for rapid response to emerging infectious diseases.

Broader Implications for mRNA Technology: Beyond infectious diseases, the technology is being explored for cancer vaccines, personalized cancer treatments, and other therapeutic applications, showcasing the versatility of mRNA-based strategies.

Increased Investment in Biotechnology: The success of mRNA vaccines has led to increased funding and investment in biotechnology companies focusing on mRNA and other novel therapeutic approaches, potentially accelerating the development of new treatments.

Global Health Impact: The deployment of mRNA COVID-19 vaccines has had a profound impact on controlling the pandemic, saving millions of lives and highlighting the importance of vaccine equity and global access to life-saving technologies.

Renewed Focus on Fundamental Research: The story of Karikó and Weissman underscores the value of basic scientific research and the unexpected ways in which fundamental discoveries can lead to transformative technologies and solutions to global health challenges.

Impact and Products

Educational Outreach and Public Awareness: The story of mRNA vaccine development, featuring Karikó and Weissman's pivotal contributions, has become a key educational tool, highlighting the importance of mRNA technology and its impact on public health. This narrative is being used in academic curricula, public lectures, and scientific outreach programs to inspire future generations of scientists.

New Research Initiatives: The success of mRNA vaccines has catalyzed new research initiatives aimed at exploring the full potential of mRNA technology, including its application in treating a wide array of diseases beyond COVID-19, such as cancer, autoimmune diseases, and genetic disorders.

Policy and Funding Shifts: Recognizing the critical role of mRNA technology in addressing the COVID-19 pandemic, governments and philanthropic organizations worldwide have increased funding for research and development in mRNA technology and vaccine distribution infrastructure, aiming to ensure global health security against future pandemics.

Technological Innovations: The need for cold chain logistics in mRNA vaccine distribution has spurred innovations in refrigeration and supply chain management, leading to improved methods that may benefit the distribution of other temperature-sensitive medical supplies.

Collaborations and Partnerships: The development and deployment of mRNA vaccines have fostered unprecedented collaborations between biotech companies, pharmaceutical giants, governments, and international health organizations, setting a new standard for global cooperation in facing public health challenges.

Katalin Karikó and Drew Weissman's groundbreaking research on mRNA technology has revolutionized vaccine development, offering a swift and effective response to the COVID-19 pandemic and potentially altering the course of future vaccine and therapeutic development.

THE NOBEL LEGACY

A Personal Perspective

REFLECTION ON THE ACHIEVEMENTS OF NOBEL LAUREATES IN MEDICINE

The Nobel Prize in Medicine, established by Alfred Nobel's will in 1895, honors individuals whose discoveries have conferred the greatest benefit to humankind. Since its inception in 1901, the prize has celebrated breakthroughs that span the breadth of medical science, from understanding diseases to developing treatments that save millions of lives.

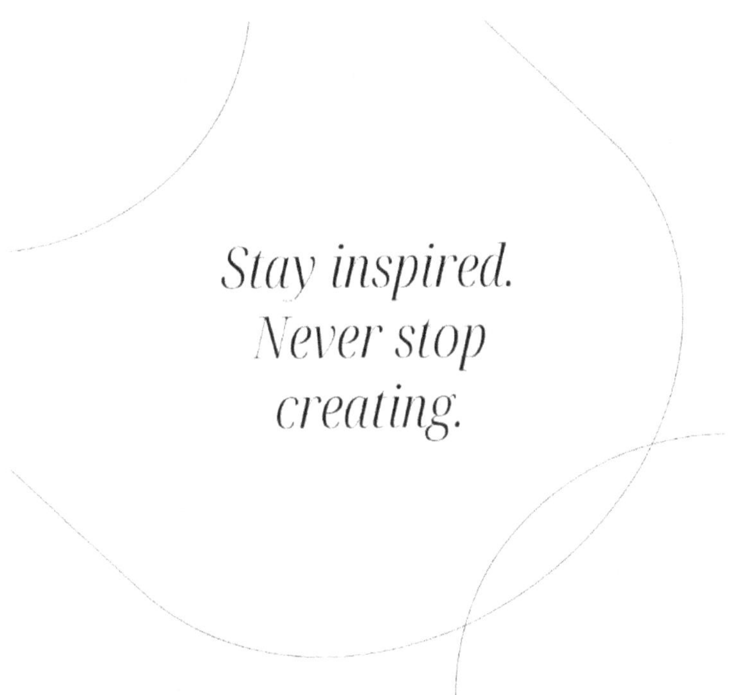

The first Nobel Prize in this category was awarded to Emil von Behring for his serum therapy against diphtheria, marking the beginning of a new era in medical science with a powerful tool against illness and death. Over the years, the Nobel Prize has acknowledged a wide array of monumental discoveries. These include Ronald Ross's work on malaria, which laid the foundation for combating this deadly disease, and Niels Ryberg Finsen's innovation in treating lupus with concentrated light radiation, which opened new avenues for medical treatment.

The discovery of insulin by Frederick Banting and John Macleod in 1923 transformed diabetes from a fatal disease to a manageable condition, illustrating the Nobel Prize's role in highlighting discoveries that significantly improve human health. The awards have also recognized advancements in understanding the human body and disease mechanisms, such as Karl Landsteiner's discovery of human blood groups, which made blood transfusions safe and effective.

In recent times, the prize has continued to acknowledge groundbreaking work that addresses pressing global health challenges. The development of an effective COVID-19 vaccine by Katalin Karikó and Drew Weissman is a prime example of how Nobel laureates have continued to push the boundaries of science to produce innovations that not only advance our understanding of biology but also offer real-world solutions to global pandemics.

The Nobel Prize in Medicine reflects the ever-evolving landscape of biomedical research, celebrating discoveries that have fundamentally transformed medical science and healthcare. From unraveling the mysteries of the genetic code to pioneering new treatments for diseases, Nobel laureates have laid the groundwork for future research and opened new doors to therapeutic possibilities, embodying the spirit of innovation and dedication that defines the medical field.

Each laureate's journey underscores a collective quest for knowledge and a relentless pursuit of solutions to humanity's most daunting challenges, embodying the essence of scientific inquiry and its profound impact on society. As we look to the future, the stories of these laureates inspire continued exploration and innovation in the quest to improve human health and well-being.

The long list of Nobel Prize winners and what they've done shows how powerful science is and how it can make big changes. When we think about these successes, we remember how crucial it is to back scientific studies and create a place where new ideas can grow. This helps new discoveries happen that will keep helping people.

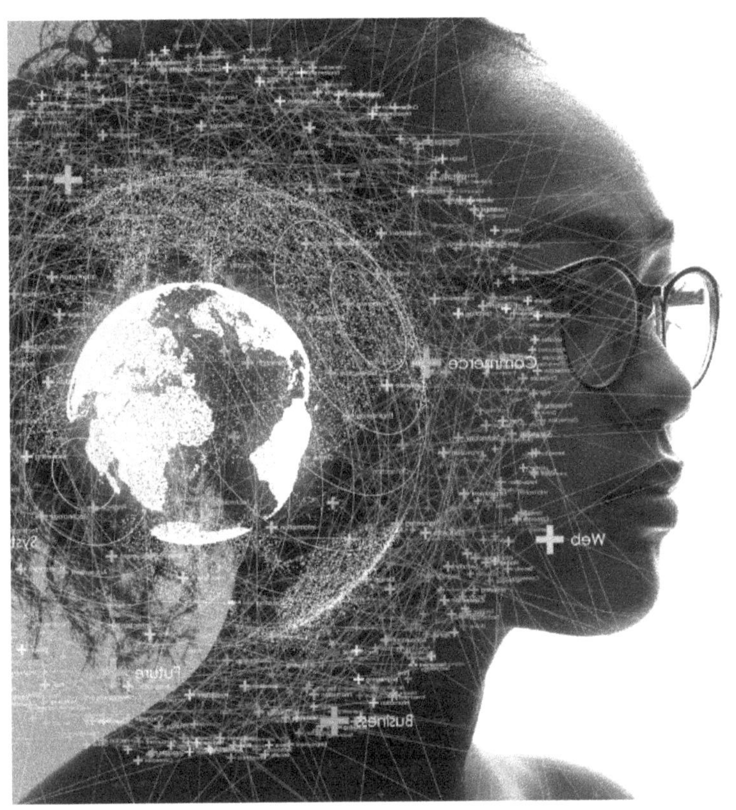

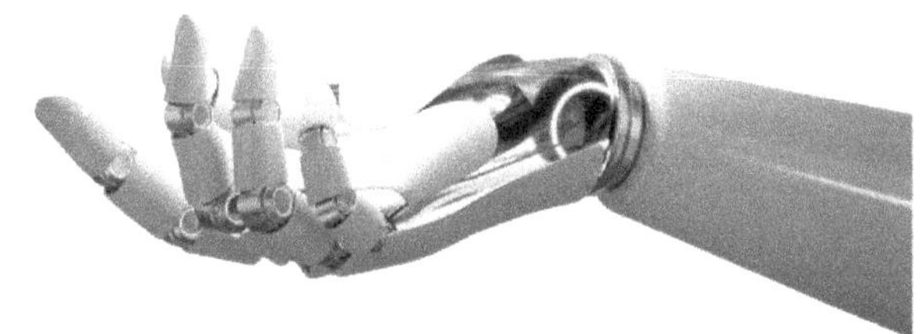

The Life-Changing Discovery of Insulin

One of the most profound anecdotes in medical history is the discovery of insulin and its impact on diabetes treatment. Before insulin was discovered in 1921 by Frederick Banting and Charles Best, a diagnosis of diabetes was essentially a death sentence. The only treatment available was a strict diet that could prolong life by a few years at most, but often led to starvation. The first successful administration of insulin to a human, Leonard Thompson, a 14-year-old boy, in 1922, dramatically changed the prognosis for people with diabetes. Within 24 hours of receiving insulin, Thompson's dangerously high blood glucose levels dropped to near-normal levels. This event marked the beginning of a new era in diabetes management, turning a lethal disease into a manageable condition.

The journey from this initial discovery to the insulin we know today has been marked by continuous innovation and improvement. Early insulin was derived from animal sources, often causing allergic reactions and requiring careful dose calculation to avoid the risks of hypoglycemia. Advances in biotechnology led to the development of human insulin in the late 1970s, significantly improving safety and efficacy. Today, insulin analogs and delivery methods such as insulin pumps provide people with diabetes greater control over their condition, dramatically improving their quality of life.

The Ripple Effect on Society and Healthcare

The impact of the discovery of insulin extends beyond individual health benefits. It revolutionized the field of endocrinology and opened new avenues for biomedical research. The story of insulin's discovery and development is a testament to the power of scientific inquiry and collaboration. It highlights the importance of research and innovation in addressing healthcare challenges, offering hope and inspiration for the treatment of other diseases.

The development of insulin also underscores the critical role of patient access to essential medicines. As research continues to advance, making these innovations available to all who need them remains a priority. The history of insulin reflects ongoing efforts to improve diabetes management technologies and reduce the burden on individuals living with this disease. Looking to the future, scientists are exploring even more sophisticated forms of insulin and delivery systems, aiming to mimic the body's natural glucose regulation more closely and ultimately improve the lives of people with diabetes worldwide.

The discovery of insulin is more than a medical breakthrough; it's a story of hope, perseverance, and the relentless pursuit of knowledge. It serves as a powerful example of how scientific discovery can profoundly impact human health and society, offering lessons that extend far beyond the field of medicine.

The Revolutionary Impact of Penicillin

Following the transformative discovery of insulin, another groundbreaking development that has had a profound impact on human health and society is the discovery of penicillin by Alexander Fleming in 1928. Penicillin's journey from a laboratory curiosity to a life-saving antibiotic showcases the immense potential of scientific research to change lives.

Fleming's accidental discovery of the antibiotic properties of the Penicillium notatum mold marked the beginning of the antibiotic era. However, it was the concerted efforts of Howard Florey, Ernst Chain, and their team at the Sir William Dunn School of Pathology at Oxford University that transformed penicillin into a practical therapeutic agent. They overcame significant challenges to purify and produce penicillin in quantities sufficient for clinical use, despite the resource constraints imposed by World War II. Their innovative production techniques and the decision to share the discovery with pharmaceutical companies in the United States significantly accelerated the mass production of penicillin.

The Global Influence of the Nobel Prize

The Nobel Prize, since its inception, has played a pivotal role in fostering international collaboration and serving as an inspiration for future generations of scientists and researchers. Its influence extends far beyond the individual achievements of the laureates, impacting the global scientific community, public health, and the broader discourse on medicine and science.

Catalyst for International Collaboration

The Prize has historically acted as a bridge, bringing together researchers from diverse backgrounds and nations towards common goals. Initiatives like CERN, supported by UNESCO, underscore the significance of such collaborative efforts. Founded in 1954 with the goal of exploring atomic energy's peaceful uses, CERN has emerged as a beacon of international scientific cooperation, hosting scientists, engineers, and students from various countries. This collaborative environment not only fosters groundbreaking research, such as the discovery of the Higgs boson but also cultivates a culture of peace and shared progress among nations with disparate political ideologies.

Moreover, the International Centre for Theoretical Physics (ICTP), established with UNESCO's backing, further illustrates the Nobel Prize's ethos by supporting scientists from developing countries, thereby democratizing access to cutting-edge scientific knowledge and fostering a global scientific community that transcends geopolitical barriers.

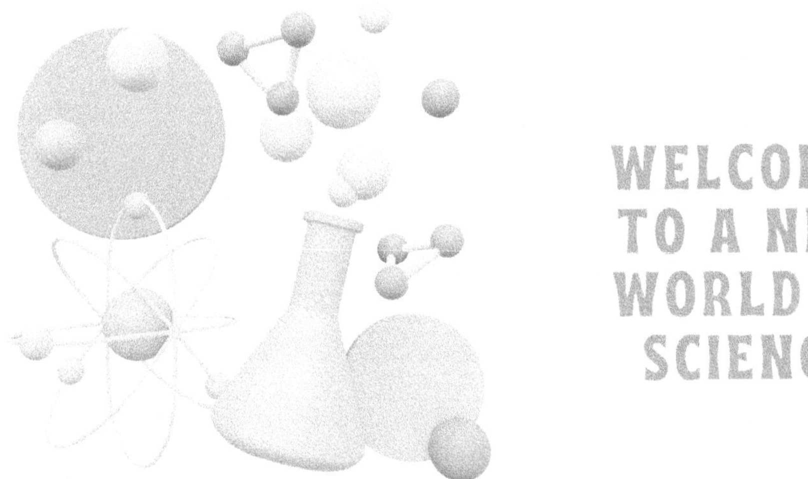

Through its annual recognition of groundbreaking achievements, the Prize brings to the fore the latest advancements and stimulates conversation and interest among scientists, healthcare professionals, policymakers, and the general public alike.

Elevating Scientific Achievements to the Public Eye

One of the most significant impacts of the Nobel Prize is its ability to bring complex scientific concepts into the public sphere, making them more accessible and understandable. By awarding researchers for their contributions to medicine, the Prize not only acknowledges their work but also educates the public about the importance of ongoing research in tackling diseases, improving health outcomes, and enhancing the quality of life. This increased awareness can lead to greater public support for scientific research, influencing funding priorities and policy decisions at both national and international levels.

Stimulating Scientific Inquiry and Research

The announcement of Nobel laureates often sparks interest and curiosity within the scientific community, encouraging further research in related fields. By highlighting specific areas of study, the Nobel Prize can direct attention to pressing health challenges and under-explored domains, fostering a collaborative and competitive spirit among researchers to push the boundaries of what is known and possible.

Influencing Policy and Funding

The recognition of certain research areas by the Nobel Committee can also have a profound impact on health policy and funding allocations. Breakthroughs deemed Nobel-worthy often receive increased visibility, which can, in turn, attract more investment from government bodies, private sector entities, and philanthropic organizations. This can accelerate the development of new treatments, vaccines, and diagnostics, ultimately benefiting public health on a global scale.

Encouraging Ethical and Societal Reflections

Nobel Prize in Medicine often prompts ethical and societal reflections on the implications of scientific discoveries. As the Prize draws attention to the latest advancements, it also invites public discourse on the ethical considerations surrounding new technologies and treatments, such as genetic editing, stem cell research, and AI in medicine. This helps to ensure that the development and application of medical innovations are guided by ethical principles and societal values.

Contemporary Challenges and Future Directions

Contemporary challenges in medicine is diverse, reflecting the complex interplay between emerging health threats, technological advancements, and ethical considerations. Addressing these challenges requires a multidisciplinary approach, focusing not only on scientific innovation but also on ensuring equitable access to healthcare advancements.

Global Health Issues and Emerging Diseases

Global health faces numerous challenges, including the management and prevention of emerging diseases. The COVID-19 pandemic underscored the importance of rapid vaccine development, with mRNA technology emerging as a pivotal innovation. This has set a precedent for future responses to pandemics but also highlights the need for global collaboration in surveillance, research, and vaccine distribution to address health disparities and ensure that all populations benefit from scientific progress.

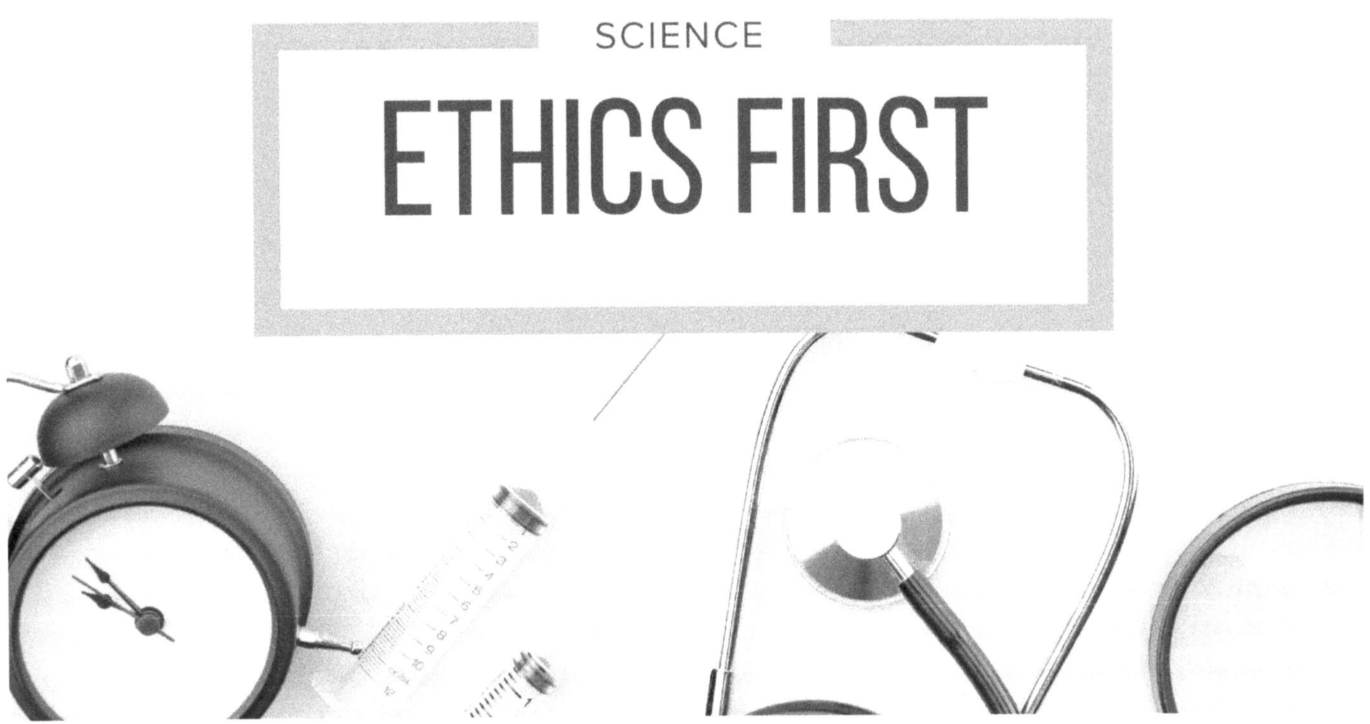

Ethical considerations in medical research and practice are increasingly prominent. Precision medicine, for example, offers personalized treatment options but raises questions about privacy, data security, and the potential for health inequities. The inclusion of diverse populations in genomic research and clinical trials is critical for developing effective, broadly applicable treatments. However, historical mistrust and systemic barriers to participation for underrepresented minority communities necessitate a concerted effort to rebuild trust and ensure that precision medicine benefits all segments of society.

Technological Advancements and Future Directions

Technological advancements present promising areas for future Nobel-worthy discoveries. Cell and gene therapies are evolving to treat diseases at their root cause, offering hope for conditions previously considered untreatable. Synthetic biology's potential to redesign biological entities could revolutionize not only medicine but also agriculture and manufacturing, addressing challenges like food security and environmental sustainability.

Xenotransplantation and AI-enhanced precision medicine represent the cutting edge of medical science, potentially solving organ shortage crises and personalizing patient care to unprecedented levels. However, these advancements also necessitate ethical considerations, particularly regarding the long-term implications of integrating technology into human health and the environment.

The Legacy and Continuing Relevance of the Nobel Prize

The Nobel Prize, established by Alfred Nobel's will in 1895, carries a legacy that extends far beyond the annual ceremonies and accolades. Nobel, known for his invention of dynamite, intended the prizes to honor those who conferred the "greatest benefit to humankind" in Physics, Chemistry, Medicine, Literature, and Peace. Over time, the Nobel Prize has become a global symbol of excellence in medical and scientific research, recognizing groundbreaking discoveries that have fundamentally changed our understanding of life and disease.

The impact of the Nobel Prize on medical and scientific research is profound. By highlighting exceptional contributions to science, the Prize not only celebrates individual achievement but also promotes a broader appreciation of the scientific method and the pursuit of knowledge. The recognition brings attention to research areas that are often at the forefront of tackling global health challenges, pushing the boundaries of what is scientifically possible, and inspiring future generations of researchers to dream big and pursue new discoveries.

Furthermore, the Nobel Prize plays a crucial role in shaping the direction of scientific inquiry and public interest. Winning research often sets the agenda for future studies, drawing talent and funding to promising fields. It signals to the scientific community and the public the importance of sustained investment in research that can lead to revolutionary advances in medicine, such as new treatments for diseases, vaccines, and understanding of complex biological processes.

The ongoing relevance of the Nobel Prize lies in its ability to adapt to the changing landscape of science while maintaining its commitment to excellence. As new areas of research emerge and interdisciplinary approaches become more critical, the Nobel Committees have recognized achievements that cross traditional boundaries, reflecting the evolving nature of scientific discovery. This adaptability ensures that the Prize remains a contemporary and forward-looking celebration of contributions that have the potential to improve the human condition.

CONCLUDING THOUGHTS AND A DREAM

"Knowledge without character & science without humanity is an ultimate social sin"

Mahatma Gandhi

In reflecting on the Nobel Prize and its laureates, it's clear that these celebrated figures are a source of inspiration for young scientists across the globe. Despite occasional controversies, narrow misses, and debates over credit, the Nobel Prize stands as the ultimate accolade for scientists. This book, while primarily a collection of facts about Nobel laureates, aims to spark a passion for science in young minds by showcasing the incredible achievements of these distinguished individuals.

The journey through the lives and discoveries of over 100 Nobel laureates since the Prize's inception reveals the vast expanse of innovation that has marked significant milestones in medical science and profoundly impacted human health. It's fascinating to observe the instances of cross-disciplinary inventions, particularly between physics and medicine, that have revolutionized our understanding and treatment of health conditions. For example, Wilhelm Roentgen's discovery of X-rays, which earned him the first Nobel Prize in Physics in 1901, laid the groundwork for medical imaging technologies such as the CT scan. Similarly, Marie Curie's pioneering work with radioactive isotopes, for which she received the Nobel Prize in Physics in 1903, has been instrumental in developing modern radiotherapy techniques.

A notable mention is Dr. Bernard Lown, a Harvard cardiologist known for inventing the first effective heart defibrillator. In 1985, he was awarded the Nobel Peace Prize not for his medical invention but for his efforts to combat nuclear warfare as a co-founder of the International Physicians for the Prevention of Nuclear War. This award highlights the Nobel Committee's recognition of contributions that, while outside traditional medical achievements, significantly benefit human health and global peace.

Do we need look beyond molecular and Nano science?

Reflecting on the Nobel Prize in the context of contemporary medical science raises an important question: Should we expand our horizons beyond molecular and nano science? Currently, the Nobel Prize in Medicine often celebrates discoveries emerging from advanced research laboratories, showcasing the pinnacle of scientific achievement. While there is no doubt that such breakthroughs are monumental, considering medical science from a broader social perspective suggests a potential for the Nobel Committee to revisit and possibly broaden its criteria for awarding this prestigious honor.

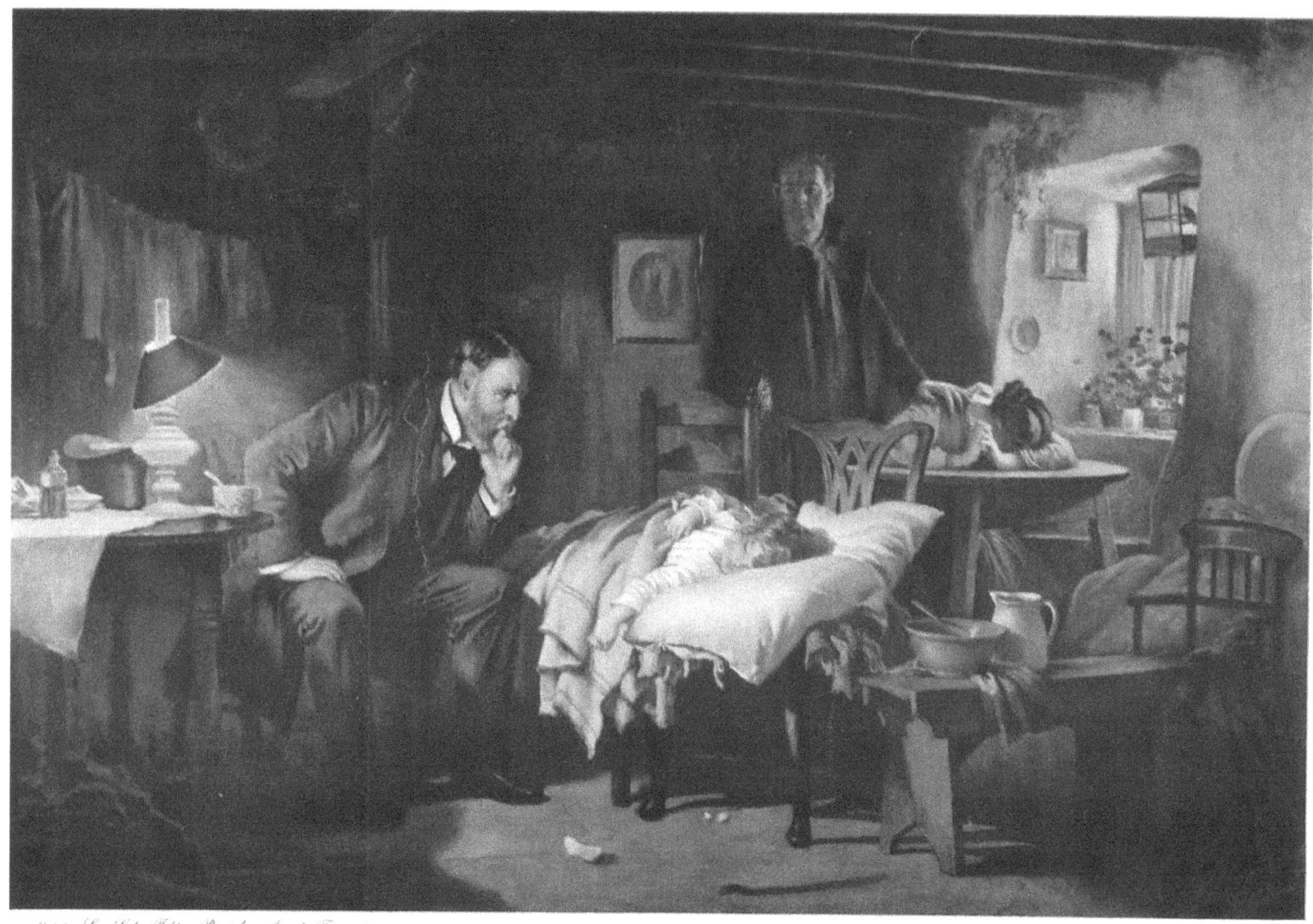

THE DOCTOR

This is an Immortal Image of a Victorian era doctor, who watches helplessly, a dying child with Typhoid fever after exhausting all treatments he could administer at that time. Inches away, we can see the grieving child's mother and loving father. This Image is surviving in every corridors of medical schools just for the haunting depiction of care and concern of the Doctor, towards his ailing patient. This canvas was drawn by British Painter by Sir Luke Fildes in 1891. It will continue to remind the generation next the true meaning and the driving force of noble profession. Does it sound unreasonable to expect a Doctor with such qualities too deserves a Nobel in current times?

Medical science is not just about groundbreaking laboratory discoveries; it encompasses the art of healing, social responsibility, moral considerations, and a strong emphasis on prevention. In a world increasingly influenced by commercial interests and non-academic influences, there's a compelling argument for global entities like the Nobel Committee to recognize contributions that extend beyond traditional scientific research. This approach could have a profound impact on humanity, aligning with the World Health Organization's inclusion of socio-economic factors such as poverty, war, and violence in the International Classification of Diseases (ICD) as conditions affecting human health.

The Nobel Prizes in Peace and Literature have historically been awarded for achievements that reflect profound philosophical and societal contributions. This raises the question: why hasn't the Nobel Prize in Medicine similarly recognized contributions that address the broader determinants of health?

To date, preventive health measures and medical interventions that have broad societal impacts have seemingly been overlooked by the Nobel Committee in Medicine. For instance, while the Nobel Peace Prize has honored organizations for their contributions to global healthcare, the World Health Organization (WHO), despite its extensive efforts to improve health outcomes worldwide, has not received Nobel recognition for its work.

The hope is that, in the future, the Nobel Prize in Medicine might evolve to include awards for achievements in medical ethics, recognition for doctors and organizations that operate on a not-for-profit basis, or for programs tackling significant global health challenges. Such an expansion would not only honor the multifaceted nature of medical science but also highlight the importance of addressing the full spectrum of factors that influence human health. This broader perspective could serve as a powerful reminder of the Nobel Prize's foundational goal: to recognize contributions that confer the greatest benefit to humankind.

I propose that the Nobel committee broaden its focus from deep molecular science to encompass a more tangible, societal, ethical, and administrative aspect of modern healthcare periodically. Ultimately, the true success of any medical breakthrough lies in its proper utilization.

I dream for a day when Alfred Nobel is brought back to life to chair a special meeting of the Nobel committee, approving these proposals. This act would address the current concerns in the rapidly expanding field of medical science lacking meaningful control.

Let the Nobel Prize keep inspiring all the budding scientists and sustain the curiosity, hope and respect.

CAN WE EVER GRADE THE NOBEL PRIZES?

May be, we should not. But under no circumstances can any Nobel invention be judged solely on its attention it created, rather by true merit and impact. Each of them holds a unique history, struggle, value, and impact. If I were to select the top 10, this would be the ranking.

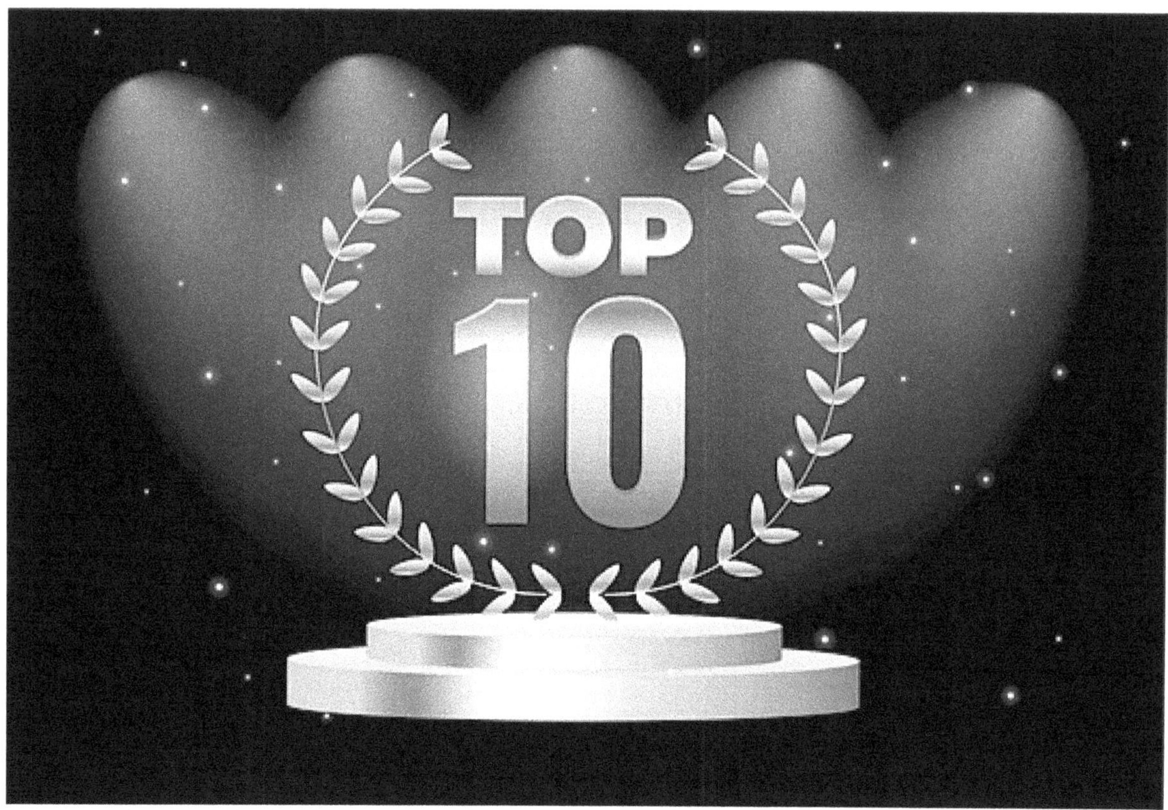

1. **In Vitro Fertilization – Robert G. Edwards (2010):** Robert G. Edwards was honored for his revolutionary development of in vitro fertilization (IVF). This marked a monumental stride in assisted reproductive technology, symbolizing humanity's capability to foster life beyond natural conception.
2. **Science of Vaccination – Emil von Behring (1901):** Awarded the first Nobel Prize in Medicine, Behring's work on serum therapies for diphtheria laid the groundwork for the science of vaccination, continuing to have a profound impact on medical science.
3. **Penicillin – Alexander Fleming, Ernst Boris Chain, and Sir Howard Florey (1945):** The development of penicillin as a life-saving antibiotic marked the dawn of the antibiotic era, transforming the treatment of bacterial infections.

4. **Citric Acid Cycle and Intracellular Metabolism – Hans Krebs and Fritz Lipmann (1953):** Their foundational work in biochemistry has impacted numerous discoveries and innovations in medicine and biology.

5. **Cardiac Catheterization – André Cournand, Werner Forssmann, and Dickinson Richards (1956):** Their development of cardiac catheterization techniques and insights into circulatory system pathology have profoundly influenced cardiology, allowing for the treatment of complex heart diseases.

6. **Neurophysiology – Joseph Erlanger and Herbert Gasser (1944):** Erlanger and Gasser were the first to explain hormone action through the concept of receptors, studying single nerve fibers. Their insights into electrical signals advanced neurophysiology and paved the way for critical drug developments like beta-blockers.

7. **Organ and Cell Transplantation – Joseph Murray and E. Donnall Thomas (1990):** Their pioneering work in organ and cell transplantation has been a monumental leap in treating human diseases, expanding the possibilities of modern medicine.

8. **Magnetic Resonance Imaging – Paul Lauterbur and Sir Peter Mansfield (2003):** Lauterbur and Mansfield revolutionized medical diagnostics with MRI technology, enabling detailed visualization of internal body structures without invasive methods or radiation, surpassing traditional X-rays and CT scans in safety and efficacy.

9. **Structure of DNA and Nucleic Acid – Francis Crick, James Watson, and Maurice Wilkins (1962):** Their discovery of the molecular structure of nucleic acids and its significance in the transmission of genetic information remains a cornerstone in understanding the essence of life.

10. **RNA Interference – Andrew Z. Fire and Craig C. Mello (2006):** The 2006 Nobel Prize was awarded to Fire and Mello for uncovering RNA interference (RNAi). This process allows double-stranded RNA to silence specific genes, offering a significant shift in drug development and gene therapy applications.